2018

ADVANCES IN
MOLECULAR PATHOLOGY

EDITOR-IN-CHIEF

Gregory J. Tsongalis, PhD, HCLD, CC

SECTION EDITORS

Ahmad N. Abou Tayoun, PhD, FACMG

Kevin Alby, PhD, D(ABMM)

Andrea Ferreira-Gonzalez, PhD, HCLD(ABB), CC(ABB), FACB

Todd W. Kelley, MD

Christopher Korch, PhD

Ann M. Moyer, MD, PhD

Jeremy P. Segal, MD, PhD

ELSEVIER

Director, Continuity Publishing: Taylor Ball
Editor: Lauren Boyle
Developmental Editor: Laura Fisher

Reprints: For copies of 100 or more of articles in this publication, please contact the Commercial Reprints Department, Elsevier Inc., 360 Park Avenue South, New York, NY 10010-1710. Tel: 212-633-3874; Fax: 212-633-3820; E-mail: reprints@elsevier.com.

Printed in the United States of America.

Editorial Office:
Elsevier, Inc.
1600 John F. Kennedy Blvd,
Suite 1800
Philadelphia, PA 19103-2899

International Standard Serial Number: 2589-515X
International Standard Book Number: 13: 978-0-323-63965-1

CONTRIBUTORS

APRIL N. ABBOTT, PhD, D(ABMM)
Department of Laboratory Medicine, Deaconess Hospital, Evansville, Indiana, USA

DARA L. AISNER, MD, PhD
Associate Professor, Department of Pathology, Director, Colorado Molecular Correlates Laboratory, Aurora, Colorado, USA

JORGE ANDRADE, PhD
Director of Bioinformatics, Center for Research Informatics, Research Assistant Professor, Department of Pediatrics, Knapp Center for Biomedical Discovery, The University of Chicago, Chicago, Illinois, USA

RANJANA ARORA, MD, MPH, FCAP
Director, Hematology Molecular Clinical Services, Associate Director, Clinical Molecular and Genomics Laboratory, Assistant Professor, Department of Pathology and Laboratory Medicine, University of Kentucky, Lexington, Kentucky, USA

ESTHER BABADY, PhD, D (ABMM)
Director of Clinical Operations, Associate Attending Microbiologist, Clinical Microbiology Service, Department of Laboratory Medicine, Infectious Disease Service, Department of Medicine, Memorial Sloan Kettering Cancer Center, New York, New York, USA

MAXIME CADIEUX-DION, PhD
Department of Pathology and Laboratory Medicine, Center for Pediatric Genomic Medicine, Children's Mercy Kansas City, University of Missouri-Kansas City, School of Medicine, Kansas City, Missouri, USA

AMANDA CAPES-DAVIS, MB BS, BSc(Med), PhD
Honorary Scientist, CellBank Australia, Children's Medical Research Institute, The University of Sydney, Westmead, New South Wales, Australia

GERALD A. CAPRARO, PhD, D(ABMM)
Director, Clinical Microbiology Laboratory, Carolinas Pathology Group, Atrium Health, Charlotte, North Carolina, USA

LARISA H. CAVALLARI, PharmD
Associate Professor, Department of Pharmacotherapy and Translational Research, Associate Director, Director, Center for Pharmacogenomics, University of Florida, Gainesville, Florida, USA

SUZANNE M. COX, PhD, MPH
Senior Director of Health and Human Sciences Education, Graham School of Continuing Liberal and Professional Studies, The University of Chicago, Chicago, Illinois, USA

MICHAEL DATTO, MD, PhD
Associate Professor, Department of Pathology, Duke University Medical Center, Durham, North Carolina, USA

MARK D. EWALT, MD
Assistant Professor, Department of Pathology, University of Colorado, Aurora, Colorado, USA

EMILY FARROW, PhD, MS, CGC
Department of Pediatrics, Center for Pediatric Genomic Medicine, Children's Mercy Kansas City, University of Missouri-Kansas City, School of Medicine, Kansas City, Missouri, USA

ERIN H. GRAF, PhD, D(ABMM)
Department of Pathology and Laboratory Medicine, Children's Hospital of Philadelphia, Perelman School of Medicine, University of Pennsylvania, Philadelphia, Pennsylvania, USA

LIMIN HAO, PhD
Senior Bioinformatician, Bioinformatics and Laboratory of Molecular Medicine, Partners Personalized Medicine, Cambridge, Massachusetts, USA

SUSAN J. HSIAO, MD, PhD
Assistant Professor, Department of Pathology and Cell Biology, Columbia University Irving Medical Center, New York, New York, USA

YUAN JI, PhD, FACMG
Department of Pathology, ARUP Laboratories, University of Utah School of Medicine, Salt Lake City, Utah, USA

SABAH KADRI, PhD
Division of Genomic and Molecular Pathology, Department of Pathology, The University of Chicago, Chicago, Illinois, USA

CHRISTOPHER KORCH, PhD
Assistant Clinical Professor, International Cell Line Authentication Committee (ICLAC) Member, Division of Medical Oncology, University of Colorado Cancer Center, University of Colorado Anschutz Medical Campus, Aurora, Colorado, USA

BRYAN L. KROCK, PhD
Department of Pathology and Laboratory Medicine, Children's Hospital of Philadelphia, Perelman School of Medicine, University of Pennsylvania, Philadelphia, Pennsylvania, USA

MATTHEW S. LEBO, PhD, FACMG
Director, Bioinformatics and Laboratory of Molecular Medicine, Partners Personalized Medicine, Cambridge, Massachusetts, USA; Assistant Professor, Pathology, Harvard Medical School, Brigham and Women's Hospital, Boston, Massachusetts, USA

CHIAO-FENG LIN, PhD
Senior Bioinformatician, Bioinformatics and Laboratory of Molecular Medicine, Partners Personalized Medicine, Cambridge, Massachusetts, USA

STEPHANIE L. MITCHELL, PhD, D(ABMM)
Department of Pathology and Laboratory Medicine, UPMC Children's Hospital of Pittsburgh, Department of Pathology, University of Pittsburgh, School of Medicine, Pittsburgh, Pennsylvania, USA

RAYMOND WHITING NIMS, PhD
Senior Consultant, RMC Pharmaceutical Solutions, Inc, Longmont, Colorado, USA

JAY L. PATEL, MD, MBA
Associate Professor, Department of Pathology, University of Utah, Medical Director, Molecular Hematopathology, ARUP Laboratories, Salt Lake City, Utah, USA

KEYUR P. PATEL, MD, PhD
Associate Professor, Department of Hematopathology, The University of Texas MD Anderson Cancer Center, Houston, Texas, USA

VICTORIA M. PRATT, PhD
Director, Pharmacogenomics and Molecular Genetics Laboratories, Department of Medical and Molecular Genetics, Indiana University School of Medicine, Indianapolis, Indiana, USA

HOLGER PROKISCH, PhD
Institute of Human Genetics, Klinikum rechts der Isar, Technische Universität München, Ismaninger Munich, Germany; Institute of Human Genetics, Helmholtz Zentrum München, Ingolstaedter Neuherberg, Germany

SARAH RAPISARDO, PhD
Assistant Professor, Department of Pathology, Duke University Medical Center, Durham, North Carolina, USA

KALPANA S. REDDY, MD
Assistant Professor, Department of Pathology and Laboratory Medicine, Division of Hematopathology, Zucker School of Medicine at Hofstra/Northwell, Lake Success, New York, USA

RYAN F. RELICH, PhD, D(ABMM), MLS(ASCP)SM
Division of Clinical Microbiology, Indiana University Health Pathology Laboratory, Indiana University Health and Indiana University School of Medicine, Indianapolis, Indiana, USA

CAROL J. SAUNDERS, PhD, FACMG
Department of Pathology, Center for Pediatric Genomic Medicine, Children's Mercy Kansas City, University of Missouri-Kansas City, School of Medicine, Kansas City, Missouri, USA

REBECCA E. SCHWEPPE, PhD
Division of Endocrinology, Metabolism, and Diabetes, University of Colorado Cancer Center, University of Colorado Anschutz Medical Campus, Aurora, Colorado, USA

SIDDHARTHA SEN, MD, PhD
Pathology Resident (PGY2), Department of Pathology, Duke University Medical Center, Durham, North Carolina, USA

ANTONIA R. SEPULVEDA, MD, PhD
Department of Pathology and Cell Biology, Columbia University Irving Medical Center, New York, New York, USA

MARYAM SHIRAZI, MD
Department of Pathology and Cell Biology, Columbia University Irving Medical Center, New York, New York, USA

ARTI SINGH, MS
Bioinformatics Data Engineer, Bioinformatics and Laboratory of Molecular Medicine, Partners Personalized Medicine, Cambridge, Massachusetts, USA

SARAH L. STENTON, MBChB, MPhil
Institute of Human Genetics, Klinikum rechts der Isar, Technische Universität München, Ismaninger Munich, Germany; Institute of Human Genetics, Helmholtz Zentrum München, Ingolstaedter Neuherberg, Germany

ISABELLE THIFFAULT, PhD, FACMG
Department of Pathology, Center for Pediatric Genomic Medicine, Children's Mercy Kansas City, University of Missouri-Kansas City, School of Medicine, Kansas City, Missouri, USA

PRIYANKA UPRETY, MSPH, PhD
Department of Pathology and Laboratory Medicine, Children's Hospital of Philadelphia, Perelman School of Medicine, University of Pennsylvania, Philadelphia, Pennsylvania, USA

MARILEILA VARELLA-GARCIA, PhD
Clinical Professor, Division of Medical Oncology, University of Colorado Cancer Center, University of Colorado Anschutz Medical Campus, Aurora, Colorado, USA

SAMUEL L. VOLCHENBOUM, MD, PhD
Director of the Center for Research Informatics, Associate Professor, Department of Pediatrics, Knapp Center for Biomedical Discovery, The University of Chicago, Chicago, Illinois, USA

ADVANCES IN MOLECULAR PATHOLOGY

CONTENTS

VOLUME 1 • 2018

Infectious Disease

Pharmacogenomics

Informatics

Advances in Molecular Pathology 1 (2018) xv–xvi
ADVANCES IN MOLECULAR PATHOLOGY

Preface

Molecular Pathology: Beyond the Base-ics of Clinical Genomics

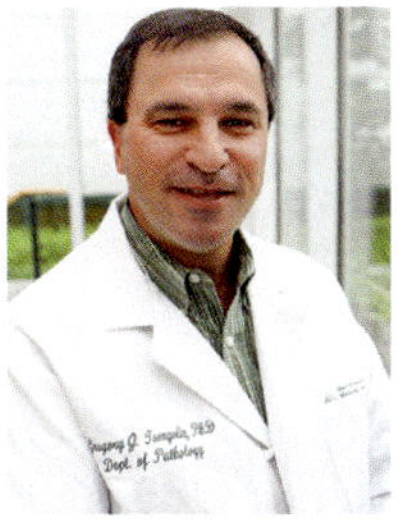

Gregory J. Tsongalis, PhD, HCLD, CC
Editor

While many advances were made in the field of molecular biology and genomic medicine since the description of the DNA double helix in 1954, the most remarkable, however, began in 1989 at the Banbury Conference to discuss the potential of sequencing the human genome. The Human Genome Project proposed that the end results would be better diagnostic testing, better prognostic testing, advanced abilities to predict who may be at risk for developing disease, and the development of novel targeted therapies based on genomic profiles. While many of these have come to fruition, the field of translational or precision medicine continues to develop at a rapid pace driven by new technologies and therapeutic management strategies.

The universal nature of the technologies used to identify nucleic acids and/or variants in genes of interest has evolved from rudimentary gel electrophoresis techniques to high throughput, highly complex massively parallel sequencing assays. Along with the many technical advances that allow for the detection and quantification of not only human gene variants but also microbial gene targets have resulted in unprecedented clinical testing applications. The added value of molecular test results to patient management strategies provides a significant opportunity for clinical laboratorians to become active members of the health care delivery team in every medical discipline.

In this inaugural issue of *Advances in Molecular Pathology*, we highlight some of the newest developments in molecular testing for genetic diseases, hematologic diseases, infectious diseases, pharmacogenomics, solid tumors and identity testing that has recently occurred. In addition, we have included several articles dedicated to informatics as this has become an additional area of expertise we will need to acquire. The practice of clinical genomics in an era of precision-based medicine is dependent upon molecular pathology to assure the highest level of performance for clinical tests that will impact all facets of our health care delivery system and the patient to whom the tests are directed.

https://doi.org/10.1016/j.yamp.2018.08.001
2589-4080/18/

Our dedication to enhancing patient outcomes and better understanding human disease through molecular diagnostic testing is something we will always strive for. I am grateful to those friends and colleagues who agreed to becoming section editors and to all of the authors who contributed articles to this issue as the advances in this field continue to occur at a record pace.

Happy reading!

Gregory J. Tsongalis, PhD, HCLD, CC
DHMC–Department of Pathology and Laboratory Medicine
1 Medical Center Drive
Lebanon, NH 03756, USA

E-mail address: Gregory.j.tsongalis@hitchcock.org

Genetics

Advances in Molecular Pathology 1 (2018) 1–8
ADVANCES IN MOLECULAR PATHOLOGY

Coming up to Speed on Whole Genome Sequencing in Critically Ill Children

Isabelle Thiffault, PhD[a], Emily Farrow, PhD, MS, CGC[b], Carol J. Saunders, PhD[a,*], Maxime Cadieux-Dion, PhD[c]

[a]Department of Pathology, Center for Pediatric Genomic Medicine, Children's Mercy Kansas City, University of Missouri-Kansas City, School of Medicine, 2401 Gillham Road, Kansas City, MO 64108, USA; [b]Department of Pediatrics, Center for Pediatric Genomic Medicine, Children's Mercy Kansas City, University of Missouri-Kansas City, School of Medicine, 2401 Gillham Road, Kansas City, MO 64108, USA; [c]Department of Pathology and Laboratory Medicine, Center for Pediatric Genomic Medicine, Children's Mercy Kansas City, University of Missouri-Kansas City, School of Medicine, 2401 Gillham Road, Kansas City, MO 64108, USA

KEYWORDS

- Whole exome sequencing (WES) • Whole genome sequencing (WGS) • Rapid sequencing • Pediatric
- Molecular diagnosis

KEY POINTS

- To date, whole genome sequencing (WGS) has largely been confined to the research space, likely due to cost, storage, and reimbursement concerns because WGS cost is 5-fold higher than exome; rapid WGS is 25-fold more.
- WGS produces even coverage than whole exome sequencing (WES), enables sequencing of noncoding targets, copy number variation detection, and has easier workflow for laboratories.
- The clinical utility is well established for WES; WGS is as good if not better for most cases. Exceptions to this are encountered due to mosaicism and other situations where higher depth of coverage is needed.
- There are many anecdotes describing patients who benefitted from rapid sequencing but outcome studies are lacking. It is intuitive that rapid sequencing may be cost-effective in some children, but it has not been established which patients will benefit.

INTRODUCTION

Genetic testing in critically ill infants is now standard of care but still can be a time-consuming and costly approach. Until recently, analysis had been largely targeted to defined genes, but pan-genomic approaches, such as microarrays, next-generation sequencing (NGS)-based gene panel testing, and whole exome sequencing (WES), are prevailing. To date, there are ~5200 genetic diseases with known gene associations [1]. These are individually rare but collectively frequent and explain a significant fraction of infant mortality, particularly in intensive care settings [2–6]. Standard molecular and cytogenetic testing aims to identify large structural copy number variations (CNVs), such as microdeletions and duplications, as well as sequencing for the detection of smaller insertion-deletions (indels) and single-nucleotide variants (SNVs) in individuals with suspected monogenic disorders. However, the still common tiered approach to genetic testing has been associated with a lower diagnostic rate and longer

Disclosure: The authors have nothing to disclose.

*Corresponding author, *E-mail address:* csaunders@cmh.edu

https://doi.org/10.1016/j.yamp.2018.06.002
2589-4080/18/

time to diagnosis than WES or whole genome sequencing (WGS) [2–15].

Despite the fact that critically ill infants with suspected genetic disorders are often evaluated by clinical geneticists, the differential diagnosis for many patients, particularly infants, may include hundreds of genes. As such, standard sequential testing often occurs, each with variable turnaround times ranging from less than a week to several months, which collectively may become years if multiple, consecutive tests are ordered and results are inconclusive.

WGS has the potential to detect multiple types of clinically relevant variants with an increased diagnostic rate of up to 2- to 4-fold over chromosomal microarray analysis [4,16]. The ability to provide an accurate molecular diagnosis in a timely manner can result in optimal clinical management for these patients by guiding treatment, initiation of appropriate subspecialty follow-up, addressing prognosis, allowing redirection of care, and assessing recurrence risk. However, there are only a few prospective and retrospective studies, limiting clear evidence for indications for rapid clinical NGS-based testing and the diagnostic superiority of WGS to WES [2–15]. Moreover, challenges remain to demonstrate the diagnostic utility of rapid WGS (rWGS) given the availability of rapid WES, which has demonstrated similar performance [6]. The premise of genotype-differentiated treatment or benefits realized from cost-effective clinical management remains substantially anecdotal. Nonetheless, the practicality of rapid NGS-based testing cannot be dissociated from its economic impact on clinical laboratories, including substantial needs for highly skilled personnel, bioinformatics resources, instrumentation, and institution-based cost concerns, because reduced turnaround time is associated with significantly higher cost of testing. Furthermore, interpretation of sequence data remains challenging, especially in young critically ill infants with atypical or unrecognized presentations. The need for a rapid comprehensive genetic diagnosis has clinical value, but additional studies are needed to clarify the type of medical indications that benefit from shorter time to diagnosis and the true impact on outcomes, or health care utilization.

GENOME OR EXOME?

Ordering physicians frequently ask which test, WGS or WES, is better for their patients. In the authors' experience, the diagnostic rate is the same in an unbiased patient population. WGS offers the potential of a single test with the ability to capture nearly all genomic variations in an unbiased manner, due to even coverage throughout the genome. This advantage includes exonic SNVs missed as a consequence of WES coverage and enrichment methods, deep intronic SNVs, SNVs in noncoding RNA, as well as the potential for small and large structural variant detection. However, the interpretation of variants in the coding regions of well-characterized genes remains challenging; in the absence of functional studies based on RNA or gene expression, the inclusion of deep-intronic and noncoding variants is futile. As long as the "exomized" genome is analyzed instead of a true whole genome, the full potential will not be realized, including the analysis of deep intronic variants that could affect splicing and other noncoding variants that affect gene expression. Over time, the ability to interpret variants in these regions will improve through functional genomics and lead to an eventual diagnostic advantage of WGS over WES.

WGS is the most comprehensive method for analyzing the genome, providing a high-resolution, base-by-base view of the genome (with the exception of certain complex sequences), with even coverage due to very limited DNA amplification and no capture step for enrichment. Unlike targeted gene panels and WES, library preparation for whole genomes is simpler and faster because it does not require targeted enrichment of coding regions and multiple cycles of PCR amplification (Fig. 1). A genome with 30× coverage generally has sufficient representation of clinically relevant exons compared with WES [17–19]. The very small fraction of exons not well covered in a typical WGS experiment is also often missed by WES and may be filled in via Sanger sequencing on an as-needed basis. Moreover, WGS is less sensitive to guanine-cytosine (GC) content, contributing to more uniform coverage but with an average of depth of coverage less than half WES. Indeed, when optimized, WGS with 65× average depth of coverage completely covered all Refseq coding exons (100%) at $\geq$13× versus 98.15% in WES at 154× [20]. Similar performance was observed in the coverage of exons in which potential disease-causing variants have been reported in the Human Gene Mutation Database (100% in WGS vs 98.2% in WES), suggesting that WES may fail to detect 0.42% of the known coding variants versus WGS [20]. In addition, WES coverage is variable among the exons of an individual and interindividuals due to enrichment efficiency, run variability, and other factors. On the other hand, the lower average depth of coverage in WGS may affect detection of low-percentage variants, such as somatic variants from tumor tissue, heteroplasmic mitochondrial variants, and germline mosaic variants [21].

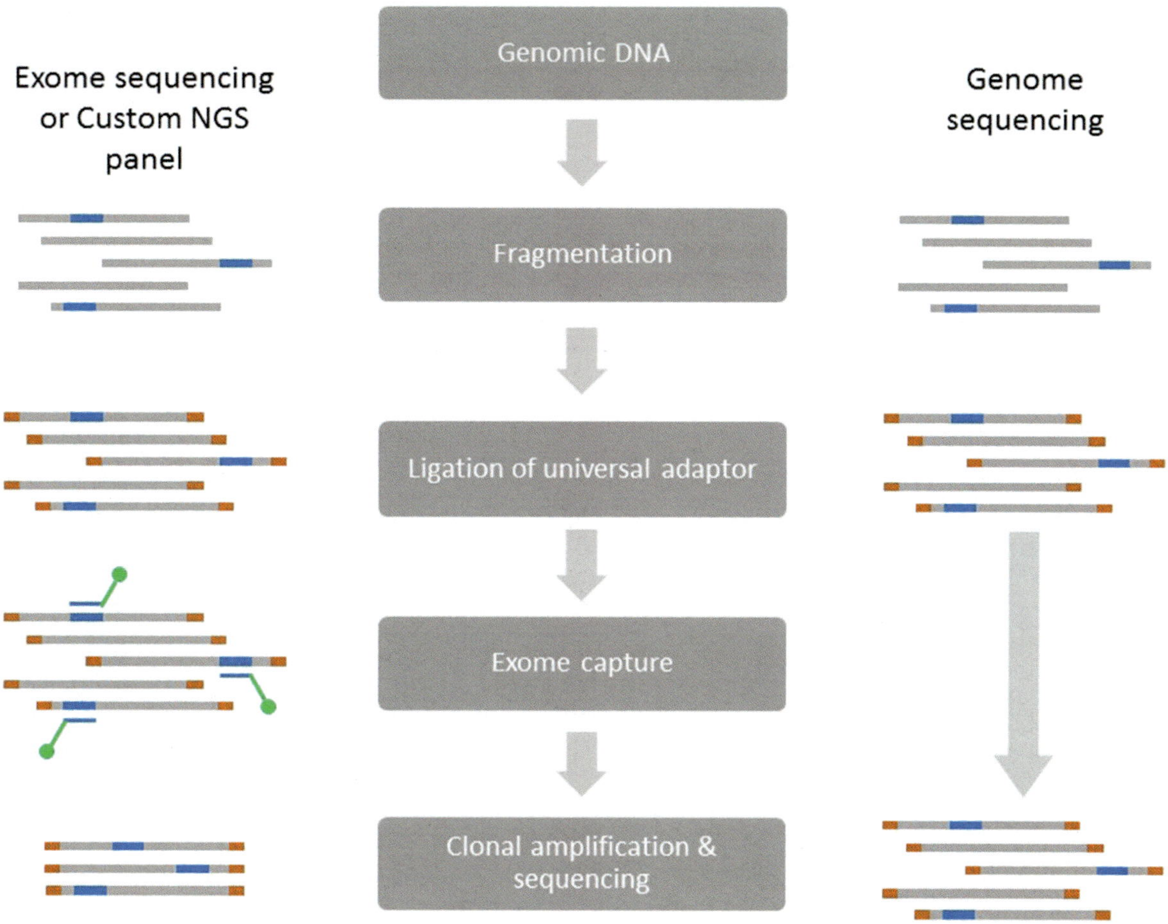

FIG. 1 Laboratory steps in targeted NGS versus genome sequencing.

From a laboratory wet-bench perspective, WGS has the advantage of significantly decreased technician time for sample preparation, which may be completed easily within a few hours as opposed to WES, which requires samples to be batched and depending on the enrichment workflow may take up to 3 days, before samples are ready for sequencing. In some aspects, genomes are also easier to sequence because the increased data requirements result in fewer samples per flow cell.

Cost remains the predominant disadvantage for WGS. Although the 1000 USD genome is here for those laboratories with new instrumentation, costs are still 5-fold amount higher than an exome. Furthermore, running rWGS costs significantly more than standard WGS (3- to 5-fold dependent on instrumentation; Tables 1 and 2). Regardless of run mode, the amount of data for WGS is 10× more, resulting in much higher storage costs. In addition, whether running WGS or WES, there are hidden costs of the testing beyond the actual sequencing costs that must be considered, such as laboratory time, genetic counseling time, clinician's time to discuss results, including explaining incidental findings to families, variant identification (bioinformatics), confirmatory testing, confirming disease presence, and data storage. Clinical Laboratory Improvement Amendment (CLIA) regulations require storage of analytical systems records and test reports for at least 2 years. In addition, the American College of Medical Genetics and Genomics recommends a minimum of 2-year storage of a file type that would allow regeneration of the primary results as well as reanalysis

TABLE 1
Comparison of Rapid and Standard Sequencing Costs

	HiSeq2500	HiSeq2500	HiSeq4000	NovaSeq6000	NovaSeq6000
Run mode	Rapid	v4 Chemistry	Standard	S1-rapid	S4
Sequencing capacity (Gb)/flow cell	40	400	750	833	6000
Read length (bp)	2 × 100	2 × 125	2 × 150	2 × 100	2 × 150
Run time	<1 d	~6 d	~3 d	~19 h	~40 h
Genome(s) per flow cell	0.5	4	8	3	33
Approximate cost per genome	$5600	$2900	$1600	$2600	$950

with improved analytical pipelines (eg, bam or fastq files with all reads retained) [22]. Cloud-based solutions are beginning to address storage needs; however, the cost associated with storage is still substantial and has yet to undergo the same price decline as sequencing [23,24].

Reanalysis of previously generated WGS data can result in diagnoses of disease with newly discovered gene associations, of which around 40 such genes are added to OMIM (Online Mendelian Inheritance in Man) each month [1]. In addition, updates to variant interpretation may result in a new diagnosis following reanalysis, such as a variant of unknown significance being upgraded to pathogenic. Indeed, multiple studies have demonstrated that data reanalysis after ~1 to 2 years can lead to new diagnoses in 10% to 24% undiagnosed cases following the reclassification of variants of unknown significance as well as the reporting of new disease-gene associations [9,25–27]. The future understanding of noncoding variants, which would not be represented in WES, would tip the scale in favor of WGS reanalysis. However, reanalysis is a labor- and time-intensive strategy that is often only performed upon request in clinical setting.

DETECTION OF COPY NUMBER VARIATION FROM NEXT-GENERATION SEQUENCING

Variants that currently elude reliable, prospective detection by short read technology include triplet repeat expansions, and variants in homologous regions. A CNV was originally defined as a duplicated or deleted DNA segment of >1 kb; however, NGS technologies have redefined this as greater than 50 base-pairs, enabling detection of exonic indels. Larger deletions, duplications, and inversions were previously grouped into the

TABLE 2
Comparison of Leading Sequencers in Clinical Laboratories Using Sequencing by Synthesis

	MiSeq	HiSeq2500	HiSeq4000	NovaSeq6000
Sequencing capacity (Gb)	15	150–180	13,000–15,000	6000
Read length (bp)	2 × 300	2 × 150	2 × 150	2 × 150
Run time	<56 h	<1–3.5 d	<1–3.5 d	19–40 h
Reads per run	n.a.	2.5–5 billion	2.5–5 billion	1.4–20 billion
Sample per run	1 exome/<12 gene panel	6–12	6–12	4–48
Relative cost per sample	Higher cost	Mid cost	Mid cost	Lower cost
Relative price per instrument	Lower cost	Mid cost	Mid cost	Higher cost
Key applications in clinical setting	Small gene panels	Gene panels, WES, WGS	Gene panels, WES, WGS	Gene panels, WES, WGS

category of what is not detectable by sequencing; however, analysis of WGS for CNV has been reported at least on a research basis [6,16,21,28,29].

WGS has the potential to detect most types of clinically relevant variants, SNVs and insertion/deletions (indels), and CNVs with an increased diagnostic rate of up to 2- to 4-fold over chromosomal microarray analysis and targeted panels [4,16]. WGS could ultimately reduce health care costs by reducing the need for other tests, such as karyotyping, chromosomal microarrays, and/or exome sequencing. In addition, it has the potential to detect more CNVs, including deletion/duplications of single exons, unbalanced changes, and more areas of homozygosity than microarray, including allele-specific CNVs. However, there are greater than 50 algorithms for structural variant detection from sequence data, but currently no widely accepted method, filtering strategy, quality control metrics, and deletion breakpoint accuracy.

Four main methods for detecting CNVs with NGS data include mate-pair, split-read, read-depth, and de novo assembly. Although mate-pair methods can detect medium-sized insertions and deletions from mapped data, they are insensitive to small insertion, or deletion events. The split-read method uses reads from paired end sequencing where only one read of the pair has reliable mapping and the other one either completely or partially fails to map to the genome. The unique aspect of this method is the ability to detect precise break points, within 10 bp in some studies, which are often intronic and not covered by WES [30]. Previous studies have shown high reproducibility and accuracy of clinically relevant CNV detection using the WGS read depth method [4,31,32]. As the name implies, this method is based on the premise that there is a correlation between depth of coverage of a genomic region and the copy number of the region. Compared with the other methods, read depth can detect the position of the potential CNVs with the exact number of copies and may be more sensitive for large CNVs. Overall, the workflow of the read depth method comprises 3 steps: (1) reads aligned to a reference genome and counted using a predefined window, (2) counts normalized to remove potential bias (ie, GC content, repeat regions), (3) segmentation algorithm and statistical significance of the CNV calls. Last, the de novo assembly methods generate contig (assembly) before comparison with the reference genome. As such, de novo assembly is rarely used because of the highly complex computational resources needed and poor CNV detection performance.

Newer bioinformatics methods for the analysis of copy number variants from WGS, WES, or even panels promise to level the playing field in terms of detecting copy number variants. The recent development of algorithms prompted the integration of multiple methods and tools to improve sensitivity and specificity. Indeed, several commercial laboratories currently offer copy number variant detection from NGS data. However, the development of professional standards and guidelines to assist clinical laboratories with the validation, performance parameters, quality control procedures, and reporting to assure the quality of NGS-based CNVs detection are still emerging.

INTERPRETATION CHALLENGES

Interpretation of sequence data remains challenging, especially in young infants with atypical or unrecognized presentations of genetic disorders. A phenotype-driven analysis may result in low diagnostic yield as the broad phenotypic presentations in many monogenetic disorders have been underascertained in many cases, particularly critically ill neonates. Relaxing filters in undiagnosed cases can result in the identification of a diagnostic genotype; however, careful selection of genes and vigilant discussions with a multidisciplinary team are essential to respect the primary reason of referral and make a critical appraisal of potentially positive results.

Cohorts investigated for rapid research NGS-based testing have been all highly clinically heterogeneous [2,3,5–7]. Most diagnoses were autosomal dominant due to de novo variants, highlighting the advantage of trio analysis. Most autosomal recessive diagnoses arose from homozygous variants in consanguineous families.

In clinical laboratories, NGS implementation must be in compliance with requirements from the College of American Pathologist/CLIA, thereby different than NGS in research settings. It is not practical as well as cost prohibitive to store every file generated by NGS analysis; however, a minimum of 2 years storage is required to comply with CLIA. Stored DNA sequence may be reevaluated following additional symptoms, variant reclassification, and discovery of new genes or reinterpretation in the context of familial segregation. Such revelation requires reanalysis ordered clinically or through an integrated translational strategy between standard diagnostic procedures and research initiatives.

DEMONSTRATION OF UTILITY AND EFFICACY AS A DIAGNOSTIC PROCEDURE

Molecular genetic testing is often reported long after patients are discharged from the hospital, making the results irrelevant in the clinical management of acute cases. An initial proof-of-concept study demonstrating the potential for using rWGS (50 hours) for the diagnosis of pediatric intensive care patients led the way for emulation by clinical reference laboratories and additional retrospective research studies. The first of these involved a highly selected group of 35 infants under 4 months of age in the neonatal intensive care unit (NICU) with diverse presentations reflective of suspected genetic conditions in whom rWGS was diagnostic in 20 (57%) [2]. Although every inheritance pattern was observed, as with other studies, a high rate of de novo variants was detected, again emphasizing the importance of sequencing parent-child trios. Several diagnoses were or could have been made clinically or with routine testing; however, 9 (45%) were diagnosed with conditions not mentioned in the differential at the time of patient enrollment. Reasons for this include atypical phenotypes and/or exceedingly rare or newly characterized genes. A second larger retrospective study reported the use of exome sequencing in 278 infants within the first 100 days of life in the intensive care unit [6]. The diagnostic rate was 36.7% and was reported to affect medical management in 52%. A subgroup of 63 infants underwent critical trio exome sequencing, with a mean turnaround time of 13 days and diagnostic rate of 50.8% (32/63).

Commonalities in various studies include high de novo rates, a higher death rate in patients with genetic diagnoses, and a high clinical impact [2,6,11]. A prospective study looking at the use of targeted genomics in the rapid diagnosis of critically ill children reported a diagnostic rate of 30% by analyzing 3426 known genes from a WGS in children less than 1 year of age in whom no diagnosis was found after routine clinical evaluation and testing. They concluded that rapid targeted genomics combined with copy number variant detection adds important value in the neonatal and pediatric intensive care setting [5].

A prospective study funded by the NSIGHT (Newborn Sequencing in Genomic medicine and public HealTh) collaborative sought to explore the use of genomic sequence information in newborns and included a randomized blinded study of the utility of rWGS in 65 NICU infants <4 months of age suspected to have a genetic condition. Thirty-two infants were randomized to receive rWGS plus standard genetic tests (which included standard WGS and other NGS-based tests), and 33 received standard tests alone. Five in the control group were crossed over to receive rWGS for compassionate care. Of note, 5 of 15 diagnoses in the standard group (33%) would not have been detected by rWGS because the diagnostic variant was either a structural variant or an abnormal methylation, indicating the continued importance of other tests in the absence of accurate CNV calling for NGS-based testing. Although the median age to diagnosis was certainly shorter in the rWGS, all patients in this group were also eventually diagnosed by standard methods, which took 2.5×longer. Although it follows that a quicker test will give quicker results, studies are needed to show whether the money spent for a rapid diagnosis results in measureable outcome changes.

Avoiding invasive and painful diagnostic procedures and putting an end to the expensive diagnostic odyssey is certainly beneficial. Frequently this leads to other benefits such as increased certainty about diagnosis that often promotes discussions about redirection of care toward palliative care, as well as benefits to families, such as more accurate genetic counseling that may influence future reproductive decisions. However, these rapid diagnoses rarely lead to the sorts of beneficial changes in management that proponents of precision medicine have heralded. In fact, one of the most powerful and important findings of the study is that there was no difference in mortality or length of hospital stay between control and rWGS [3].

Another prospective study evaluated the application of WGS compared with conventional genetic testing in a cohort of 103 children with a suspected underlying genetic disorder [16]. They found that WGS resulted in a diagnosis in 41% of participants, compared with 24% by conventional testing. Not surprisingly, the increased diagnostic rate in the WGS was partially due to the detection of CNV and intronic SNV.

TECHNOLOGICAL ADVANCEMENTS

Advancements in technology have been the foundation for the rapid integration of NGS into clinical testing. Both the time and the cost of WGS have dramatically decreased; indeed, with the newest instrumentation (NovaSeq 6000, Illumina), 66 WGS can be run on a single instrument in 3 days for less than $1000 each. As sequencing costs continue to decline, combined with increasing choices for data storage and processing, more laboratories will likely begin offering clinical WGS. Building on advancements in sample throughput and costs, new advancements in genome sequencing are also beginning to address the current diagnostic limitations of short read sequencing. Linked reads, whereby long pieces of DNA are barcoded before short read sequencing, allow for the phasing of most variants, and increased detection of copy number variants.

Linked reads can be particularly helpful in cases whereby biological parents are unavailable for phasing; however, it does not negate the need for parents to detect de novo variants. Current sequencing also performs poorly in repetitive regions, regions with high homology, and GC-rich regions. True long read sequencing offers the promise of variant phasing, increased detection of insertions/deletions and CNVs, and the detection of triplet repeat expansions. Similar to short read technology, the cost of long read sequencing is decreasing and throughput is increasing, albeit at a much slower rate [33]. Nonetheless, sequencing reads are increasing in length, and it is only a matter of time before true long read sequencing moves into production.

Rapid changes in technology bring up an important consideration when discussing the time to store sequencing results. Storing large amounts of raw data for future analysis requires significant resources [23]. Perhaps more importantly, a genome run 5 years ago is not equivalent to today's genome. Not only should reanalysis be discussed in the setting of nondiagnostic testing, but also, at some point, as significant advancements are made in sequencing technology, resequencing should be considered. The reality is that a combination of data archival with resequencing will need to be used to ensure that reanalysis and new analyses can be completed.

The ultimate goal of technological advances is not just to sequence more for less, but rather to develop sequencing technology that will fully realize the potential of precision medicine. As increasing numbers of genomes are sequenced, the understanding of a genome will also increase, allowing for the interpretation of additional variants not only in Mendelian disease but also in common-complex diseases that are poorly understood. This understanding is the ultimate goal of multiple national and international Precision Medicine Initiatives (eg, All of Us Research Program, National Institutes of Health United States, and 100,000 Genomes Project–Genomics England).

SUMMARY

The widespread use of WGS in routine clinical service is no longer a distant proposition. Although there are certainly cases whereby a rapid diagnosis may be beneficial, health outcome studies are lacking as to which patients should receive this testing.

Over time, the ability to interpret deep intronic and regulatory variants will improve, increasing the diagnostic advantage of WGS over WES. Until then, WES remains a more cost-effective option.

REFERENCES

[1] Online Mendelian Inheritance in Man. McKusick-Nathans Institute of Genetic Medicine. Baltimore (MD): Johns Hopkins University; 2018.

[2] Willig LK, Petrikin JE, Smith LD, et al. Whole-genome sequencing for identification of Mendelian disorders in critically ill infants: a retrospective analysis of diagnostic and clinical findings. Lancet Respir Med 2015;3: 377–87.

[3] Petrikin JE, Cakici JA, Clark MM, et al. The NSIGHT1-randomized controlled trial: rapid whole-genome sequencing for accelerated etiologic diagnosis in critically ill infants. NPJ Genom Med 2018;3:6.

[4] Stavropoulos DJ, Merico D, Jobling R, et al. Whole genome sequencing expands diagnostic utility and improves clinical management in pediatric medicine. NPJ Genom Med 2016;1 [pii:15012].

[5] van Diemen CC, Kerstjens-Frederikse WS, Bergman KA, et al. Rapid targeted genomics in critically ill newborns. Pediatrics 2017;140 [pii:e20162854].

[6] Meng L, Pammi M, Saronwala A, et al. Use of exome sequencing for infants in intensive care units: ascertainment of severe single-gene disorders and effect on medical management. JAMA Pediatr 2017;171:e173438.

[7] Saunders CJ, Miller NA, Soden SE, et al. Rapid whole-genome sequencing for genetic disease diagnosis in neonatal intensive care units. Sci Transl Med 2012;4: 154ra135.

[8] Charng WL, Karaca E, Coban Akdemir Z, et al. Exome sequencing in mostly consanguineous Arab families with neurologic disease provides a high potential molecular diagnosis rate. BMC Med Genomics 2016;9:42.

[9] Costain G, Jobling R, Walker S, et al. Periodic reanalysis of whole-genome sequencing data enhances the diagnostic advantage over standard clinical genetic testing. Eur J Hum Genet 2018;26(5):740–4.

[10] Powis Z, Farwell KD, Alamillo CL, et al. Diagnostic exome sequencing for patients with a family history of consanguinity: over 38% of positive results are not autosomal recessive pattern. J Hum Genet 2016;61:173–5.

[11] Soden SE, Saunders CJ, Willig LK, et al. Effectiveness of exome and genome sequencing guided by acuity of illness for diagnosis of neurodevelopmental disorders. Sci Transl Med 2014;6:265ra168.

[12] Tan TY, Dillon OJ, Stark Z, et al. Diagnostic impact and cost-effectiveness of whole-exome sequencing for ambulant children with suspected monogenic conditions. JAMA Pediatr 2017;171:855–62.

[13] Trujillano D, Bertoli-Avella AM, Kumar Kandaswamy K, et al. Clinical exome sequencing: results from 2819 samples reflecting 1000 families. Eur J Hum Genet 2017;25: 176–82.

[14] Valencia CA, Husami A, Holle J, et al. Clinical impact and cost-effectiveness of whole exome sequencing as a diagnostic tool: a pediatric center's experience. Front Pediatr 2015;3:67.

[15] Yang Y, Muzny DM, Reid JG, et al. Clinical whole-exome sequencing for the diagnosis of mendelian disorders. N Engl J Med 2013;369:1502–11.

[16] Lionel AC, Costain G, Monfared N, et al. Improved diagnostic yield compared with targeted gene sequencing panels suggests a role for whole-genome sequencing as a first-tier genetic test. Genet Med 2018;20(4):435–43.

[17] Lelieveld SH, Spielmann M, Mundlos S, et al. Comparison of exome and genome sequencing technologies for the complete capture of protein-coding regions. Hum Mutat 2015;36:815–22.

[18] Meynert AM, Ansari M, FitzPatrick DR, et al. Variant detection sensitivity and biases in whole genome and exome sequencing. BMC Bioinformatics 2014;15:247.

[19] Wang Q, Shashikant CS, Jensen M, et al. Novel metrics to measure coverage in whole exome sequencing datasets reveal local and global non-uniformity. Sci Rep 2017;7:885.

[20] Meienberg J, Bruggmann R, Oexle K, et al. Clinical sequencing: is WGS the better WES? Hum Genet 2016; 135:359–62.

[21] King DA, Sifrim A, Fitzgerald TW, et al, Deciphering Developmental Disorders Study. Detection of structural mosaicism from targeted and whole-genome sequencing data. Genome Res 2017;27:1704–14.

[22] Rehm HL, Bale SJ, Bayrak-Toydemir P, et al, Working Group of the American College of Medical Genetics and Genomics Laboratory Quality Assurance Commitee. ACMG clinical laboratory standards for next-generation sequencing. Genet Med 2013;15:733–47.

[23] Stephens ZD, Lee SY, Faghri F, et al. Big data: astronomical or genomical? PLoS Biol 2015;13:e1002195.

[24] Weymann D, Laskin J, Roscoe R, et al. The cost and cost trajectory of whole-genome analysis guiding treatment of patients with advanced cancers. Mol Genet Genomic Med 2017;5:251–60.

[25] Reanalysis of clinical whole-exome sequence data yields multiple new diagnoses: a time-intensive but successful strategy highlights the benefits of data sharing and international collaborations. Am J Med Genet A 2018;176:264–5.

[26] Nambot S, Thevenon J, Kuentz P, et al. Clinical whole-exome sequencing for the diagnosis of rare disorders with congenital anomalies and/or intellectual disability: substantial interest of prospective annual reanalysis. Genet Med 2018;20(6):645–54.

[27] Zhu X, Petrovski S, Xie P, et al. Whole-exome sequencing in undiagnosed genetic diseases: interpreting 119 trios. Genet Med 2015;17:774–81.

[28] Dong Z, Ye L, Yang Z, et al. Balanced chromosomal rearrangement detection by low-pass whole-genome sequencing. Curr Protoc Hum Genet 2018;96: 8.18.1–18.18.16.

[29] Wilfert AB, Sulovari A, Turner TN, et al. Recurrent de novo mutations in neurodevelopmental disorders: properties and clinical implications. Genome Med 2017;9:101.

[30] Nguyen HT, Boocock J, Merriman TR, et al. SRBreak: a read-depth and split-read framework to identify breakpoints of different events inside simple copy-number variable regions. Front Genet 2016;7:160.

[31] Yuen RK, Thiruvahindrapuram B, Merico D, et al. Whole-genome sequencing of quartet families with autism spectrum disorder. Nat Med 2015;21:185–91.

[32] Gilissen C, Hehir-Kwa JY, Thung DT, et al. Genome sequencing identifies major causes of severe intellectual disability. Nature 2014;511:344–7.

[33] Jain M, Koren S, Miga KH, et al. Nanopore sequencing and assembly of a human genome with ultra-long reads. Nat Biotechnol 2018;36(4):338–45.

Advances in Molecular Pathology 1 (2018) 9–26
ADVANCES IN MOLECULAR PATHOLOGY

Bioinformatics in Clinical Genomic Sequencing

Matthew S. Lebo, PhD[a,b,c,*], Limin Hao, PhD[a], Chiao-Feng Lin, PhD[a], Arti Singh, MS[a]
[a]Bioinformatics and Laboratory of Molecular Medicine, Partners Personalized Medicine, 65 Landsdowne Street, Cambridge, MA 02139, USA; [b]Pathology, Harvard Medical School, 25 Shattuck Street, Boston, MA 02115, USA; [c]Pathology, Brigham and Women's Hospital, 75 Francis Street, Boston, MA 02115, USA

KEYWORDS

• Genome sequencing • Exome sequencing • Alignment • Variant calling • Annotation • Filtration • Validation • Bioinformatic infrastructure

KEY POINTS

- Clinical bioinformatics encompasses generating raw sequence data from the machine through identifying reportable variants.
- Throughout the process, important quality control metrics are tracked based on the data, including the completeness of coverage across the region of interest for the assay.
- The process starts by taking raw sequence data, aligning it to a reference genome, and identifying variants based on the quality of the reads and the base pair calls.
- Variants are then annotated and filtered using a variety of features, including gene, transcript, Human Genome Variation Society nomenclature, population frequency, and presence in databases.
- In a clinical setting, a thorough validation of each of the components of the bioinformatics pipeline is critical, as is a detailed understanding of infrastructure, privacy, and security requirements.

INTRODUCTION

With the onset of high-throughput sequencing technologies, molecular genetic pathology has emerged from a visual-based specialty to an informatics-driven specialty. The increasing capabilities and reduced costs of sequencers, data computation, and data storage have enabled large-scaled sequencing (exomes and genomes) to be accessible to a wide range of patients. These include diagnosis of rare genetic conditions, in depth analysis of tumor–normal pairs, and screening of ostensibly healthy individuals. The increasing amount of data has also raised the profile of the burgeoning field of clinical bioinformatics. This article details the processes underlying clinical bioinformatics in the current molecular genetics workflow and provides the reader with a basic framework of the requirements needed to implement clinical bioinformatics in genomic sequencing.

SIGNIFICANCE

Although informatics is important in many aspects of laboratory testing, this article is focused on the computation, parsing, and analysis from sequencing machines through a final filtered set of variants. On the front end, the descriptions are most relevant for high-throughput genomic sequencing technologies (often referred to as next-generation sequencing [NGS]), although traditional sequencing machines have some commonalities.

Disclosure: The authors have nothing to disclose.

*Corresponding author, *E-mail address:* mlebo@bwh.harvard.edu

https://doi.org/10.1016/j.yamp.2018.06.003

On the back end, this article stops short of the process of variant interpretation, although the software required for variant interpretation may depend on the clinical bioinformatics processes that come before it.

Overall Workflow

The typical clinical bioinformatics process can be seen in Fig. 1. The process can roughly be broken down into primary, secondary, and tertiary analysis. Primary analysis refers to the algorithms associated to the sequencing machines that convert the raw sequence reads to a string of As, Cs, Ts, and Gs. Secondary analysis details the mapping, or alignment, of these sequence reads onto the reference genomic sequence and then variant calling, or the identification of differences between the individual's sequence and the reference genome. Tertiary analysis involves the steps needed to properly interpret the sequence variants identified, and includes annotating and filtering the identified variants to find clinically relevant variation. Underlying all steps within the clinical bioinformatics process are the quality control metrics that determine the completeness, robustness, and reliability of the generated data.

Primary Analysis

Primary analysis algorithms are provided by the sequencing manufacturer to transform the raw data generated from the sequencing machine into interpretable sequence. Because the raw data are imperfect, the algorithms also contain associated quality metrics detailing the likelihood of each base call being correct. Different sequence manufacturers, techniques, and chemistries have different error patterns and error rates. Therefore, the error composition may not be identical from one sequence vendor to another. The sequence data are typically returned as fastq or ubam files (Table 1). These file types contain information on the sequence identified in each read, a per-base assignment of the quality of that variant, as well as data corresponding with the sequence read itself. Note that some techniques sequence 2 sides of a smaller sequencing fragment. This method, called paired-end sequencing, can help with alignment and accuracy of the sequences. For the purposes of primary analysis, it is critical for these files to include information on the mate-pair to best use these additional data.

Secondary Analysis

Secondary analysis involves the taking the original sequencing data, processing it using a variety of statistical algorithms, and producing a set of sequence reads mapped to a genome and identifying difference between the individual and the reference. As mentioned, this stage depends on a reference genome. The reference genome is a

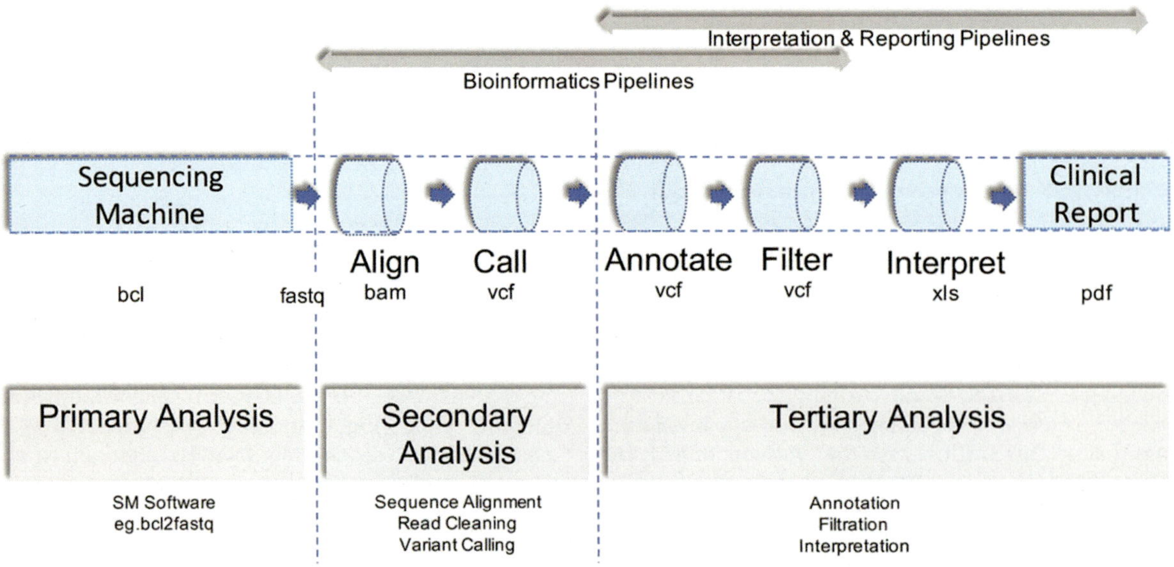

FIG. 1 Overview of bioinformatics processes in clinical genomic sequencing. This figure outlines the process for a data sample from the sequencing machine to clinical report. Detailed are the key steps in the process as well as some of the standard file types used in the pipeline.

TABLE 1
Common Data File Formats Used in Clinical Bioinformatics Tools

File Type	Link to Standard	Uses
FASTA	https://fasta.bioch.virginia.edu/fasta_www2/fasta_intro.shtml	Originally the format of the input file for FASTA, which "Compares a protein sequence to another protein sequence or to a protein database, or a DNA sequence to another DNA sequence or a DNA library." It is most commonly used for storing reference genome sequences.
FASTQ	http://maq.sourceforge.net/fastq.shtml	It stores sequences and Phred qualities in a single file.
SAM (Sequence Alignment Map)	https://samtools.github.io/hts-specs/SAMv1.pdf	It is a tab-delimited text format consisting of a header section, which is optional, and an alignment section.
BAM/BAI	http://samtools.github.io/hts-specs/SAMv1.pdf	Binary form of SAM. BAI is BAM index file.
uBAM (unmapped BAM)	https://gatkforums.broadinstitute.org/gatk/discussion/6484	Similar to BAM, because it maintains metadata, but with raw unmapped read sequences.
CRAM/CRAI	https://samtools.github.io/hts-specs/CRAMv3.pdf	CRAM is a more compressed version of aligned reads than BAM. Use of a CRAM file requires accessing the reference genome the reads were aligned to. CRAI is CRAM index file.
VCF/BCF	https://samtools.github.io/hts-specs/VCFv4.2.pdf	It contains metainformation lines, a header line, and then data lines each containing information about a position in the genome. The format also can contain genotype information on samples for each position. BCF is binary form of VCF.
BED (browser extensible data)	http://genome.ucsc.edu/FAQ/FAQformat#format1	Originally designed for displaying annotation data on a genome browser. It became widely used for describing features over sequence intervals. Not to be confused with PLINK BED, which is binary ped for individual genotype data.

standard set of sequence contigs for a species that define the current knowledge of the most likely consensus sequence, represented as a fasta file (see Table 1). It provides both a standard and a coordinate system to ensure the downstream components are referencing the same position. Typically, clinical laboratories currently use either hg19/GRCh37 or GRCh38 (Box 1, Table 2).

Once a defined reference sequence is selected, the secondary analysis pipeline typically involves the following components (Table 3 provides examples of commonly used software):

- Alignment—The process of mapping the specific reads found in the sequencer to the reference genome. This step uses the quality metrics present in the sequence read as well as the uniqueness or redundancy of the genomic sequence to determine the quality of the alignment.
- Sequence read cleanup—Depending on the sequencer and/or downstream algorithms, the original mapped reads may be adjusted or removed. Typical examples include removing duplicate reads that may be sequencing artifacts or using a more specialized local alignment within some of the reads.
- Variant calling—Using the mapped reads, algorithms look for differences between these reads and the reference genome. These differences may be single nucleotides, or large structural variants, depending on the sequencing methodology. The quality of these variant calls is determined using the quality and abundance of the sequence reads.

Alignment

During the alignment phase, the sequence reads are mapped to the reference genome. These alignment algorithms use data from the quality of the specific base calls as well as specific parameters allowing for both mismatches and gaps as compared with the reference.

BOX 1
Discussion of Genomic Reference Sequences

The human genome reference sequence is critical to the underlying clinical genomic bioinformatics process, because it provides both the template for alignment and a coordinate system for ensuring proper annotation and comparison of variants. There are 2 major genome builds currently in use today (GRCh37 [also referred to as hg19] and GRCh38). The GRC sequences are maintained by the Genome Reference Consortium (h referring to human), which releases both the reference genome build and patches to the build. Although the GRCh38 is a few years old, GRCh37 is still primarily used in clinical laboratories as the underlying annotation sources are being aligned against GRCh38 (see Table 5). There is also numerous software available that will liftover, or translate, between the 2 coordinate systems for resources that are only available on a single build [34–36].

Many research laboratories and some clinical laboratories have migrated to using GRCh38. There are some advantages to doing this, including fixing of errors in the underlying genome build. Additionally, GRCh38 has a large increase in the number of alternative loci. These loci are large regions of the genome in which there are multiple common haplotypes. These alternative loci may help to increase the accuracy of alignment for individuals who have these haplotypes, although they can also cause further confusion downstream in terms of annotation and variant calling. However, alignment and variant calling software have been updated to deal with these alternative loci. It is up to the laboratory to determine which genome build they will use in their assays and a thorough understanding of the pros and cons for either build is important in making this decision.

Related to genome build is the underlying transcript coordinate system used (see Table 2). RefSeq and Ensembl are 2 of the major sources for transcripts, but take different approaches. RefSeq is independent of the genome build, but then contains differences where there might be discrepancies. Ensembl transcripts are mapped to the genome build, but then depend on the genome build being used. Choosing which transcript system is most applicable for your laboratory should also consider these differences.

In this regard, a longer sequence read tends to map more accurately, because it enables less ambiguity in the alignment as well being able to handle more individual-specific variation against the reference genome. Furthermore, mapping from paired-end sequences can use 1 read with a high likelihood of aligning to a particular region to anchor the other read that may have similarity with multiple regions of the genome. Alignment software also gives a statistical likelihood that the read maps to the genomic region predicted, and is often represented as mapping quality (Table 4 provides definitions of quality metrics). Mapping quality represents the uniqueness of the region in the reference genome to which the read aligns, with regions not being able to uniquely map given a lower mapping quality score. See Box 2 for a discussion of difficult genomic regions.

Sequence read cleanup

There are often additional tools used after the alignment step to further process and clean the reads that have been mapped. Examples include the following.

- Aligned reads will get sorted by genomic position to enable faster processing in the downstream steps.
- For some methods, reads that are exact copies are likely to be duplicates of the original raw data and could skew variant calling if more than 1 read is included.
- Many algorithms realign certain regions, including around suspected indels, where the default settings in the alignment step may not be reliable.
- Some algorithms will adjust quality metrics using a set of variant calls most likely to be real.

Variant calling

Variant calling is perhaps both the most critical step in the clinical bioinformatics process as well as the biggest black box and most reliant on statistical modeling. The goal of variant calling is to identify all the instances where the individual's sequence is different as compared with the reference genome. These differences may be small (eg, single nucleotide variants [SNVs]) or may be very large (eg, multiple megabase deletions). Variant calling algorithms are often targeted to a class of variant (see examples elsewhere in this article and in Table 3), and even to a specific type of sequencing assay (eg, genome vs exome copy number variant calling). Detailed herein are some of the common variant types and approaches seen in genomic sequencing.

Single nucleotide variants and small insertion/deletions. SNVs and small insertion and/or deletion events (indels) are the smallest type of change identified in genomic sequencing assays. In this process, differences against the reference sequence are identified in the individual sequence reads. The quality metrics of the individual reads are combined for each of the reads overlapping that position to generate confidence in the call. In germline sequencing, heterozygous calls should have roughly one-half the reads with the variant call

TABLE 2
Community Resources in Clinical Bioinformatics

Type	Name	Link
Reference genome	GRCh37 (hg19)/GRCh38	https://www.ncbi.nlm.nih.gov/grc
Transcript/Gene	Ensembl	http://ensembl.org/info/genome/genebuild/genome_annotation.html
	RefSeq/Entrez	https://www.ncbi.nlm.nih.gov/refseq/
	LRG	http://www.lrg-sequence.org/
	CCDS	https://www.ncbi.nlm.nih.gov/projects/CCDS/CcdsBrowse.cgi
	UCSC	https://genome.ucsc.edu/cgi-bin/hgTables
Official Gene Names and Symbols	HUGO	https://www.genenames.org
Variant Nomenclature	HGVS	http://varnomen.hgvs.org/

and homozygous calls should have all reads with the variant call. Owing to random stochastic processes, especially at low coverage depth, low-quality sequence reads, ambiguities in mapping, and challenges with indel detection, the actual fraction of reads with a variant call may be different.

In general, variant calling for SNVs is highly accurate (>99.5% sensitivity and specificity) [1]. Indels, however, can prove more difficult. The longer the insertion/deletion event, the more challenging it is to map the read accurately. Additionally, if the indel even gets called at the end of the read, it is difficult for the aligner to know if this is a true variant or due to the reduced accuracy, in general, of nucleotide calls at the ends of reads. Other reasons may lead to more difficulty in calling SNVs/indels include the following.

- The variant lies in a challenging genomic region. For instance, regions with high homology are difficult to accurately map reads against. See Box 2 for more details.
- The variant is near or part of a homopolymer stretch. This positioning can cause issues with alignment and changes in the homopolymer stretches may appear as SNVs.
- Complex insertion deletion events can often look to the aligner like separate variants.

Copy number variants and structural variants. Genomic sequencing can also detect copy number variation (gains or losses of genomic sequence) and other types of structural variation (translocations, copy neutral insertions, inversions, fusions, chromothripsis, etc). These events can range from single exon copy number changes to megabase-sized events. However, the ability and methodologies used to detect these events depends entirely on the type of sequencing assay, the method for capturing genomic sequence, and other upstream sequencing assays [2]. For instance, exome and panel sequencing assays typically use one type of data (read depth) for calling copy number variants because breakpoints typically lie in intronic or intergenic sequences and they cannot use other methods that make use of breakpoint data. Similarly, exome- and panel-based assays do not detect other balanced structural variations, unless the assay is designed specifically to detect them (ie, fusion events in cancer or known, recurrent deletions), whereas genome sequencing can make use of both breakpoint and paired-end analysis to find these events.

Regions of homozygosity. Depending on the size of the sequencing panel, one may be able to identify large stretches of the genome where the individual seems to only have homozygous variation (also referred to absence of heterozygosity or loss of heterozygosity). Although this may occur sporadically owing to the presence of only common variation in that region, larger stretches may in fact reflect disease-causing variation, for instance, uniparental disomy or an underlying rare homozygous pathogenic variant. Additionally, summing up these homozygosity stretches can indicate both degrees of consanguinity (in germline sequencing) and tumor progression (in somatic sequencing).

Genotyping from sequencing. The benefit of high-throughput sequencing lies in the ability to scan large genomic regions for variation, including novel

TABLE 3
Examples of Popular Software Used in Secondary Analysis

Software Class	Name	Use	Ref
Alignment	BWA-SW	Alignment for shorter reads	Li & Durbin [42], 2009
	BWA-MEM	Alignment for longer reads (>100 bp)	Li & Durbin [43], 2010
	Novoalign	Commercial alignment software	[44]
Manipulating mapped sequence read files	Picard Tools [45], Samtools [46], and GATK [47] were all developed very early when next-generation sequencing was not so pervasive. They have been kept up to date with the advancement of sequencing technology and data processing best practices. They overlap on functions for frequently used manipulation. Samtools was implemented in C and Picard and GATK in Java.		
Manipulating and analyzing VCF files	Both BCFtools [48] and VCFtools [49] accept BCF and VCF files. The two have a highly overlapping set of functions yet each has its distinctive analytical features.		
SNV and indel calling	BCFtools/Samtools	Its variant calling is not used as widely as its other versatile features.	Li [45], 2011
	GATK—UnifiedGenotyper	Earlier version of GATK variant caller. Gradually gives way to HaplotypeCaller.	McKenna et al, [46] 2010
	GATK—HaplotypeCaller	Its local de novo assembly made the local realignment step that was required for UnifiedGenotyper redundant and intrinsically phases genotype calls to some extent.	Poplin et al, [47] 2017
	Freebayes	Bayesian haplotype-based. Its ability to use prior information and nonuniform genome-wide ploidy provided by users makes it more effective in analyzing genomes having particular properties.	Garrison & Marth [48], 2012
SV and CNV calling	Pindel	Detects large deletions and medium insertions by finding breakpoints in the unmapped pair-end read.	Ye et al, [49] 2009
	BreakDancer	One of very early SV callers. Detects SV by analyzing anomalous mapped read pairs.	Fan et al, [50] 2014
	GenomeStrip	Requires ≥20 samples. Analyzes a combination of read depth, read length, and read mate-pairing.	Handsaker et al, [51] 2015
	Manta	Illumina's SV and medium indels caller for germline and somatic analysis.	Chen et al, [52] 2016
	XHMM	CNV calling for exome data.	Fromer & Purcell [53], 2014
	VisCap	CNV calling for panel data.	Pugh et al, [54] 2016
Manipulating genomic intervals	bedtools	Touted as a Swiss Army Knife of tools for genome arithmetical, it is particularly useful for manipulating multiple bed (or other genomic interval format) files.	Quinlan [55], 2014
Variant call comparison	vcfeval	Can compare 2 different variant call files. Useful for validation.	Cleary et al, [56] 2015

(*continued on next page*)

TABLE 3
(*continued*)

Software Class	Name	Use	Ref
Obtaining quality control metrics	FastQC	Provides metrics useful for assessing sequencing quality. Supports multiple platforms.	[57]
	verifybamID	Detects sample contaminations and swaps.	Jun et al, [58] 2012
	Picard Tools	Provides quality control metrics for various stages of secondary analysis.	[59]

Abbreviations: CNV, copy number variant; SNV, structural variant.

variation, and not being limited to previously discovered variation. However, there are times when it is critical to know not only if the individual has the variant, but also exactly what their genotype is at a specific position. Common examples here include pharmacogenomic variation and instances where the disease-associated variant is the reference allele (often seen in risk alleles, eg, the factor V Leiden allele in GRCh37). A standard vcf file will just contain variation against the reference, so the downstream processes may not be able to determine whether the absence of a call is due to lack of data or if the individual is truly homozygous reference. Therefore, genotyping these specific positions off the sequencing data can provide further confidence into the individual's exact genotype.

TABLE 4
Examples of Quality Metrics in Secondary Analysis

Name	Abbreviation	Definition
Read depth	DP	Depth of sequencing coverage at that position
Mapping quality	MQ	Mapping quality of specific position
Strand bias	SB	Measure of strand bias at that position
Variant call quality by depth	QD	Variant call quality normalized by depth
Quality score	QUAL	Confidence of any call at that position
Genotype call quality	GQ	Confidence in the genotyping call in an individual
Allele depth	AD	Coverage of specific variants at genomic position

Tertiary Analysis

During tertiary analysis, the identified sequence variants are placed more broadly into the genomic and clinical context. Whereas secondary analysis ends with the identification of a genomic change (ie, a difference against the genomic reference), tertiary analysis enables the downstream systems and users to appropriately interpret the exact difference. This factor makes the process both difficult and critically important to make robust and complete, and provides its own challenges in validation (discussed elsewhere in this article).

Tertiary analysis can involve the following components.

- Annotation—The process of adding details to the identified genomic change, including gene, transcript, and nomenclature information. This gives the specific context and available knowledge for the variant of interest.
- Filtration/prioritization—In genomic sequencing, depending on what was targeted, one can identify hundreds, thousands, or even millions of variants. Filtration involves the process of using bioinformatic approaches and annotations to limit the number of variants that require manual review.
- Interpretation—Although the actual process of variant interpretation falls outside of the purview of clinical bioinformatics, the data and systems used for interpretation are entirely within scope. Thus, it is critical for this component to follow standard bioinformatic practices.

Annotation

After variant calling, the variants need to be annotated to assess their effects in biology, physiology, and clinical relevance. This analysis involves extracting available

> **BOX 2**
> **Challenging Genomic Regions in Clinical Sequencing**
>
> There are certain regions of the genome that are complex and challenging to interrogate with the current sequencing modalities. These regions can cause decreases in accuracy during sequencing and are important to understand upfront in the assay development process. Difficult genomic regions are normally described as the following categories.
>
> - Low complexity DNA regions can be simple repeats (microsatellites where a unit of 2 or 3 nucleotides repeat many times), poly-purine (strings of guanine or cytosine)/poly-pyrimidine (adenine or thymine) stretches, or regions of extremely high AT or GC content.
> - Segmental duplication are large-scale chromosomal duplications. They can be remnants of whole genome duplication. Such regions have high similarity (homology).
> - Low mappability. Mappability describes how sequence reads can be uniquely mapped/aligned to a region. This factor can vary depending on read lengths. The longer the reads are, the greater the overall mappability of a genome is.
> - High or low guanine-cytosine (GC) content.
>
> These categories can be somewhat related. For instance, both low-complexity regions and segmental duplications can lead to low mappability. Genomic regions with particularly high GC content are difficult to sequence owing to the stronger base pairing between G (guanine) and C (cytosine) than that of A (adenine) and T (thymine). This can lead to insufficient coverage. The Genome in a Bottle Consortium and the Global Alliance for Genomics and Health have defined a set of these regions that can be useful during benchmarking and validation of pipelines [37] and a similar resource has identified stretches of homology in clinically relevant genes that could cause issues in sequencing [38].

knowledge at the gene, transcript, protein, and regulatory levels from biological databases, as well as a detailed knowledge of the variant at the population and evolution levels to predict the effects and function of a variant. Prior clinical data and published literature are also mined to identify previous genetic information that may indicate disease association.

Gene/transcript annotation and Human Genome Variation Society nomenclature. Clinical genomic interpretation today remains focused on coding content. Thus, at its basis, a variant is annotated with regard to the genes and transcripts in which it lies. These annotations place the variant in the context of the coding portion of the gene, and include variant effect (silent, nonsense, missense, frameshift, etc), variant location (exon, intron, untranslated region), and variant nomenclature. A gene can be expressed in multiple forms (transcripts) by alternative splicing. The position of a variant in a gene could affect all or only some of the transcripts. Different laboratories use different resources for determining transcripts (see Table 2) and different policies for determining the major transcript (ie, longest, most highly expressed, historic, or transcript with most clinically relevant variants).

Regarding variant nomenclature, the Human Genome Variation Society has developed and iterated on a sequence variant nomenclature system and its recommendations have been widely accepted as the standard, which provides a consistent and unambiguous description of sequence variants [3]. The representation of variants by these recommendations is described at the most basic DNA level and in relation to an accepted reference sequence. The type of reference sequences used is indicated by 6 letter prefixes—g, c, m, n, r, and p—corresponding with genomic DND, cDNA, mitochondrial DNA, noncoding RNA, RNA, and protein sequences. The more detailed recommendations can be seen at http://varnomen.hgvs.org/.

Population frequency. Minor allele frequency is ratio of the count of a nonreference allele to total number of alleles of the same locus in a population. A low allele frequency implies rarity of the variant, which is usually thought as linked to disease, although this is not always the case. The aggregation of genome sequencing data (eg, 1000 Genome Project, Exome Aggregation Consortium, and Genome Aggregation Database) [4–6] allows the integration of hundreds of thousands of individuals to compute variant frequencies across different ethnicities. So far, variant frequencies have been computed in more than 20 races that are further clustered into subpopulations, such as Black, American, Ashkenazi Jewish, East Asian, non-Finnish European, Finnish, and South Asian. Laboratories will use the maximum of these minor allele frequencies across the subpopulations as an aid in filtration, with the assumption that a particular population does not have an increased incidence of a certain disease that would cause a higher subpopulation frequency.

The sequencing depth, also known as coverage, is an important indicator to evaluate the sequencing quality. It determines if absence of a variant is real or due to poor coverage at genomic location. Although the aggregated data provided precise allele frequency among human races, an average coverage data will facilitate assessing the quality of variant frequency.

Variant databases. To annotate variants accurately and precisely, high-quality and reliable data sources are essential. These data sources can be public or commercially available. A list of datasets and databases is included in Table 5, which are selected by laboratories based on their availability, quality, and reliability. These resources often contain information on variant classification, disease association, relevant literature, and case history. They are crucial to determining the previous genetic information known about a variant.

TABLE 5
Datasets and Databases for Variant Annotation

Dataset/ Database	Description	Features	GRCh37	GRCh38
dbSNP	A central repository for both SNP/indel polymorphisms.	Variant ID, location.	Yes	Yes
Human Gene Mutation Database (HGMD)	Repository for all known (published) gene lesions responsible for human inherited disease.	It provides gene symbol, cDNA sequence, genomic coordinates, HGVS nomenclature, missense/nonsense, splicing, regulatory, deletions/insertions, complex rearrangements, repeat variations.	Yes	Yes
ClinVar	Repository of human variants related to phenotypes with supporting evidence.	It provides identifiers, attributes of phenotype, description of the genotype/phenotype relationship, submission information, represented evidence, integrated data from multiple sources.	Yes	Yes
LOVD	Repository of gene-centered DNA variations, as well as storage of patient-centered data and NGS data.	It provides gene symbol, genomic position of variants, variants on genes, variants on transcripts, variants in a patient, all diseases associated with a gene, all screenings for a gene.	NA	NA
1000 Genome	A project to find genetic variants with frequencies of $\geq$1%.	Population frequency.	Yes	Yes
gnomAD	A resource aggregating both exome and genome sequencing data from a wide variety of large-scale sequencing projects.	Population frequency, coverage.	Yes	No
ExAC	Same as gnomAD.	Population frequency, coverage.	Yes	No
Alamut	A database that integrates NCBI, EBI, UCSC, HGVS nomenclature.	It provides annotations such as variant effect, splicing prediction, protein domain, functional prediction.	Yes	Yes
dbNSFP	A lightweight database of human nonsynonymous SNPs and their functional predictions.	It compiles prediction scores from SIFT, Polyphen2, LRT, MutationTaster, PhyloP and other related information for every potential nonsynonymous variant in the human genome. It also provides annotations of conservation values, function prediction.	Yes	Yes

Abbreviations: HGVS, Human Genome Variation Society; NGS, next-generation sequencing; SNP, single nucleotide polymorphism.

Computational prediction algorithms and conservation. There are many algorithms available that attempt to computationally predict the effect that a variant may have on a protein (ie, MutationAssessor, MutationTaster, PolyPhen2, REVEL [7–10]). Initial methods aimed to determine the potential impact of missense variation on a protein, whereas more recent, sophisticated algorithms attempt to predict the effect of any genomic change. In general, these algorithms predict benign variation better than pathogenic variation and still suffer from a high number of false calls. These tools often make use of conservation of the nucleotide or amino acid across species, where high conservation can be reflective of positive selection and thus likely functional consequence.

To implement variant annotation, a few software tools (ANNOVAR, SnpEff, VEP, Oncotator), among a long list of bioinformatics genome annotation tools, are commonly used (Table 6) [11–14]. A more integrated annotation tool named WGSA was relatively recently developed which integrates the outputs of other annotation approaches and combines other prediction scores, conservations scores, and knowledge of regulator region-centric resources to annotate variants [15]. The procedure of variant annotation for a sample is shown in Fig. 2.

TABLE 6
Commonly Used Software of Variant Annotation

Software	Description	Functionality	Ref
ANNOVAR	An efficient software tool to use update-to-date information to functionally annotate genetic variants.	Gene-based, region-based, filter-based annotation.	Wang et al, [11] 2010
SnpEff	A variant annotation and effect prediction tool.	It annotates and predicts the effects of variants on genes.	Cingolani et al, [13] 2012
VEP	A variant effect predictor.	VEP determines the effect of variants on genes, transcripts and protein sequence, as well as regulatory regions.	McLaren et al, [12] 2016
Oncotator	A web application for annotating human genomic point mutations and indels with data relevant to cancer researchers.	Annotations are aggregated from Genomic Annotations, protein annotations, cancer variants annotations, and noncancer variant annotations.	Ramos et al, [14] 2015
WGSA	WGSA is an annotation pipeline for human genome resequencing studies, to facilitate the functional annotation step of whole genome sequencing.	It integrates the outputs from ANNOVAR, SnpEff, and VEP for gene-model based annotation. It also integrates multiple prediction scores, conservation scores, allele frequencies and disease related database for SNV-centric resources, as well as integrates multiple epigenomics projects for regulatory region-centric resources.	Liu et al, [15] 2016
CADD	CADD is a tool for scoring the deleteriousness of SNP/indels variants in the human genome.	It integrates multiple annotations into one metric by contrasting variants that survived natural selection with simulated mutations. It is an algorithm designed to annotate both coding and noncoding variants.	Kircher et al, [60] 2014
DANN	A deep learning approach for annotating the pathogenicity of genetic variants.	Same as CADD.	Quang et al, [61] 2014

Abbreviations: CADD, combined annotation-dependent depletion; SNP, Single nucleotide polymorphism; SNV, single nucleotide variant; WGSA, WGS Annotator.

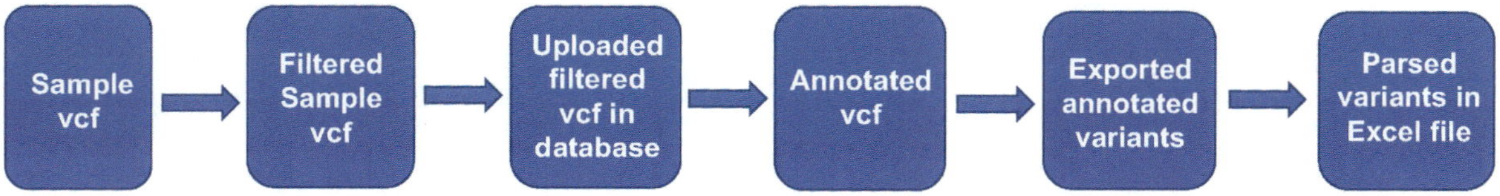

FIG. 2 Key steps of variant annotation. A sample vcf file is filtered through a bed file with regions of interest. The filtered vcf file is then uploaded into database and annotated. The annotated variants can then be managed in the software, or can be exported and examined externally, such as in Excel.

Gene-level annotations. The clinical effect of a variant is principally through affecting expression and function of the gene. If a protein plays a known function in human physiology, loss or alteration of the protein's function could lead to phenotypic consequences. It is, therefore, important to determine the likelihood that altering a protein will affect biological function. This analysis can be done by evaluating the evidence of a gene–disease association. The Clinical Genome Reference (ClinGen) has produced a framework and a team of curators for this task [16]. Additionally, it is important to know whether a gene can tolerate variation, particularly whether it can tolerate a loss-of-function variation, to know the likelihood of a specific variant having an impact. Computational resources examining how constrained a gene is against variation, including loss-of-function variation, have been developed and are widely used [4,17,18].

Filtration/prioritization

After annotating the identified variants, one is left with thousands, tens of thousands, or even millions of variants to sort through. This scenario is obviously too challenging to perform manually and thus the bioinformatics processes must make use of the structured annotation data generated. The goal of the filtration component is to get to the minimal set of variants required to interpret for the assay (Fig. 3). In panel-based sequencing, this may be every variant identified in the regions or genes of

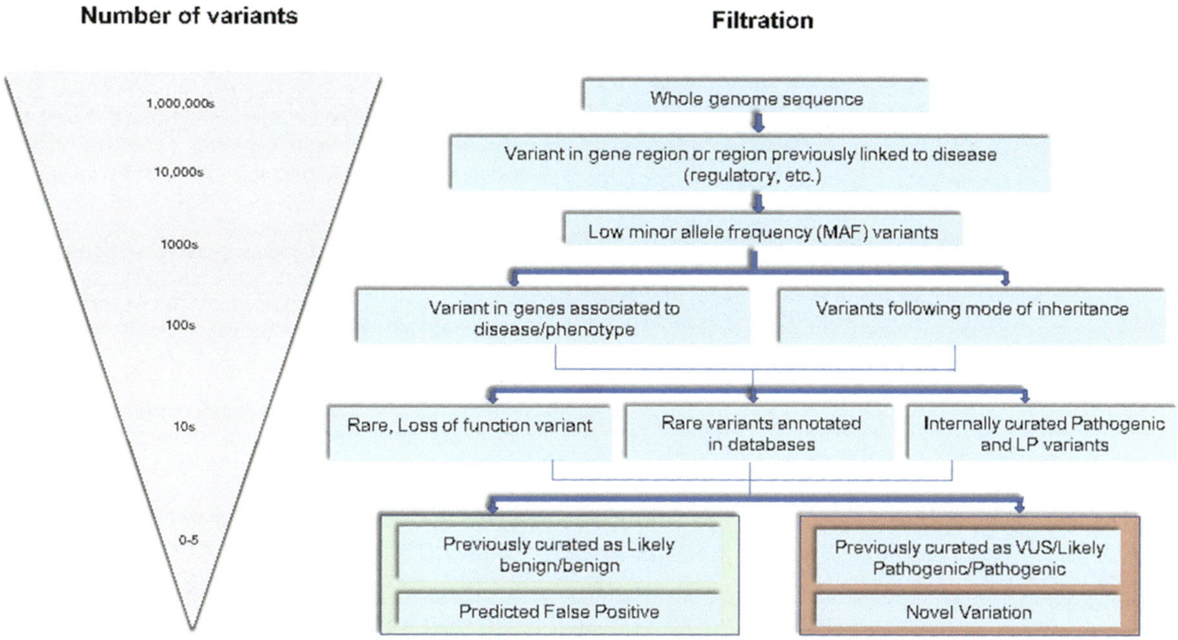

FIG. 3 Genomic sequencing filtration process. Example of a filtration workflow for identifying disease-associated variants from genomic sequencing. As more filters are applied, the smaller the number of variants that are kept for review. After variants are filtered in, they may have different classifications based on previous interpretation or quality metrics. Variants in green should be reviewed quickly, but can be discarded quickly. Variants in red will need a more thorough review process to determine if they meet reporting criteria. LP, likely pathogenic; VUS, variant of uncertain significance.

interest, whereas in exome or genome sequencing this may be the smaller set of variants most likely to have clinical relevance.

The simplest filter mechanism, and the one used in nearly every assay, is to limit the variants to exons, genes, and/or regions of interest. These regions may be predefined by the assay or defined on the fly based on the individual's presentation. Either way, the goal is to limit the reviewed variants to those most likely to correspond with the indication for testing. A similar approach is to limit variants in exome and genome sequencing to the medical exome, or the set of approximately 2000 to 4500 genes with evidence of having a disease association.

Other common types of filtration approaches include the following. Often, multiple filters or combinations of filters are applied in each case. A more in-depth discussion on the tools used in tertiary analysis can be found in Box 3 and some challenges can be found in Box 4.

BOX 3
Resources for Tertiary Analysis

There are numerous bioinformatic software solutions for the tertiary sequencing component of clinical genomics. These software solutions may do part of the process or may even extend into other areas, including secondary analysis and clinical reporting. At a minimum, it is important for these solutions to contain a genomic database that can store the annotations in a robust way and that efficient searching or filtering can be performed against it. It is important to remember that, whether these systems are vendor supplied, open source, or developed in house, the molecular geneticist/pathologist and the clinical bioinformaticians are responsible for ensuring their accuracy. It is also critical to have a thorough understanding of how they work, including which data they are using, how that data have been parsed, and how they are performing their exact filtrations.

Another important aspect to consider for these softwares is that they offer a continuous learning environment. Typically, variants that are either parsed during a triage process or fully interpreted are seen on multiple cases. It is important to get these variant classifications back into the system so they can be used in the filtering or review of the next case. It is also useful to have the date of the initial interpretation to make sure the classification is up to date with the most recent knowledge. Similarly, it is useful to maintain a repository of all individuals who have been identified with a variant. This way, when a variant classification changes, it can be properly reflected in each of the previous cases and communicated to the clinicians if necessary.

BOX 4
Challenges in Annotation and Variant Nomenclature

Although annotation of variants in genomic sequencing is critical, there are often difficulties of which the molecular geneticist/pathologist needs to be aware. One of the most challenging aspects that can cause issues in annotation involved variant nomenclature and how variants are represented in different standards. For instance, although the Human Genome Variation Society provides rules for variant nomenclature, some of the rules are ambiguous, allow for multiple options, or have changed over time. Similarly, HUGO, the resource responsible for determining gene names and symbols, is often updating these symbols in real time, causing gene nomenclature to become inaccurate and obsolete. This factor makes accurately mapping the change identified in an individual to a change previously reported difficult at times.

One way to solve this issue is to ensure that all annotations involve the same standard. For instance, a common approach is to use vcf files to add annotations, because this approach can normalize the information to a single genomic change. However, this also can cause challenges. Namely, the vcf standard for indels is different than the Human Genome Variation Society standard for indels. Often, an indel occurs at a region where there is similar sequence context, because the variant cannot be unambiguously placed at one specific location (Fig. 4). In this case, the vcf standard is to shift the indel to the 5′ most position on the genomic reference (left align). The Human Genome Variation Society standard, however, has the indel shifted to the 3′ most position on the transcript (right align). Therefore, when the transcript is on the top (or positive) strand, the indels will be represented by different genomic positions. The Human Genome Variation Society standard also may use duplication or repeat nomenclature, which is not part of the vcf standard. Furthermore, the vcf standard does not allow for blank values for either the reference (ref) or variant (alternative; alt) fields, causing insertion and deletion events to be shifted by another position to account for the upstream nucleotide that is not part of the event. Accounting for these issues in the bioinformatics pipeline are possible, so it is important that the molecular geneticist/pathologist knows how they were implemented.

- Genetics-based filtration—This includes sequencing a trio (proband and parents) and looking for compound heterozygous or homozygous variants in recessive conditions, or de novo variation in sporadic cases; sequencing multiple affected individuals to find variants in common; and sequencing a tumor/normal pair to identify somatically derived variation.

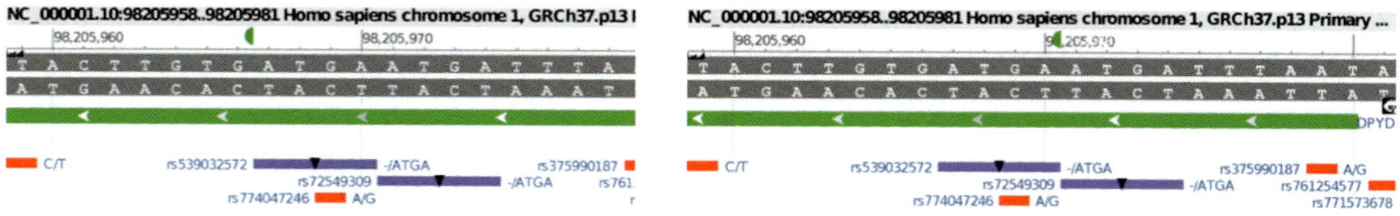

	Variant ID	Location	Variant type	Gene	Molecular consequences	Most severe clinical significance	ExAC MAF	Publications
▸	rs539032572	98,205,967 - 98,205,970	deletion	DPYD	frameshift variant		- = 9.1e-5	
▸	rs72549309	98,205,971 - 98,205,974	deletion	DPYD	frameshift variant			1

FIG. 4 A variant cannot be unambiguously placed at 1 specific location. A deletion of 1 unit (ATGA) of tandem repeats can be placed at 2 locations, which are represented by 2 database of single nucleotide polymorphisms (dbSNP) entries: (1) rs539032572: NC_000001.10:g.98205967_98205970delATGA and (2) rs72549309: NC_000001.10:g.98205971_98205974delATGA. Both result in a frameshift. Deletion of either unit would be annotated as rs539032572 (*left align*) in vcf, whereas rs72549309 (right align) per Human Genome Variation Society (HGVS) guidelines. rs72549309 is cited in 1 publication on pharmacogenes. A researcher looking for its allele frequency in ExAC would not find any frequency information because the same ATGA deletion is represented by rs539032572 in ExAC, whose variants are natively stored in vcf. (*Adapted from* National Center for Biotechnology Information. Variation viewer. Available at: https://www.ncbi.nlm.nih.gov/variation/view/. Accessed April 17, 2018.)

- Phenotype-based filtration—As mentioned, limiting the variant calls to those previously associated with the disease or present in genes with established disease causation. The gene-based approach captures all potential variation in the gene, whereas the variant-based approach relies on previously published information present in curated variant databases (eg, ClinVar [19]).
- Variant-based filtration—This filtration strategy may be unbiased. It relies on using structured annotations to extract variants with certain features, including:
    - Rarity (low frequency or absence) in population databases;
    - Type of variation (ie, nonsense, missense mutations);
    - Location of variant (ie, near splice site); and
    - In silico predicted effects on function, structure, or evolutionary conservation.

Interpretation

The final stage in the clinical genomics workflow before reporting is providing a full interpretation of the identified variants, which entails using all available evidence to determine a variant's association with disease. Recent guidelines have detailed approaches for classifying both germline and somatic variation [20,21]. Although the actual interpretation falls outside of the purview of clinical bioinformatics, the software and resources used are often heavily driven by the informatics infrastructure, especially reliable and complete annotation of the data [22]. Therefore, an understanding of the interpretation workflow is critical to clinical bioinformatics. The number of possible annotations is often too numerous to completely consume manually and the bioinformatics workflow is responsible for paring those down into clinically meaningful subsets.

In the genomic workflow, there are often multiple different approaches to interpretation. As mentioned, the number of variants that come out of the pipeline cannot be all reviewed manually for each case. Therefore, filtration and other methods are needed to be able to parse through these variants while maintaining a high clinical rigor. This process includes the following.

- Preclassifying variation before identifying it in the laboratory. One use case would be relatively common pathogenic variation that one is likely to encounter during testing. Another use case would be variants that have high population frequency and no evidence for pathogenicity that can be classified as benign or likely benign.
- Triaging variants that come out of the filtration process. Even though the filtration process is geared toward extracting variants that are most likely to have clinical relevance, often variants get pulled in whose evidence is limited. These variants can be parsed through more quickly, assuming they do not meet requirements to be included on the clinical report.
- Full assessment of variant pathogenicity. For variants that may have clinical relevance, it is important to

use a tool that pulls in all potentially relevant data and enables the molecular geneticist/pathologist to perform a thorough review and approve the final variant classification.

Quality Control Measures

The clinical bioinformatics process for genomic sequencing focuses on identifying and interpreting variation, but includes numerous additional components. Chief among these are analyzing the data at various steps for quality control measures, including what was done during the upstream laboratory process. The quality control metrics can help to determine the accuracy and completeness of the sequencing assay. Some common metrics can be found in Table 7. More specific use cases during the quality control process are detailed herein.

Coverage

In a NGS assay, coverage (often represented by depth) is a measure of the number of reads overlapping a position. Although the overall raw coverage of a base can be useful, most clinical metrics view coverage in terms of usable data or data that would be used to make a variant call. In this regard, coverage is often reduced to those reads where both the mapping quality of the entire read is high and the base quality for the specific position within that read is high. Coverage also often gets defined by 2 metrics:

- Average coverage—Across all positions within the region of interest, the average number of usable reads that align; and
- Percent completeness—For a given coverage depth (ie, 15×), the percent of bases within the region of interest that have at least that coverage

These metrics can be measured at an exon, gene, panel, exome, or genome level. Typically, completeness is more informative owing to differences in sequencing ability because it more accurately reflects the overall ability to call variants.

Contamination

Owing to the generally high depth within clinical sequencing assays and the size of the sequencing assays, it is also possible to detect low level contamination in samples. This contamination may be due to other clinical samples in the laboratory, or my even be due to bacteria and other organisms. Depending on the specific assay and library preparation methods, it may be important to

TABLE 7
Common Quality Control Metrics

Type	Metric	Definition
Coverage	Average coverage	Average depth across all bases within ROI
	% completeness	% of bases within ROI at a minimum depth of coverage (ie, 15×)
	% low covered regions	% of regions not meeting target coverage level
Sample identity	Contamination	Estimate of the number of reads that come from another individual or another species, such as bacteria
	% identity	Uniqueness of sample as compared with an orthogonal genotyping assay
Sequencing metrics	Total number of reads	Total number of raw read associated to the sample
	% reads passing filters	% of raw reads that pass filter metrics for being of sufficient quality
	% reads mapped	% of raw reads that map to reference genome
	% reads on target	% of raw reads that map to capture region (not used in genome sequencing)
	Insert size	In paired-end sequencing, the average distance between the 2 ends of the sequence
Variant metrics	Total number of variants	Total number of variants identified in ROI; should reflect control samples in ROI
	Ti/Tv ratio	Ratio of transitions to transversions. Should reflect control samples in ROI
	SNV/Indel ratio	Ratio of SNV to indel calls. Should reflect control samples in ROI
	Het/Hom ratio	Ratio of heterozygous variants to homozygous variants. Should reflect control samples in ROI

Abbreviations: ROI, region of interest; SNV, single nucleotide variant.

monitor sequencing runs for contamination, because a small amount may compromise variant calling.

Identity checking

Similarly, it is also important to ensure that the data from the sequencer and against which variant calling is occurring is correctly associated with the right individual. In this regard, it is possible to use both the sheer number of variants called and rare variation. Using the population frequency of potential variants, one can determine the uniqueness of a sample. Combining this information with a previous a separately run dataset (often a genotyping array or small sequencing assay), one can determine that the data they are reviewing is from the individual from which it is suspected to have come.

Validation

Perhaps the most unique aspects in clinical bioinformatics as compared with research sequencing is the deep validation that needs to be performed before launching of the clinical assay. In typical NGS guidelines, the bioinformatics component of the validation has not been thoroughly detailed. However, some publications, including the checklists provided by the College of American Pathologists and the recent guidelines specifically on bioinformatics pipelines by the Association of Molecular Pathologists, provide much more detail into how to think about assay validation in terms of the bioinformatics components [23–25].

For typical clinical assays, sensitivity and specificity are common metrics to analyze during validation. However, in sequencing assays, most positions are not expected to have a variant and, thus, sensitivity is less meaningful. Laboratories therefore often think about sensitivity and positive predictive value. Determining these values for the sequencing assay can be difficult. The recent Association of Molecular Pathologists guidelines suggest at least 59 variants tested per variant type (SNV, small indel, large indel, complex variant, etc). Although this strategy is useful for challenging variants, in practice it may be underpowered to evaluate true sensitivity and positive predictive value. However, there are resources to help the laboratory reach the required number of variants, including the following.

- NIST Genome in a Bottle—A series of very well-characterized genomes that have been sequenced across multiple technologies to be used for comparison purposes. Corresponding samples are also available [26].
- Illumina Platinum Genomes—High-coverage genome sequencing of 17 members from a CEPH family [27].
- The Centers for Disease Control and Prevention's Get-RM program—Includes regions orthogonally validated by external laboratories, including a detailed pharmacogenomic characterization of 137 samples [28,29].
- Synthetic cell lines—Provided by a variety of vendors, these samples are engineered to contain multiple variants in 1 sample and, thus, can be good to test a high number of variants in a single run
- In silico–derived variation—There are numerous tools that take raw sequence data and use in silico algorithms to insert variation into the sample [30–32]. These tools can serve as a good proxy for difficult variation, but should not supplement actual samples.

These datasets, as well as internal and external samples with known variation, can help the laboratory to properly set thresholds for determining false-positive calls. Similarly, these samples can help the laboratory to determine the threshold for high-confidence true positives, that is, variants that may not need orthogonal confirmation. For further detail, see Box 5.

In addition to sensitivity and positive predictive value, it is important for the laboratory to properly version each pipeline and to capture the exact pipeline

BOX 5
Orthogonal Confirmation of Genomic Variants

Typically, especially in germline molecular genetics, reported variants identified by genomic sequencing are confirmed by an orthogonal method. However, this can cause both increased costs and a delayed turn-around time, specifically in exome and genome sequencing where the primer pairs may need to be developed on the fly. To minimize this occurrence, some laboratories have implemented policies to not confirm variants based on classes (ie, likely benign and benign variants, or carrier status variants). With the high accuracy of most next-generation sequencing data (excluding the difficult regions discussed in Box 2), it may not be necessary to do this for every variant.

Indeed, some laboratories have shown high enough accuracy to either reduce or eliminate confirmation with Sanger sequencing of the identified single nucleotide variants and indels [1,39–41]. Although these publications did not contain many false-positive calls on which to set their metrics, they did show that the general framework exists. Confirmation of low-quality calls or calls in difficult regions may still be necessary, but using specific metrics to identify only high-quality true positives that do not need confirmation will add a direct benefit to the laboratory, providers, and patients.

through which a specific sample was run. Changes to the pipeline need to be revalidated. The scope of revalidation should coincide with the scope of the changes. For instance, a new variant calling pipeline should dictate a complete revalidation, whereas updating an interpretation database may just require a simple equivalency check. It is up to the molecular geneticist/pathologist to determine the scope of revalidation and, thus, is a further reason why a thorough understanding of the process is required.

Infrastructure and Storage Policy

The discussion of bioinformatics in clinical genomic sequencing is incomplete without a basic understanding of information infrastructure and current computing paradigms used to plan and manage infrastructure for computation and analysis of vast amount of NGS data. This field is fast evolving, but there are 3 general approaches a laboratory or an organization can take.

- On Premises—This is the traditional way of implementing information and computing infrastructure. This strategy usually is a combination of HPC and grid computing implementation with analysis and bioinformatics pipeline software installed and implemented within an organization's firewall.
- Cloud—This technology is an emerging way of doing large-scale computation and analysis without spending unnecessary amounts of money and time on infrastructure outright. It is usually the way smaller organizations and startups implement their infrastructure.
- Hybrid—Most large organizations tend to lean toward hybrid approach, which is a combination of both approaches mentioned, mostly owing to various regulatory and systems requirements and considerations.

As with the need for infrastructure plan, there is a need to create policies that take systems view of bioinformatics data to ensure the bioinformatics processes run with efficiency, optimizing data processing and storage, and in adherence to regulatory requirements. Box 6 goes over some common topics to consider for data policy implementation.

BOX 6
Common Topics to Consider for Data Policy Implementation

Some important topics to consider while planning for implementation of data policy for an organization or a research group include data format used, data compression, metadata, storage, backup, Intellectual Property/Patient Health Information, data life cycle, and retention periods, in addition to data organization and data quality assurance. Setting best practices to be followed by the bioinformatics team is critical here, to be able to track and maintain original and reported data and to keep storage costs within budget. Another critical aspect of clinical bioinformatics is maintaining data security. This goal can be achieved by implementing measures to ensure data integrity, for instance, by appropriately understanding roles, ownership, and end users of clinical data. Similarly, the data policy needs to adhere to regulatory considerations, such as the Health Insurance Portability and Accountability Act, Clinical Laboratory Improvement Amendments, and state regulations, that an organization's data may fall under. It is good practice in next-generation sequencing data management to have regular data audits with the team to ensure that best practices and data policy items are implemented. Designing and implementing these policies upfront is critical to the long-term success of the organization, including designing a data architecture and integration platform that is not just for current needs but flexible enough to handle future challenges.

FUTURE DIRECTIONS

Genome-scale sequencing is on the cusp of being the routine assay for not only diagnostics, but also for the screening of healthy individuals and even newborns. There are numerous advances in algorithms, technology, and computation that will enable faster, more accurate, and more complete genomic sequencing. These advances include the following.

- Longer read sequencing that will enable better resolution of the genome and more accurate alignment.
- GPU-based software that will enable increased parallelization and faster computation.
- A graph-based reference genome that will enable a true complete genome path and more accurate alignment, especially for underrepresented ethnicities.

Genomic sequencing is also starting to make use of general advances in computation, specifically around big data. There are already examples of using machine learning approaches in variant calling [33] and similar machine learning and natural language processing approaches will be able to increase the accuracy of variant interpretation as well. There is also promising work extending the laboratory beyond its silo and better integrating laboratory findings with deep mining of clinical data and patient phenotypes. This data integration will also enable interpretation of the full genome, without being limited to the coding regions, which are the main focus of current clinical interpretation workflows. Taken together, these advances will help to unleash the potential of an individual's genome within the continuum of clinical practice.

SUMMARY

Genomic sequencing is increasingly becoming part of clinical practice and the size and scope of the data generated relies more and more heavily on bioinformatics. Although the underlying algorithms and pipelines may seem complex, it is crucial for the molecular geneticist/pathologist to have a thorough understanding of the bioinformatics tools' purpose, outputs, and main underlying assumptions. This understanding includes each of the steps in the process, important quality control metrics and criteria, and validation approaches. Having a broad knowledge of the clinical bioinformatics process can enable the molecular geneticist/pathologist to ensure that the genomic assay is complete, robust, and accurate for clinical practice.

REFERENCES

[1] Baudhuin LM, Lagerstedt SA, Klee EW, et al. Confirming variants in next-generation sequencing panel testing by sanger sequencing. J Mol Diagn 2015;17:456–61.

[2] Mason-Suares H, Landry L, Lebo MS. Detecting copy number variation via next generation technology. Curr Genet Med Rep 2016;4:74–85.

[3] den Dunnen JT, Dalgleish R, Maglott DR, et al. HGVS recommendations for the description of sequence variants: 2016 update. Hum Mutat 2016;37:564–9.

[4] Lek M, Karczewski KJ, Minikel EV, et al. Analysis of protein-coding genetic variation in 60,706 humans. Nature 2016;536:285–91.

[5] 1000 Genomes Project Consortium, Auton A, Brooks LD, Durbin RM, et al. A global reference for human genetic variation. Nature 2015;526:68–74.

[6] gnomAD browser. Available at: http://gnomad.broadinstitute.org/. Accessed April 16, 2018.

[7] Schwarz JM, Rödelsperger C, Schuelke M, et al. MutationTaster evaluates disease-causing potential of sequence alterations. Nat Methods 2010;7:575–6.

[8] Reva B, Antipin Y, Sander C. Predicting the functional impact of protein mutations: application to cancer genomics. Nucleic Acids Res 2011;39:e118.

[9] Adzhubei I, Jordan DM, Sunyaev SR. Predicting functional effect of human missense mutations using PolyPhen-2. Curr Protoc Hum Genet 2013;Chapter 7: Unit7.20.

[10] Ioannidis NM, Rothstein JH, Pejaver V, et al. REVEL: an ensemble method for predicting the pathogenicity of rare missense variants. Am J Hum Genet 2016;99:877–85.

[11] Wang K, Li M, Hakonarson H. ANNOVAR: functional annotation of genetic variants from high-throughput sequencing data. Nucleic Acids Res 2010;38:e164.

[12] McLaren W, Gil L, Hunt SE, et al. The ensemble variant effect predictor. Genome Biol 2016;17:122.

[13] Cingolani P, Platts A, Wang le L, et al. A program for annotating and predicting the effects of single nucleotide polymorphisms, SnpEff: SNPs in the genome of Drosophila melanogaster strain w1118; iso-2; iso-3. Fly (Austin) 2012;6:80–92.

[14] Ramos AH, Lichtenstein L, Gupta M, et al. Oncotator: cancer variant annotation tool. Hum Mutat 2015;36: E2423–9.

[15] Liu X, White S, Peng B, et al. WGSA: an annotation pipeline for human genome sequencing studies. J Med Genet 2016;53:111–2.

[16] Strande NT, Riggs ER, Buchanan AH, et al. Evaluating the clinical validity of gene-disease associations: an evidence-based framework developed by the clinical genome resource. Am J Hum Genet 2017;100:895–906.

[17] Samocha KE, Robinson EB, Sanders SJ, et al. A framework for the interpretation of de novo mutation in human disease. Nat Genet 2014;46:944–50.

[18] Petrovski S, Wang Q, Heinzen EL, et al. Genic intolerance to functional variation and the interpretation of personal genomes. PLoS Genet 2013;9:e1003709.

[19] Landrum MJ, Lee JM, Benson M, et al. ClinVar: improving access to variant interpretations and supporting evidence. Nucleic Acids Res 2017;46:D1062–7.

[20] Li MM, Datto M, Duncavage EJ, et al. Standards and guidelines for the interpretation and reporting of sequence variants in cancer: a joint consensus recommendation of the association for molecular pathology, American Society of Clinical Oncology, and College of American Pathologists. J Mol Diagn 2017;19:4–23.

[21] Richards S, Aziz N, Bale S, et al. Standards and guidelines for the interpretation of sequence variants: a joint consensus recommendation of the American College of Medical Genetics and Genomics and the Association for Molecular Pathology. Genet Med 2015;17:405–24.

[22] Yohe SL, Carter AB, Pfeifer JD, et al. Standards for clinical grade genomic databases. Arch Pathol Lab Med 2015; 139:1400–12.

[23] Roy S, Coldren C, Karunamurthy A, et al. Standards and guidelines for validating next-generation sequencing bioinformatics pipelines: a joint recommendation of the association for molecular pathology and the College of American Pathologists. J Mol Diagn 2018;20:4–27.

[24] Aziz N, Zhao Q, Bry L, et al. College of American Pathologists' laboratory standards for next-generation sequencing clinical tests. Arch Pathol Lab Med 2015; 139(4):481–93. Available at: https://www.ncbi.nlm.nih.gov/pubmed/25152313. Accessed April 16, 2018.

[25] College of American Pathologists (CAP). Accreditation checklists. Available at: http://www.cap.org/web/home/lab/accreditation/accreditation-checklists. Accessed April 16, 2018.

[26] Zook JM, Catoe D, McDaniel J, et al. Extensive sequencing of seven human genomes to characterize benchmark reference materials. Sci Data 2016;3:160025.

[27] Eberle MA, Fritzilas E, Krusche P, et al. A reference data set of 5.4 million phased human variants validated by genetic inheritance from sequencing a three-generation 17-member pedigree. Genome Res 2017;27:157–64.

[28] Pratt VM, Everts RE, Aggarwal P, et al. Characterization of 137 genomic DNA reference materials for 28 pharmacogenetic genes: a GeT-RM collaborative project. J Mol Diagn 2016;18:109–23.
[29] Genetic Testing Reference Materials Coordination Program (GeT-RM) - Home. Available at: https://wwwn.cdc.gov/clia/Resources/GetRM/. Accessed April 16, 2018.
[30] Duncavage EJ, Abel HJ, Merker JD, et al. A model study of in silico proficiency testing for clinical next-generation sequencing. Arch Pathol Lab Med 2016;140:1085–91.
[31] Duncavage EJ, Abel HJ, Pfeifer JD. In silico proficiency testing for clinical next-generation sequencing. J Mol Diagn 2017;19:35–42.
[32] Escalona M, Rocha S, Posada D. A comparison of tools for the simulation of genomic next-generation sequencing data. Nat Rev Genet 2016;17:459–69.
[33] Poplin R, Newburger D, Dijamco J. Creating a universal SNP and small indel variant caller with deep neural networks. bioRxiv 2016. https://doi.org/10.1101/092890.
[34] Zhao H, Sun Z, Wang J, et al. CrossMap: a versatile tool for coordinate conversion between genome assemblies. Bioinformatics 2014;30:1006–7.
[35] Lift genome annotations. Available at: http://genome.ucsc.edu/cgi-bin/hgLiftOver. Accessed April 17, 2018.
[36] Coordinate remapping service: NCBI. Available at: https://www.ncbi.nlm.nih.gov/genome/tools/remap. Accessed April 17, 2018.
[37] ga4gh. ga4gh/benchmarking-tools. GitHub. Available at: https://github.com/ga4gh/benchmarking-tools. Accessed April 16, 2018.
[38] Mandelker D, Schmidt RJ, Ankala A, et al. Navigating highly homologous genes in a molecular diagnostic setting: a resource for clinical next-generation sequencing. Genet Med 2016;18:1282–9.
[39] Mu W, Lu H-M, Chen J, et al. Sanger confirmation is required to achieve optimal sensitivity and specificity in next-generation sequencing panel testing. J Mol Diagn 2016;18:923–32.
[40] Beck TF, Mullikin JC, Biesecker LG, on Behalf of the NISC Comparative Sequencing Program. Systematic evaluation of sanger validation of next-generation sequencing variants. Clin Chem 2016;62:647–54.
[41] Strom SP, Lee H, Das K, et al. Assessing the necessity of confirmatory testing for exome-sequencing results in a clinical molecular diagnostic laboratory. Genet Med 2014;16:510–5.
[42] Li H, Durbin R. Fast and accurate short read alignment with Burrows-Wheeler transform. Bioinformatics 2009;25:1754–60.
[43] Li H, Durbin R. Fast and accurate long-read alignment with Burrows-Wheeler transform. Bioinformatics 2010;26:589–95.
[44] NovoAlign | Novocraft. Available at: http://www.novocraft.com/products/novoalign/. Accessed April 16, 2018.
[45] Li H. A statistical framework for SNP calling, mutation discovery, association mapping and population genetical parameter estimation from sequencing data. Bioinformatics 2011;27:2987–93.
[46] McKenna A, Hanna M, Banks E, et al. The genome analysis toolkit: a MapReduce framework for analyzing next-generation DNA sequencing data. Genome Res 2010;20:1297–303.
[47] Poplin R, Ruano-Rubio V, DePristo MA, et al. Scaling accurate genetic variant discovery to tens of thousands of samples. BioRxiv 2017. https://doi.org/10.1101/201178.
[48] Erik Garrison, Gabor Marth. Haplotype-based variant detection from short-read sequencing. arXiv, 2012; 1207.3907
[49] Ye K, Schulz MH, Long Q, et al. a pattern growth approach to detect break points of large deletions and medium sized insertions from paired-end short reads. Bioinformatics 2009;25:2865–71.
[50] Fan X, Abbott TE, Larson D, et al. BreakDancer: identification of genomic structural variation from paired-end read mapping. Curr Protoc Bioinformatics 2014;45:15.6.1–15.6.11.
[51] Handsaker RE, Van Doren V, Berman JR, et al. Large multiallelic copy number variations in humans. Nat Genet 2015;47:296–303.
[52] Chen X, Schulz-Trieglaff O, Shaw R, et al. Manta: rapid detection of structural variants and indels for germline and cancer sequencing applications. Bioinformatics 2016;32:1220–2.
[53] Fromer M, Purcell SM. Using XHMM software to detect copy number variation in whole-exome sequencing data. Curr Protoc Hum Genet 2014;81:7.23.1-21.
[54] Pugh TJ, Amr SS, Bowser MJ, et al. VisCap: inference and visualization of germ-line copy-number variants from targeted clinical sequencing data. Genet Med 2016;18:712–9.
[55] Quinlan AR. BEDTools: the Swiss-army tool for genome feature analysis. Curr Protoc Bioinformatics 2014;47:11.12.1-34.
[56] Cleary JG, Braithwaite R, Gaastra K. Comparing variant call files for performance benchmarking of next-generation sequencing variant calling pipelines. bioRxiv 2015. https://doi.org/10.1101/023754.
[57] Babraham Bioinformatics - FastQC a quality control tool for high throughput sequence data. Available at: https://www.bioinformatics.babraham.ac.uk/projects/fastqc/. Accessed April 16, 2018.
[58] Jun G, Flickinger M, Hetrick KN, et al. Detecting and estimating contamination of human DNA samples in sequencing and array-based genotype data. Am J Hum Genet 2012;91:839–48.
[59] Picard Tools - By Broad Institute. Available at: https://broadinstitute.github.io/picard/. Accessed April 16, 2018.
[60] Kircher M, Witten DM, Jain P, et al. A general framework for estimating the relative pathogenicity of human genetic variants. Nat Genet 2014;46:310–5.
[61] Quang D, Chen Y, Xie X. DANN: a deep learning approach for annotating the pathogenicity of genetic variants. Bioinformatics 2014;31:761–3.

Advances in Molecular Pathology 1 (2018) 27–36
ADVANCES IN MOLECULAR PATHOLOGY

The Clinical Application of RNA Sequencing in Genetic Diagnosis of Mendelian Disorders

Sarah L. Stenton, MBChB, MPhil[a,b,*], Holger Prokisch, PhD[a,b]
[a]Institute of Human Genetics, Klinikum rechts der Isar, Technische Universität München, Ismaninger Straße 22, 81675, Munich, Germany; [b]Institute of Human Genetics, Helmholtz Zentrum München, Ingolstaedter Landstraße 1, 85764, Neuherberg, Germany

KEYWORDS
• RNA-seq • Genomic sequencing • Variant prioritization • Diagnostic yield

KEY POINTS

- Molecular genetic approaches have evolved at an astonishing pace resulting in increasingly routine use of whole exome sequencing in Mendelian disorder diagnosis.
- After whole exome sequencing, 50% to 75% of patients remain without a genetic diagnosis, indicating limitations in variant calling and prioritization and a role for noncoding variants.
- Whole genome sequencing has the potential to reveal all genetic variants; however, it escalates the challenge of variant prioritization owing to the vast numbers called.
- Promising approaches to aid in variant interpretation include the integration of functional genomic data such as transcriptome sequencing, which achieves diagnostic yields of 10% to 35%.
- International-scale collaboration and establishment of data repositories are paramount in accelerating the diagnosis of Mendelian disorders.

INTRODUCTION

Molecular genetic approaches have evolved at astonishing pace in capacity, capability, and application in recent years, reflected by the increasingly routine use of whole exome sequencing (WES) in Mendelian and rare disorder diagnosis [1–3] and by the approximately 160 new disease-gene discoveries documented yearly [4]. However, despite the revolutionary ascension of WES, 50% to 75% of patients remain without a genetic diagnosis (Fig. 1) [5–8] and, furthermore, more than 3000 Mendelian disorders are yet to be genetically defined [8]. This diagnostic rate may seems to be low. However, these figures must be considered in the context of the inability of WES to appreciate the impact of variation outside of the exonic regions. WES covers just 2% of the genome [9], the exonic protein-coding

Disclosure Statement: The authors have nothing to declare.
Funding: mitoNet German Network for Mitochondrial Diseases (01GM1113). GENOMIT European Network for Mitochondrial Disease (01GM1207). SOUND (Statistical Multi-Omics Understanding) EU Horizon2020 Collaborative Research Project (633974). PhD Program Medical Life Science and Technology scholarship (TUM School of Medicine).

*Corresponding author. Institute of Human Genetics (IHG), Helmholtz Zentrum München, Deutsches Forschungszentrum für Gesundheit und Umwelt (GmbH), Building 3537, Room 8128, Ingolstaedter Landstr. 1, Neuherberg D-85764, Germany.
E-mail address: sarah.stenton@helmholtz-muenchen.de

https://doi.org/10.1016/j.yamp.2018.06.004
2589-4080/18/

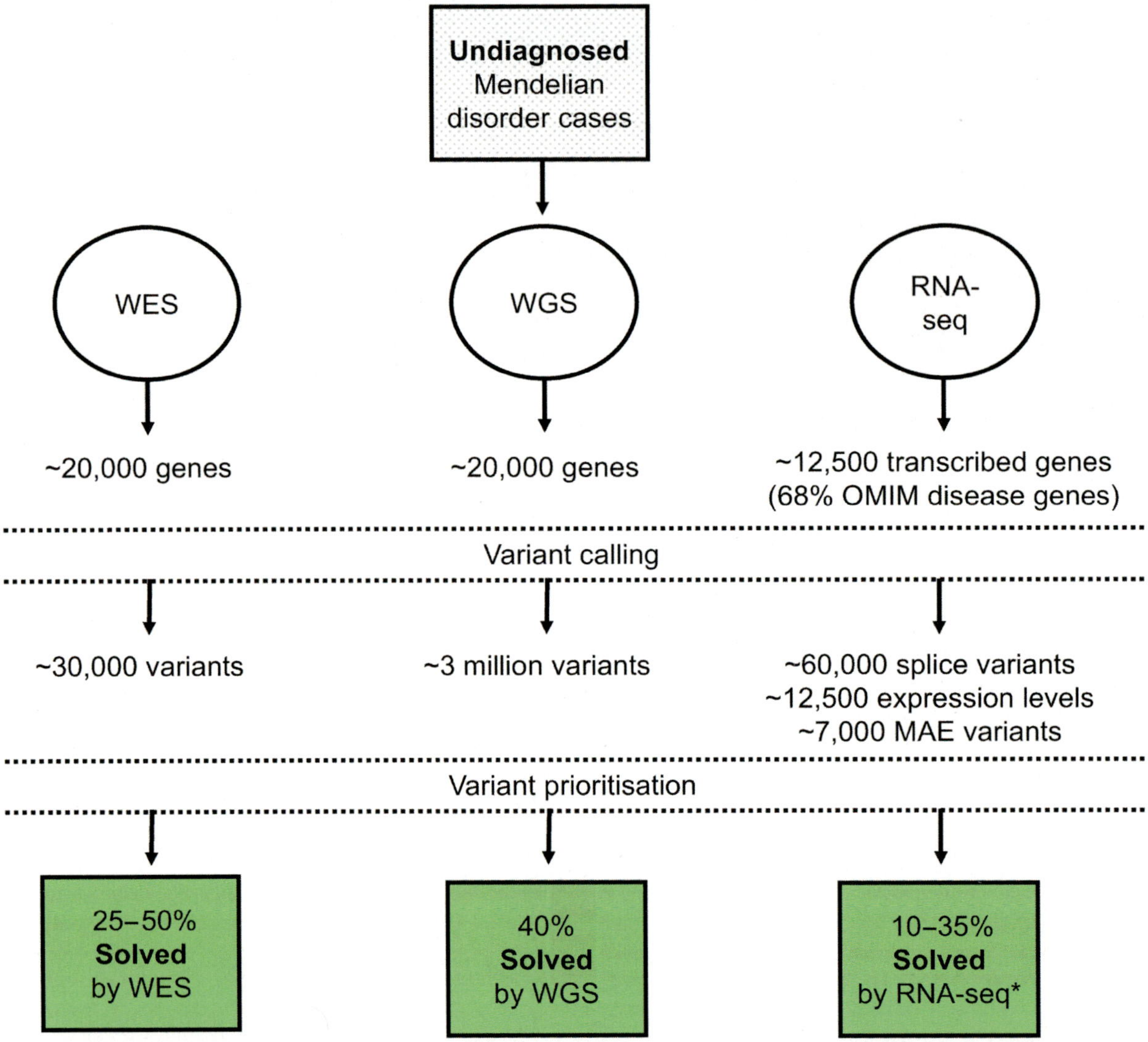

FIG. 1 Schematic of the analysis pipeline for whole exome sequencing (WES), whole genome sequencing (WGS), and transcriptome sequencing (RNA-seq) with the number of genes and variants and the currently reported diagnostic yield. *Unsolved WES cases. MAE, monoallelic expression.

regions, indicating that disease-causing variants may be harboring in the noncoding regions, such as deep intronic or regulatory variants [10].

By contrast, whole genome sequencing (WGS) has the potential to capture nearly all genomic variation in an unbiased manner, with higher sensitivity than WES for certain coding variants, indels, copy number variants, and chromosomal rearrangements [11–13]. Additionally, WGS reveals variants in the regulatory noncoding regions and more complex rearrangements, such as inversions and transposons [14]. In terms of influence on diagnostic rate, WGS has been reported to identify disease-causing variants in an additional 14% compared with WES, with an overall diagnostic yield of 41% [15].

However, WGS increases the challenge of variant prioritization owing to the sizable number of variants called (approximately 3 million) [7,16,17]. The former challenge of variant discovery has, therefore, shifted to the ability to interpret function and ultimately clinical impact of such variants [18–20], rendering numerous disease-causing variants to be variants of unknown significance (VUS).

A promising approach to aid in variant interpretation is the integration of functional genomic data such as the transcriptome [21,22]. Transcriptome sequencing (RNA-seq) has already proven useful in elucidating mechanisms of cancer and common disease [23–25], but until recently had not been systematically applied in Mendelian disorder diagnosis.

THE CHALLENGE OF VARIANT CALLING AND PRIORITIZATION

Variant calling and prioritization play central roles in genomic sequencing analysis. Sequencing error resulting in artifactual data is a common phenomenon and, owing to the diversity in variant calling algorithms and filtering strategies as well as the aspiration for high sensitivity and precision, distinguishing low-frequency potentially disease-causing variants from random sequencing errors remains a significant challenge [26]. Variant prioritization, defined as the process of determining whether identified variants have the potential to damage gene function and thus underlie disease phenotype [27], aims to ultimately identify the 1 to 2 variants responsible for a patient's Mendelian disorder. This is a classic needle in the haystack problem [28], approached by enforcing filters for inheritance model, minimum population allele frequency (according to population-scale variation databases, such as the Exome Aggregation Consortium [29], the Genome Aggregation Database, and the 1000 Genomes Project) [16] and variant effect. Numerous variant effect prediction tools can be used; however, those for noncoding variants remain less accurate than their protein-coding counterparts, owing to insufficient understanding of the regulatory machinery encrypted in noncoding DNA [27]. Thus, reinforcing the argument for integration of functional transcriptomic (RNA-seq) data.

THE TRANSCRIPTOME AND RNA-SEQ

The transcriptome describes the complete set of transcripts in a cell and their abundance for a specific snapshot in time [30]. In contrast with DNA, which is essentially identical across all cells, the actively transcribed RNA is highly dynamic, serving as a transient intermediary molecule between DNA and protein translation, therefore, revealing the link between the cellular phenotype and the underpinning genetics [25].

RNA-seq is the first genome scale sequencing methodology to allow the entire transcriptome to be surveyed in a high-throughput, quantitative, and qualitative manner. It has emerged as a part of the development of NGS technologies, with the capability to both quantify known predefined RNA species and to detect and quantify rare and novel RNA transcript variants and isoforms [31], thus, providing a direct insight into the transcriptional perturbations caused by VUS (frequently synonymous or noncoding variants) such as on RNA abundance and isoform [32].

RNA-SEQ METHODOLOGY

RNA-seq is not a single protocol, but rather a workflow of methodologies encompassing sample preparation, sequencing, and downstream computational analysis [25]. First, cells are disrupted for isolation of RNA. Owing to the inherent labile nature of RNA, degradation and subsequent low input amounts [33] are considerable challenges, addressed by optimizing protocols for the input of just 0.1 to 1.0 μg of total high-quality RNA (RNA integrity number of >8) [34]. Second, library preparation is required. An umbrella term for the purification and enrichment of messenger RNA by selection of Poly(A)+ transcripts and/or depletion of contaminating ribosomal RNA, fragmentation (necessitated by the size limitation of sequencing platforms), amplification by polymerase chain reaction (to ensure sufficient coverage of the transcriptome and to enable detection of low abundance transcripts) and finally cDNA synthesis and sequencing [25]. A non-stranded or stranded protocol can be used in the cDNA synthesis step of library preparation (Fig. 2). The more recently developed stranded methods allow retention of information on which strand the messenger RNA template originated, thus, allowing determination of expression from genes with overlapping genomic coordinates but transcription from opposite strands [35]. The leading protocol, dUTP second-strand marking, uses dUTPs instead of dTTPs during the synthesis of the second strand cDNA [36]. Marking of the second strand cDNA with uracils permits degradation with uracil-DNA-glycosylase, facilitating the preservation of strand-of-origin information during adapter ligation and library enrichment by polymerase chain reaction. After quality control measures, the short-read data require computational reconstruction of the original RNA transcript by alignment of reads to the human reference genome to detect and measure expression [37].

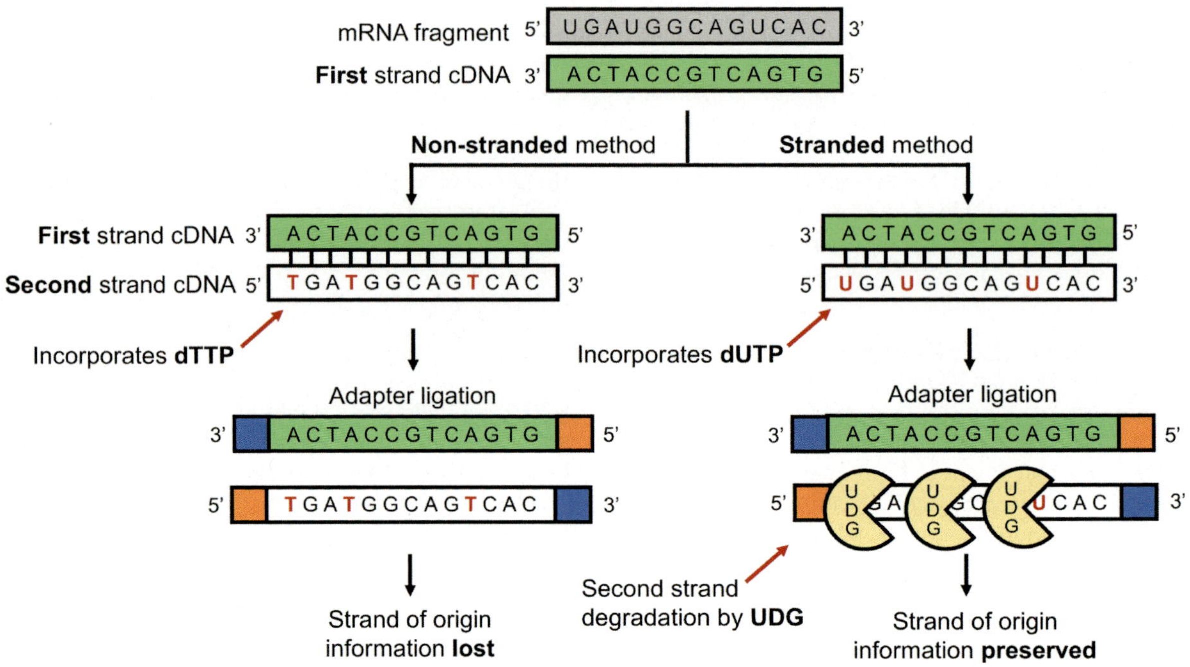

FIG. 2 Nonstranded and stranded transcriptome sequencing (RNA-seq) protocols. In the stranded protocol, during cDNA synthesis, second strand synthesis utilizes dUTPs in place of dTTPs with subsequent second strand degradation by uracil-DNA-glycosylase. This ensures that strand of origin information during adapter ligation and library enrichment by polymerase chain reaction is preserved.

INTERPRETATION OF RNA-SEQ

The analysis of RNA-seq data in the context of Mendelian disorders is a novel and developing field. At present, 3 situations can be interpreted to prioritize candidate disease-causing variants for rare Mendelian disorders [21] (Fig. 3). First, RNA-seq can reveal extreme cases of allele-specific expression, termed monoallelic expression (MAE), whereby 1 allele is silenced, leaving only the other allele expressed (see Fig. 3A). When assuming an autosomal recessive mode of inheritance, genes with a single heterozygous rare coding variant (minor allele frequency of <0.01) identified by WES analysis are not prioritized. However, MAE of such variants fits the recessive mode of inheritance assumption. Detection of MAE can thus help in reprioritizing heterozygous rare variants.

MAE can arise as a consequence of multiple mechanisms, encompassing allele-specific transcription, genomic imprinting and X-chromosome inactivation [38,39]. Genomic imprinting is the most frequent mechanism, whereby DNA methylation and histone modifications result in biased expression of an allele in a parent-of-origin–specific manner, exemplified in Angelman syndrome owing to deficient maternal allele expression of *UBE3A* in the brain [40]. Additionally, posttranscriptional mechanisms can result in MEA, such as alternative splicing causing exon skipping and MEA of variants contained within the skipped exon [41] and such as the creation of premature stop codons leading to nonsense-mediated decay of one allele and MAE of the other [21,42,43].

Second, genes with expression outside physiologic range can be identified as expression outliers (see Fig. 3B), termed aberrant expression. The cause of such aberrant expression includes rare variants in promoter and enhancer regions [44] and rare variants within both coding and intronic regions [24], in addition to posttranscriptional mechanisms.

Third, splicing of a gene can be affected (see Fig. 3C). Aberrant splicing has long been recognized as a major cause of Mendelian disorders [45–47] and, in fact, approximately 10% of exonic disease-associated alleles are found to disrupt splicing [48]. Any change in exonic sequence may disrupt or create cis-acting elements, which facilitate exon recognition, resulting in aberrant splicing. Splice-disrupting variants may also be located in the deep intronic sequence [49] and thus not covered by WES or detected by WGS, but not prioritized. Hence, direct probing of splice isoforms by RNA-seq is important and can detect an array of splice defects from exon creation, skipping, extension, and truncation to intronic inclusion, providing invaluable information about exonic and intronic positions susceptible to affect splicing. Aberrant splicing events can be detected by testing for differential splicing between an individual case and a control population. Splice sites can be annotated with reference exon annotation such as provided by GENCODE [50]. Detection of de novo splice sites, however, requires the use of annotation-free algorithms, such as provided by the LeafCutter software [51].

SYSTEMATIC ANALYSIS OF RNA-SEQ IN MENDELIAN DISORDER DIAGNOSIS

In parallel effort, 2 studies systematically investigated the use of RNA-seq for the molecular genetic diagnosis of Mendelian disorders, using near analogous approaches [21,22] (Table 1).

RNA-SEQ IN UNDIAGNOSED MITOCHONDRIAL DISORDERS

Kremer and colleagues [21] investigated the application of RNA-seq in 105 mitochondrial disorder cases, a clinically and genetically heterogeneous cohort of patients with a rare disorder, of whom only 35% to 60% [10,53–56] receive a diagnosis after WES. Mitochondrial disorders have a complex genetic architecture with more than 1500 genes implicated in healthy mitochondrial function [57] and causal defects identified in more than 300 genes implicated in mitochondrial metabolism [58]. An additional layer of complexity arises from the bigenomic control of the energy-generating oxidative phosphorylation system, primarily responsible for mitochondrial disorders, and disrupted by both mitochondrial DNA and nuclear DNA variants [59]. Despite disease manifestation occurring in the high-energy demanding tissues (such as brain, heart, muscle, and liver) for which biopsy is often

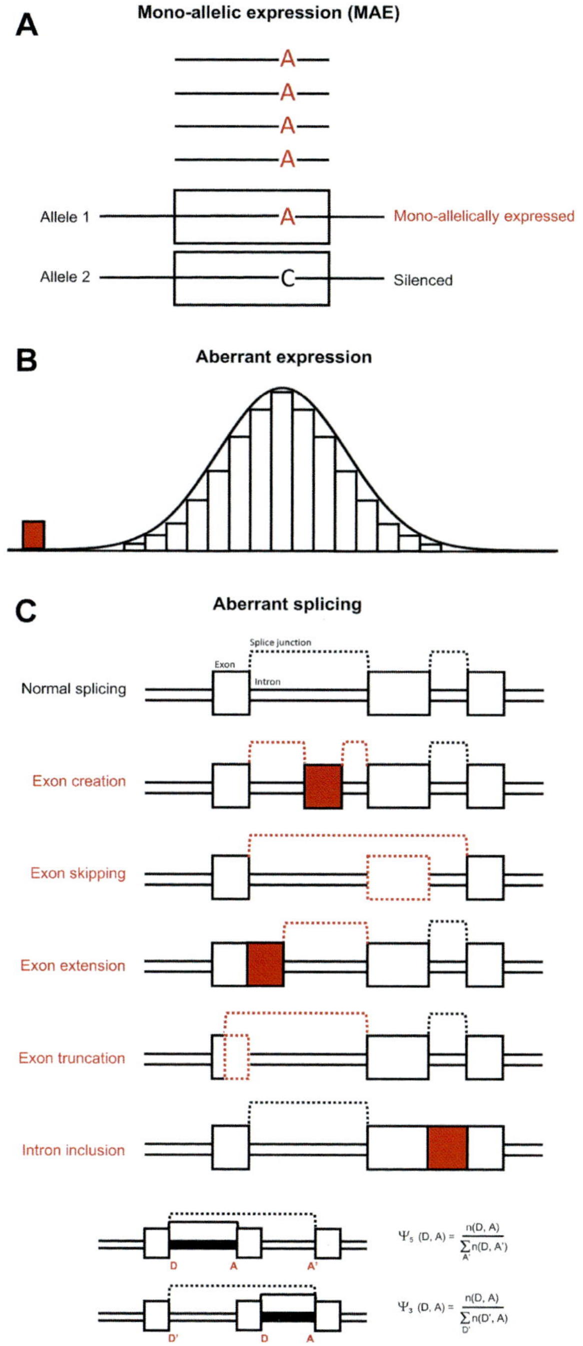

FIG. 3 Three situations interpreted in prioritization of candidate disease-causing variants for rare Mendelian disorders. (*A*) Monoallelic expression (MAE), (*B*) aberrant expression, and (*C*) aberrant splicing. Frequency of splice variants is calculated by the percent spliced in (psi) denoted by ψ. The ψ_5-splicing index defines the number of reads supporting the splicing event from D to A relative to the combined number of reads supporting splicing from D to any acceptor site A'. The ψ_3-splicing index defines the number of reads supporting the splicing event from D to A relative to the combined number of reads supporting splicing from any donor site D' to A [52]. Aberrant expression or splicing is defined as statistically significant deviation from the normal distribution of the controls.

TABLE 1
The Diagnostic Yield of WES and RNA-Seq Analyses in Mendelian Disorders

Patient Cohort	Total Cases	Undiagnosed Cases	Diagnostic Yield of WES	Diagnostic Yield of RNA-Seq
Mitochondrial disorders (Kremer et al [21], 2017)	105	48	35% to 60% [10,53–56]	5/48 (10%)
Rare muscle disorders (Cummings et al [22], 2017)	63	50	25% to 50% [5–8]	17/50 (35%)

Abbreviation: WES, whole exome sequencing.

unobtainable, skin biopsy and thus fibroblast cell lines allow mitochondrial disease mechanisms to be assayed [60]. Fibroblasts are, therefore, a readily available resource for RNA-seq analysis and for downstream rapid demonstration of the role of candidate variants by complementation assays [61].

There were 105 fibroblast cell lines that were analyzed, 48 for which WES did not yield a diagnosis. Genetically diagnosed patients were included in the analysis pipeline to increase the power for the detection of aberrant events. The study considered all transcribed genes in the fibroblast cell lines and, after filtering to remove lowly expressed genes, identified 12,680 transcribed genes. The genetic variants were systemically prioritized with 3 strategies: MAE, defined as 80% or greater of transcripts harboring the rare variant of a heterozygous single nucleotide polymorphism, aberrant expression, and aberrant splicing. Read count outliers (aberrant expression) were identified as those with an absolute Z-score of greater than 3 and statistical significance according to DESeq2, a statistical test originally developed for differential expression analysis [62] that is applied by testing each sample in turn against the remainder. The analysis of aberrant splicing used an annotation-free algorithm comparing the percentage of splice variants at each exon between one patient and the remainder to detect spice outliers from the normal distribution. This method allowed each to serve as a control for one another, a robust strategy given the genetic diversity in mitochondrial disorders [21].

The method resulted in the median detection of 6 monoallelically expressed rare variants, 1 aberrantly expressed gene, and 5 aberrant splicing events per case. Notably, among the 175 aberrantly spliced genes detected, the most abundant events were the differential expression of isoforms, exon skipping, and the creation of new exons. This resulted in an overall molecular genetic diagnosis of 10% of patients with undiagnosed mitochondriopathy (5 of 48) and a yield of promising candidate genes for 36 additional patients [21].

RNA-SEQ IN UNDIAGNOSED PRIMARY MUSCLE DISORDERS

Cummings and colleagues [22] investigated the application of RNA-seq in 63 rare muscle disorder cases, including myopathies and muscular dystrophies, for whom only 25% to 50% [5–8] receive a diagnosis after WES. RNA was sourced from 63 patients, 13 of whom had prior diagnoses with variants expected to influence transcription (such as loss-of-function or essential splice site variants), and 50 of whom were genetically undiagnosed. The undiagnosed cases included those for whom prior genetic analysis had prioritized variants predicted to alter RNA splicing or strong candidate genes, in addition to cases with no strong candidate from prior genetic analysis. RNA was isolated from muscle tissue biopsy, obtained routinely during the diagnostic evaluation of primary muscle disease patients.

Here, the study compared each patient with 184 control skeletal muscle samples available through the GTEx database [63], an RNA-seq compendium of health donors across multiple tissues. For the detection of transcript-level changes, Z-scores were computed on the logarithm of gene length normalized read counts by subtracting the mean count and dividing by the standard deviation. Expression outliers were identified as those with an absolute Z-score of greater than 3, with no test of significance performed. The expression outlier analysis did not yield any convincing candidates. To identify rare splice events, outlier events were considered that were maximal in a given sample and less than half in the next highest sample. Their approach focused on identifying transcriptional aberrations in a defined list of neuromuscular disorder–associated genes [22].

Using this approach RNA-seq (re)identified all putative disease-causing splice variants in the 13 diagnosed patients and, thus, validated the capability of this approach to identify transcriptional aberrations and enabling its use in the subsequent discovery of novel disease-causing variants in undiagnosed cases. The method results in a median of 5 potentially pathogenic splice events per samples in 190 neuromuscular disorder associated genes. Resulting in an overall diagnosis of 35% of the undiagnosed patients (17 of 50) [22]. Remarkably, 4 of 17 of these cases harbored the same recurrent de novo intronic variant in *COL6A1*, resulting in a dominantly acting splice-gain aberration and 23 further cases were identified in an external collagen VI-like dystrophy cohort, explaining approximately 25% of cases with clinically suspected collagen VI dystrophy in whom prior genetic analysis is negative.

THE KEY ADVANTAGES OF RNA-SEQ

Newly diagnosed cases in these studies highlight the key advantages of RNA-seq in rare Mendelian disorder diagnosis (Box 1). In 4 patients with a rare muscle disorder harboring an extended splice site VUS, RNA-seq confirmed splice disruption in 2 patients with no observable effect on local splicing patterns in the remaining 2 patients, emphasizing the value of RNA-seq in ruling out nonpathogenic VUS. Remarkably, RNA-seq enabled pathogenicity to be assigned to a number of putatively benign synonymous variants. Cummings and colleagues detected a synonymous variant in *RYR1* resulting in an exonic splice gain owing to strengthening of a novel splice site over that of the canonical splice site and in *POMGNT1* resulting in exon skipping secondary to disruption of a splice motif. Notably, identification of aberrant splicing not only provided pathogenic confirmation of exonic variants, but also enabled the identification of pathogenic noncoding variants. Kremer and colleagues [21] described a homozygous deep intronic variant leading to a defective splice event (creation of a pseudoexon resulting in a premature stop codon) and subsequent loss of function in *TIMMDC1*. *TIMMDC1* also appeared as an expression outlier in the analysis, presumably owing to nonsense-mediated decay. Importantly, this study also revealed the occurrence of cryptic exons arising from loci with weak background splicing (approximately 1% in the general population), termed cryptic splice sites, in 2 patients, thus, providing a valuable clue for variant prioritization because rare variants in these locations are more likely to affect splicing [21].

BOX 1
Key Advantages of Transcriptome Sequencing in Mendelian Disorder Diagnosis

- Direct insight into the transcriptional perturbations of genetic variation.
- Identification of noncoding pathogenic variants unobservable by whole exome sequencing.
- Identification of noncoding pathogenic variants too abundant to be interpreted by whole genome sequencing.
- Reprioritization of variants of unknown significance detected by whole exome sequencing and whole genome sequencing.
- Resolving pathogenicity of noncoding and coding variants of unknown significance (including synonymous variants).
- Value in ruling out nonpathogenic variants of unknown significance.
- Identifying a practicable number of strong candidates for validation.
- Discovery of new disease-associated genes.
- Provision of genetic diagnoses for undiagnosed cases.

CHALLENGES IN RNA-SEQ APPROACHES

Disease-Relevant Tissue Selection

Both studies identified tissue selection as a considerable obstacle. It is natural to question whether RNA-seq analysis of unaffected tissues can reliably aid in genetic diagnosis, owing to the presumably negligible physiologic consequence of the variant in the tissue [21]. However, Mendelian disorders frequently show specificity to selected tissue(s) which are unobtainable for RNA-seq in a premortem setting, necessitating exploration of surrogate tissues.

Because gene expression and messenger RNA isoforms vary widely across tissues types [64,65], the identification of proxy tissues using the GTEx database, with careful consideration of expression status of the relevant genes, is one proposed way to circumnavigate the potentially underpowered analysis to detect relevant transcriptional aberrations in unaffected, easily accessible tissues [22]. Reprogramming of patient cells into induced pluripotent stem cells and differentiation into disease-relevant tissues may also be used in cases of high-interest or theoretic possibility, such as the recently published use of induced pluripotent stem cells and RNA-seq to pinpoint the noncoding disease-causing variant in *TAF1* responsible for X-linked dystonia–parkinsonism [14].

In the case of mitochondrial disorders, patient fibroblast cell lines are a valuable surrogate for affected tissue, indicating that tissue specificity does not preclude RNA-seq of unaffected tissues. In fact, expression of 2574 of the 3768 disease genes (68%)

listed in OMIM could be detected in fibroblast cell lines [66]. Moreover, nonaffected tissues have the advantage that the regulatory consequences on other genes are limited and, therefore, the causal defects are more likely be detected as outliers [67]. However, in the case of rare muscle disorders, poor expression of commonly disrupted muscle disorders genes in whole blood and fibroblasts necessitated biopsy of affected tissue for correct interpretation of genetic variation [22].

Extensive Normalization and Statistical Assessments

Both studies highlight the need for closely matched, extensively normalized RNA-seq samples, requiring knowledge of technical variables, such as quality metrics (RNA integrity number), methodology (RNA extraction, library preparation), and phenotypic features, to exclude expression outliers from analysis, whether this be between patient samples [21] or with a database of public RNA-seq datasets such as GTEx [22,63]. Altogether, in this immature area, methods for detecting aberrant expression lack adequate assessment of statistical significance, use arbitrary cutoffs, and rely on manual correction for available confounders. A newly developed algorithm, OUTRIDER, addresses some of these issues (https://github.com/gagneurlab/OUTRIDER).

Future Prospects and Challenges for RNA-seq in Mendelian Disorder Diagnosis

The power of RNA-seq as a complementary tool to WES and WGS in identifying candidate variants for Mendelian disorders is clear. The flexibility and seemingly infinite methodologic and analytical options for RNA-seq present a double-edged sword, because these traits both spur discoveries while simultaneously complicating translation into the clinical diagnostic setting [32]. However, as with WES and WGS, which still uses multiple different platforms, protocols, and pipelines, we suspect that, given time and development of appropriate methodology, RNA-seq will establish itself in the clinical diagnostic pipeline for unsolved Mendelian disorders, given its increase in diagnostic yield, with blood as the likely easily accessible tissue of choice.

Multiomics Approaches and Data Sharing

With the ascension of multiomics approaches, encompassing genomics, epigenomics, transcriptomics, proteomics, and metabolomics, among others, there is an immense increase in the volume of exploitable data, giving rise to an increasingly integrated view of disease pathophysiology [30]. When these data are deposited into public databases, it becomes an invaluable resource for the broader scientific community, facilitating increase in study size and statistical power for more sophisticated data analyses [68].

SUMMARY

The successful application of RNA-seq analysis in the setting of unsolved WES cases deems RNA-seq an essential companion to genome-based diagnostics, illustrated by the ability to validate suspected splice variants and the substantial increase in diagnostic yield. Integration of RNA-seq as a standardized diagnostic assay for all Mendelian disorders, akin to DNA sequencing, is within reach. To optimally investigate the true potential of RNA-seq in the diagnosis of Mendelian disorders and to establish the accuracy required for clinical translation, it is paramount that we collaborate on an international scale via the establishment of -omics data repositories.

REFERENCES

[1] Ashley EA, Butte AJ, Wheeler MT, et al. Clinical assessment incorporating a personal genome. Lancet 2010; 375(9725):1525–35.

[2] Choi M, Scholl UI, Ji W, et al. Genetic diagnosis by whole exome capture and massively parallel DNA sequencing. Proc Natl Acad Sci U S A 2009;106(45):19096–101.

[3] Ng SB, Buckingham KJ, Lee C, et al. Exome sequencing identifies the cause of a Mendelian disorder. Nat Genet 2010;42(1):30.

[4] Boycott KM, Rath A, Chong JX, et al. International cooperation to enable the diagnosis of all rare genetic diseases. Am J Hum Genet 2017;100(5):695–705.

[5] Ankala A, da Silva C, Gualandi F, et al. A comprehensive genomic approach for neuromuscular diseases gives a high diagnostic yield. Ann Neurol 2015;77(2):206–14.

[6] Yang Y, Muzny DM, Xia F, et al. Molecular findings among patients referred for clinical whole-exome sequencing. JAMA 2014;312(18):1870–9.

[7] Taylor JC, Martin HC, Lise S, et al. Factors influencing success of clinical genome sequencing across a broad spectrum of disorders. Nat Genet 2015;47(7):717.

[8] Chong JX, Buckingham KJ, Jhangiani SN, et al. The genetic basis of Mendelian phenotypes: discoveries, challenges, and opportunities. Am J Hum Genet 2015; 97(2):199–215.

[9] Bamshad MJ, Ng SB, Bigham AW, et al. Exome sequencing as a tool for Mendelian disease gene discovery. Nat Rev Genet 2011;12(11):745.

[10] Wortmann SB, Koolen DA, Smeitink JA, et al. Whole exome sequencing of suspected mitochondrial patients in clinical practice. J Inherit Metab Dis 2015;38(3): 437–43.

[11] Gilissen C, Hehir-Kwa JY, Thung DT, et al. Genome sequencing identifies major causes of severe intellectual disability. Nature 2014;511(7509):344.

[12] Belkadi A, Bolze A, Itan Y, et al. Whole-genome sequencing is more powerful than whole-exome sequencing for detecting exome variants. Proc Natl Acad Sci U S A 2015;112(17):5473–8.

[13] Stavropoulos DJ, Merico D, Jobling R, et al. Whole-genome sequencing expands diagnostic utility and improves clinical management in paediatric medicine. NPJ Genom Med 2016;1:15012.

[14] Valente EM, Bhatia KP. Solving Mendelian mysteries: the non-coding genome may hold the key. Cell 2018;172(5): 889–91.

[15] Lionel AC, Costain G, Monfared N, et al. Improved diagnostic yield compared with targeted gene sequencing panels suggests a role for whole-genome sequencing as a first-tier genetic test. Genet Med 2018;20(4):435–43.

[16] 1000 Genomes Project Consortium, Auton A, Brooks LD, Durbin RM, et al. A global reference for human genetic variation. Nature 2015;526(7571):68.

[17] Sudmant PH, Rausch T, Gardner EJ, et al. An integrated map of structural variation in 2,504 human genomes. Nature 2015;526(7571):75.

[18] MacArthur D, Manolio T, Dimmock D, et al. Guidelines for investigating causality of sequence variants in human disease. Nature 2014;508(7497):469.

[19] Goldstein DB, Allen A, Keebler J, et al. Sequencing studies in human genetics: design and interpretation. Nat Rev Genet 2013;14(7):460.

[20] Lek M, MacArthur D. The challenge of next generation sequencing in the context of neuromuscular diseases. J Neuromuscul Dis 2014;1(2):135–49.

[21] Kremer LS, Bader DM, Mertes C, et al. Genetic diagnosis of Mendelian disorders via RNA sequencing. Nat Commun 2017;8:15824.

[22] Cummings BB, Marshall JL, Tukiainen T, et al. Improving genetic diagnosis in Mendelian disease with transcriptome sequencing. Sci Transl Med 2017;9(386) [pii: eaal5209].

[23] Jung H, Lee D, Lee J, et al. Intron retention is a widespread mechanism of tumor-suppressor inactivation. Nat Genet 2015;47(11):1242.

[24] Li YI, van de Geijn B, Raj A, et al. RNA splicing is a primary link between genetic variation and disease. Science 2016;352(6285):600–4.

[25] Cieślik M, Chinnaiyan AM. Cancer transcriptome profiling at the juncture of clinical translation. Nat Rev Genet 2018;19(2):93.

[26] Sandmann S, De Graaf AO, Karimi M, et al. Evaluating variant calling tools for non-matched next-generation sequencing data. Sci Rep 2017;7:43169.

[27] Eilbeck K, Quinlan A, Yandell M. Settling the score: variant prioritization and Mendelian disease. Nat Rev Genet 2017;18(10):599.

[28] Cooper GM, Shendure J. Needles in stacks of needles: finding disease-causal variants in a wealth of genomic data. Nat Rev Genet 2011;12(9):628.

[29] Karczewski KJ, Weisburd B, Thomas B, et al. The ExAC browser: displaying reference data information from over 60 000 exomes. Nucleic Acids Res 2016;45(D1): D840–5.

[30] Lowe R, Shirley N, Bleackley M, et al. Transcriptomics technologies. PLoS Comput Biol 2017;13(5):e1005457.

[31] Mortazavi A, Williams BA, McCue K, et al. Mapping and quantifying mammalian transcriptomes by RNA-seq. Nat Methods 2008;5(7):621.

[32] Byron SA, Van Keuren-Jensen KR, Engelthaler DM, et al. Translating RNA sequencing into clinical diagnostics: opportunities and challenges. Nat Rev Genet 2016; 17(5):257.

[33] Adiconis X, Borges-Rivera D, Satija R, et al. Comparative analysis of RNA sequencing methods for degraded or low-input samples. Nat Methods 2013; 10(7):623.

[34] TruSeq® RNA sample preparation v2 guide (Illumina). Available at: https://support.illumina.com/content/dam/illumina-support/documents/documentation/chemistry_documentation/samplepreps_truseq/truseqrna/truseq-rna-sample-prep-v2-guide-15026495-f.pdf.

[35] Zhao S, Zhang Y, Gordon W, et al. Comparison of stranded and non-stranded RNA-seq transcriptome profiling and investigation of gene overlap. BMC Genomics 2015;16(1):675.

[36] Levin JZ, Yassour M, Adiconis X, et al. Comprehensive comparative analysis of strand-specific RNA sequencing methods. Nat Methods 2010;7(9):709.

[37] Wang Z, Gerstein M, Snyder M. RNA-seq: a revolutionary tool for transcriptomics. Nat Rev Genet 2009;10(1):57.

[38] Eckersley-Maslin MA, Spector DL. Random monoallelic expression: regulating gene expression one allele at a time. Trends Genet 2014;30(6):237–44.

[39] Reinius B, Sandberg R. Random monoallelic expression of autosomal genes: stochastic transcription and allele-level regulation. Nat Rev Genet 2015;16(11): 653.

[40] Lossie AC, Whitney MM, Amidon D, et al. Distinct phenotypes distinguish the molecular classes of Angelman syndrome. J Med Genet 2001;38(12):834–45.

[41] Klimpe S, Zibat A, Zechner U, et al. Evaluating the effect of spastin splice mutations by quantitative allele specific expression assay. Eur J Neurol 2011;18(1): 99–105.

[42] Wood DL, Nones K, Steptoe A, et al. Recommendations for accurate resolution of gene and isoform allele-specific expression in RNA-seq data. PLoS One 2015; 10(5):e0126911.

[43] Rivas MA, Pirinen M, Conrad DF, et al. Human genomics. effect of predicted protein-truncating genetic

variants on the human transcriptome. Science 2015; 348(6235):666–9.

[44] Zhao J, Akinsanmi I, Arafat D, et al. A burden of rare variants associated with extremes of gene expression in human peripheral blood. Am J Hum Genet 2016;98(2): 299–309.

[45] Tazi J, Bakkour N, Stamm S. Alternative splicing and disease. Biochim Biophys Acta 2009;1792(1):14–26.

[46] Scotti MM, Swanson MS. RNA mis-splicing in disease. Nat Rev Genet 2016;17(1):19.

[47] Singh RK, Cooper TA. Pre-mRNA splicing in disease and therapeutics. Trends Mol Med 2012;18(8):472–82.

[48] Soemedi R, Cygan KJ, Rhine CL, et al. Pathogenic variants that alter protein code often disrupt splicing. Nat Genet 2017;49(6):848.

[49] Xiong HY, Alipanahi B, Lee LJ, et al. RNA splicing. the human splicing code reveals new insights into the genetic determinants of disease. Science 2015;347(6218): 1254806.

[50] Harrow J, Frankish A, Gonzalez JM, et al. GENCODE: the reference human genome annotation for the ENCODE project. Genome Res 2012;22(9):1760–74.

[51] Li YI, Knowles DA, Humphrey J, et al. LeafCutter: annotation-free quantification of RNA splicing. Nat Genet 2018;50(1):151.

[52] Pervouchine DD, Knowles DG, Guigo R. Intron-centric estimation of alternative splicing from RNA-seq data. Bioinformatics 2012;29(2):273–4.

[53] Taylor RW, Pyle A, Griffin H, et al. Use of whole-exome sequencing to determine the genetic basis of multiple mitochondrial respiratory chain complex deficiencies. JAMA 2014;312(1):68–77.

[54] Ohtake A, Murayama K, Mori M, et al. Diagnosis and molecular basis of mitochondrial respiratory chain disorders: exome sequencing for disease gene identification. Biochim Biophys Acta 2014;1840(4):1355–9.

[55] Kohda M, Tokuzawa Y, Kishita Y, et al. A comprehensive genomic analysis reveals the genetic landscape of mitochondrial respiratory chain complex deficiencies. PLoS Genet 2016;12(1):e1005679.

[56] Pronicka E, Piekutowska-Abramczuk D, Ciara E, et al. New perspective in diagnostics of mitochondrial disorders: two years' experience with whole-exome sequencing at a national paediatric centre. J Transl Med 2016;14(1):174.

[57] Elstner M, Andreoli C, Ahting U, et al. MitoP2: an integrative tool for the analysis of the mitochondrial proteome. Mol Biotechnol 2008;40(3):306–15.

[58] Wortmann SB, Mayr JA, Nuoffer JM, et al. A guideline for the diagnosis of pediatric mitochondrial disease: the value of muscle and skin biopsies in the genetics era. Neuropediatrics 2017;48(04):309–14.

[59] Gorman GS, Chinnery PF, DiMauro S, et al. Mitochondrial diseases. Nat Rev Dis Primers 2016;2:16080.

[60] Haack TB, Kopajtich R, Freisinger P, et al. ELAC2 mutations cause a mitochondrial RNA processing defect associated with hypertrophic cardiomyopathy. Am J Hum Genet 2013;93(2):211–23.

[61] Haack TB, Danhauser K, Haberberger B, et al. Exome sequencing identifies ACAD9 mutations as a cause of complex I deficiency. Nat Genet 2010;42(12):1131.

[62] Love MI, Huber W, Anders S. Moderated estimation of fold change and dispersion for RNA-seq data with DESeq2. Genome Biol 2014;15(12):550.

[63] GTEx Consortium. Human genomics. The genotype-tissue expression (GTEx) pilot analysis: multitissue gene regulation in humans. Science 2015;348(6235): 648–60.

[64] Mele M, Ferreira PG, Reverter F, et al. Human genomics. the human transcriptome across tissues and individuals. Science 2015;348(6235):660–5.

[65] Wang ET, Sandberg R, Luo S, et al. Alternative isoform regulation in human tissue transcriptomes. Nature 2008;456(7221):470.

[66] Kremer LS, Wortmann SB, Prokisch H. "Transcriptomics": molecular diagnosis of inborn errors of metabolism via RNA-sequencing. J Inherit Metab Dis 2018;41(3): 525–32.

[67] Gagneur J, Stegle O, Zhu C, et al. Genotype-environment interactions reveal causal pathways that mediate genetic effects on phenotype. PLoS Genet 2013;9(9):e1003803.

[68] Sham PC, Purcell SM. Statistical power and significance testing in large-scale genetic studies. Nat Rev Genet 2014;15(5):335.

Hematopathology

Advances in Molecular Pathology 1 (2018) 37–42
ADVANCES IN MOLECULAR PATHOLOGY

The Clinical and Laboratory Features of Clinical Hematopoiesis of Indeterminate Potential

Jay L. Patel, MD, MBA[a,b,*]
[a]Department of Pathology, University of Utah, 500 Chipeta Way, MS115-G04, Salt Lake City, UT 84108, USA; [b]Molecular Hematopathology, ARUP Laboratories, 500 Chipeta Way, MS115-G04, Salt Lake City, UT 84108, USA

KEYWORDS

• Clonal hematopoiesis of indeterminate potential (CHIP) • Clonal cytopenia(s) of undetermined significance (CCUS) • Myelodysplastic syndrome • Leukemia • Myeloid neoplasm • Myeloid malignancy • Cytopenia(s) • Mutation

KEY POINTS

- Somatic mutations in genes commonly mutated in myeloid neoplasms (eg, *DNMT3A*, *TET2*, *ASXL1*) occur with increasing frequency as a function of age in normal individuals. This phenomenon has been described as clonal hematopoiesis of indeterminate potential (CHIP).
- CHIP is associated with higher likelihood of development of a hematologic malignancy as well as an increased risk of mortality due to cardiovascular events.
- These somatic mutations may occur in the setting of cytopenic patients who do not meet criteria for a definitive diagnosis of myelodysplastic syndrome or other myeloid malignancy, in which case the term clonal cytopenia of undetermined significance (CCUS) should be used.
- Certain patterns of somatic mutations and variant allele fractions may confer a higher positive predictive value for diagnosis of an overt myeloid neoplasm versus CHIP or CCUS. As data accumulate, specific mutation patterns are increasingly likely to be codified in diagnostic criteria and prognostic scoring systems related to myeloid neoplasms.

INTRODUCTION

Technological advances in genetic profiling via next-generation or massively parallel sequencing (NGS) facilitated the landmark discovery of age-related somatic mutations in noncytopenic, otherwise ostensibly hematologically normal individuals [1,2]. The term clonal hematopoiesis of indeterminate potential (CHIP) has since been coined to describe this clinical setting. The somatic mutations in CHIP may occur in a variety of genes, which are also commonly mutated in myeloid malignancies (eg, *DNMT3A*, *TET2*, *ASXL1*), thus potentially shedding light on pathogenesis [3,4]. The overlap of CHIP-related mutations with previously characterized myelodysplastic syndrome (MDS) and acute myeloid leukemia (AML) mutational landscapes presents a diagnostic challenge. In turn, as the availability of relatively inexpensive targeted NGS panels has increased dramatically in recent years, the concept of CHIP-related mutations has become crucial to understanding the workup of patients with cytopenia or cytopenias in which myeloid neoplasm is a differential diagnostic consideration.

Disclosure Statement: The author has nothing to disclose.

*Hematopathology, 500 Chipeta Way, MS115-G04, Salt Lake City, UT 84108. *E-mail address:* Jay.Patel@path.utah.edu

https://doi.org/10.1016/j.yamp.2018.06.005
2589-4080/18/

This article reviews the clinical and genetic characteristics of CHIP and explores the relationship between this premalignant state and pathologic conditions, including clonal cytopenia of undetermined significance (CCUS), idiopathic cytopenia of undetermined significance (ICUS), and overt myeloid neoplasms such as MDS or AML.

SIGNIFICANCE

Clonal Hematopoiesis of Indeterminate Potential in the Spotlight

In 2014, 2 separate groups concurrently reported the discovery of clonal hematopoiesis using whole exome sequencing in independent population-based cohorts of individuals unselected for hematologic phenotypes and lacking cytopenias [5,6]. Both of these studies were further remarkable for their association of CHIP with increased risk of subsequent development of hematological malignancy (hazard ratio 11–12) as well as all-cause mortality (hazard ratio 1.4). More recently, CHIP has been linked with atherosclerosis apparently related to cytokine-mediated inflammation and represents a cardiovascular risk factor conferring an approximate doubling in the risk of coronary heart disease [7]. The incidence of CHIP increases as a function of age and exceeds 10% in patients aged more than 65 years, which far exceeds the prevalence of myeloid neoplasms [8].

The vast majority (nearly 95%) of individuals with CHIP demonstrated a single somatic variant with a minority (5%) showing 2 distinct variants. Exceedingly few individuals with CHIP show more than 2 distinct variants: a finding with potential diagnostic utility in the setting of myeloid neoplasms. Three of the most commonly mutated genes in individuals with CHIP as well as more broadly in myeloid malignancies are *DNMT3A*, *TET2*, and *ASXL1* (Table 1) [9,10]. These genes are generally involved in DNA methylation and epigenetic modification, and mutations confer a growth advantage, which drives clonal cell expansion [11,12]. CHIP may also involve splicing factors, such as *SF3B1*, *SRSF2*, *U2AF1*, and *ZRSR2* [13]. Less frequently, several other genes may be mutated in CHIP, surprisingly including *TP53* and *JAK2* as well as *BCOR*, *BCORL1*, *CBL*, *PPM1D*, and others. Variant allele fraction (VAF), defined as the number of reads containing the variant of interest divided by the total number of reads, associated with somatic variants can also be informative [14]. In CHIP, VAFs may show a range, but VAF significantly greater than 10% is uncommon in CHIP and should raise suspicion for underlying hematologic malignancy [15].

Clonal Hematopoiesis of Indeterminate Potential –Related Mutations and Diagnosis of the Cytopenic Patients

The recognition of CHIP and related mutations has profound consequences for diagnostic workup of MDS. MDS is a genetically heterogeneous, challenging-to-diagnose stem cell disorder characterized by ineffective hematopoiesis manifested in the form of cytopenias and subsequently bone marrow failure. It has a nonspecific clinical presentation, and current diagnostic criteria rely heavily on morphology, which suffers from poor interobserver reproducibility [16,17]. In addition, morphologic dysplasia is nonspecific and can be observed as a reactive phenomenon in cytopenic patients with conditions, including infection, autoimmune disease, and nutritional deficiency [18]. Half or more of MDS patients have a normal karyotype, underscoring

TABLE 1
Biological Characteristics of Commonly Mutated Genes in Clonal Hematopoiesis of Indeterminate Potential

Gene	Role	Variants	Mutation Phenotype
DNMT3A	DNA methylation	Loss of function frameshift or nonsense mutations, particularly at Arg882 hotspot	DNA hypomethylation due to loss of DNA methyltransferase enzyme activity
TET2	DNA demethylation	Loss of function deletions, frameshift, or nonsense mutations	DNA hypermethylation resulting from disruption of normal function of TET family of dioxygenases
ASXL1	Chromatin modification	Recurrent truncating loss of function exon 11 or 12 nonsense or frameshift mutations resulting	Abnormal epigenetic regulation via interaction with polycomb recessive complex

the difficulty of demonstrating clonality and diagnosing MDS before the advent of high throughput sequencing. More complete characterization of the genomic landscape of MDS reveals that 80% to 90% of cases show somatic mutations across the spectrum of genetic aberrations, including balanced and unbalanced translocation, copy number variation, small insertion/deletion, and single nucleotide variants [19].

Although CHIP lacks the cytopenias that are the sine qua none of MDS, an intermediate clinical scenario called CCUS exists in which somatic mutation and cytopenias are present, but diagnostic criteria for a definitive diagnosis of MDS are unfulfilled [20]. Alternatively, patients may present with unexplained cytopenias in the absence of somatic mutation, a condition referred to as ICUS. CHIP, CCUS, and ICUS are important considerations in the setting of patients being worked up for a possible diagnosis of MDS (Fig. 1).

Specific gene mutations or patterns of comutation have correlated with clinical phenotypes and thereby confer higher positive predictive value for a specific diagnosis of myeloid neoplasm. Comutation of *TET2* with *ASXL1* or spliceosome genes *SRSF2* or *ZRSR2* is characteristic of chronic myelomonocytic leukemia [10]. Mutation of the spliceosome gene *SF3B1* (particularly Lys700Glu) is closely associated with ring sideroblasts in MDS [21]. More recently, Malcovati and colleagues [22] showed that comutation of *DNMT3A*, *TET2*, or *ASXL1* (CHIP-related mutations) with a spliceosome gene (eg, *U2AF1*, *SRSF2*, *EZH2*, *SF3B1*, or *ZRSR2*) are especially closely related to myelodysplasia and carry a positive predictive value of 86% to 100%. Therefore, although spliceosome mutations do occur in the context of CHIP, specific patterns involving these gene mutations carry strong predictive value for a diagnosis of myeloid neoplasm. These data support the clinical utility of mutation profiling by NGS on peripheral blood or bone marrow samples from patients with unexplained cytopenias. Detection of these mutation patterns in cytopenic patients should increase diagnostic yield and improve overall accuracy.

Although AML remains an exceedingly genetically heterogeneous disease, comprehensive genomic profiling of AML has shed light on pathogenesis, and a model is taking shape in which CHIP-related somatic mutations occur stochastically in conjunction with function of age and set the stage for stem cell expansion [9]. Acquisition of CHIP-related mutation(s) is followed by stepwise accumulation of additional mutations that drives the leukemic phenotype [23]. This paradigm is exemplified by one of the most common mutation profiles clinically encountered in normal karyotype AML patients: comutation of *DNMT3A*, *TET2*, *NPM1*, and *FLT3* internal tandem duplication [24]. This model also has implications for follow-up or minimal residual disease testing (MRD) in AML.

Ivey and colleagues [25] showed that MRD as measured by detection of *NPM1* mutation by

	Normal	CHIP	CCUS	ICUS	MDS
Cytopenia	✗	✗	✓	✓	✓
Mutation	✗	✓	✓	✗	✓
Number of variants	N/A	1–2	1–2	N/A	≥2
VAF	N/A	Low	Low	N/A	High
Dysplasia	✗	✗	✗	✗	✓
BM Blasts	<5%	<5%	<5%	<5%	<20%

FIG. 1 CHIP can be distinguished from normal hematopoiesis, CCUS, ICUS, and MDS based on comprehensive assessment of hematologic findings (blood counts, morphologic dysplasia, bone marrow blast percentage) and genetic data (mutation status, number of variants, VAF). BM, bone marrow; N/A, not applicable.

allele-specific real-time quantitative polymerase chain reaction in *NPM1*-mutated AML is one of the most important predictors of outcome at the postinduction chemotherapy time point. Persistence of CHIP-related mutations such as DNMT3A in MRD-negative patients was observed in a subset of patients but did not affect prognosis. This finding suggests that clonal hematopoiesis in the form of CHIP-related mutations may persist following therapy but do not necessarily correlate with outcomes in AML (Fig. 2). A more recent study showed that detection of specific CHIP-related mutations in DNMT3A, TET2, or ASXL1, so-called DTA mutations, after induction therapy during complete remission does not predict relapse, whereas persistence of other "non-DTA" mutations does confer an increased risk of relapse and correlates with decreased overall survival [26].

PRESENT RELEVANCE AND FUTURE AVENUES TO CONSIDER OR TO INVESTIGATE

A working knowledge of the concept of CHIP is essential for practicing hematologists and pathologists broadly involved in the diagnosis and management of patients with cytopenias and myeloid neoplasms. Targeted panels by NGS using a panel-based approach has rapidly become an indispensable tool in the differentiation of CHIP, ICUS, CCUS, and MDS [13]. These distinctions require assessment of clinical and hematologic findings in close conjunction with genetic data. As discussed, understanding of CHIP in the context of pathogenesis of hematopoietic malignancies is also key to interpreting NGS findings correctly in special clinical settings, such as postchemotherapy or stem cell transplantation patients.

Further investigation and more data are needed in order to more comprehensively understand the natural history of CHIP and CCUS in particular. A more robust understanding of these conditions will likely allow for highly granular associations between particular gene mutations, comutation patterns, and/or VAFs with specific clinical phenotypes. The accuracy of MDS diagnosis and prognostication will thereby be improved as will clinicians' ability to rule out this condition with a high degree of confidence due to the high negative predictive value associated with lack of somatic mutation in cytopenic patients [8]. The risk of CHIP in terms of development of a myeloid malignancy also requires further study. The same genetic features that may allow increased diagnostic accuracy may allow for more precise risk stratification and could inform clinical management of individuals being followed for CHIP or asymptomatic CCUS. In addition, the relationship between

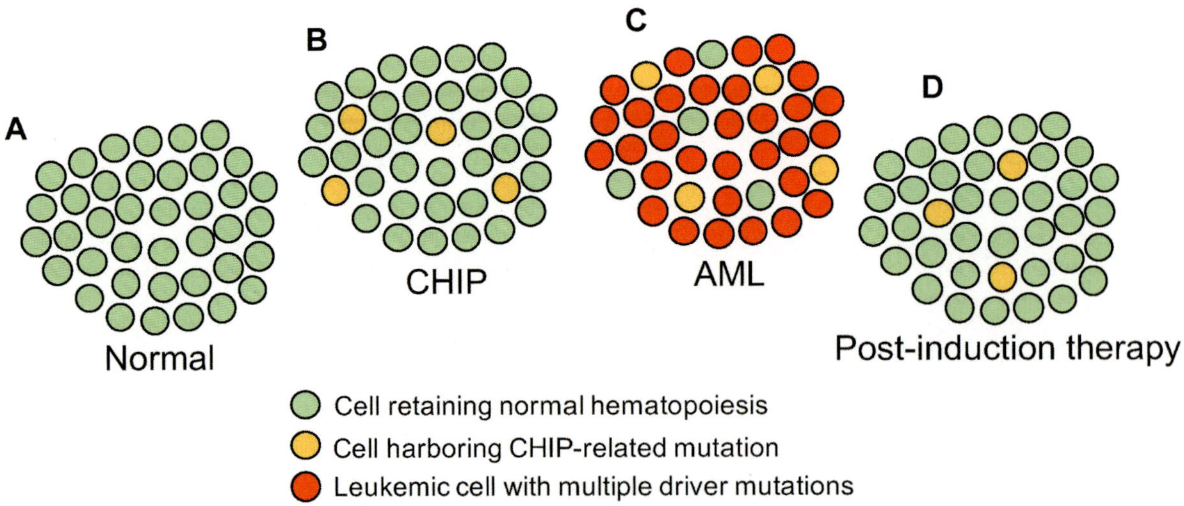

FIG. 2 (**A**) Normal hematopoiesis. (**B**) CHIP: a small subset of cells acquires somatic CHIP-related mutations such as *DNMT3A* R882H. (**C**) AML: acquisition of additional driver mutations, such as *NPM1* exon 11 tetranucleotide insertion and/or *FLT3* internal tandem duplication in combination with existing CHIP-related mutation results in a predominant population of leukemic blasts. (**D**) Induction therapy eliminates the leukemic blast population and restores mostly normal hematopoiesis, but a minor subset of cells containing CHIP-related mutations may persist.

CHIP and increased mortality requires further study, especially as it relates to other established cardiovascular risk factors and the current lack of available intervention.

SUMMARY

CHIP is a recently recognized phenomenon in which hematologically normal individuals acquire somatic mutations as a function of age in genes that are commonly mutated in myeloid malignancies. The incidence of CHIP far exceeds overt neoplasia, suggesting that CHIP is a benign but premalignant condition in the mold of established preclinical hematologic states, such as monoclonal gammopathy of undetermined significance or monoclonal B-cell lymphocytosis. Individuals with CHIP carry both an increased risk of subsequent diagnosis of a bona fide hematologic malignancy as well as higher mortality due to cardiovascular events.

The clinical utility of targeted NGS panels that provide comprehensive assessment of CHIP-related mutations is increasingly clear in the context of cytopenic patients in which a diagnosis of MDS is being considered [27,28]. Although ongoing study relating somatic mutations to clinical impact is necessary, data are accumulating that may facilitate designation of "MDS-associated somatic mutations" (or patterns of comutation) to allow for definitive diagnosis of MDS in absence of morphologic criteria similar to "MDS-associated cytogenetic abnormalities" established in current World Health Organization classification [29]. Numerous somatic mutations also carry prognostic value in MDS but have yet to be incorporated into existing prognostic scoring systems [30,31].

REFERENCES

[1] Busque L, Patel JP, Figueroa ME, et al. Recurrent somatic TET2 mutations in normal elderly individuals with clonal hematopoiesis. Nat Genet 2012;44(11):1179–81.

[2] Xie M, Lu C, Wang J, et al. Age-related mutations associated with clonal hematopoietic expansion and malignancies. Nat Med 2014;20(12):1472–8.

[3] Haferlach T, Nagata Y, Grossmann V, et al. Landscape of genetic lesions in 944 patients with myelodysplastic syndromes. Leukemia 2014;28(2):241–7.

[4] Cancer Genome Atlas Research, Network, Ley TJ, Miller C, et al. Genomic and epigenomic landscapes of adult de novo acute myeloid leukemia. N Engl J Med 2013;368(22):2059–74.

[5] Genovese G, Kähler AK, Handsaker RE, et al. Clonal hematopoiesis and blood-cancer risk inferred from blood DNA sequence. N Engl J Med 2014;371(26):2477–87.

[6] Jaiswal S, Fontanillas P, Flannick J, et al. Age-related clonal hematopoiesis associated with adverse outcomes. N Engl J Med 2014;371(26):2488–98.

[7] Jaiswal S, Natarajan P, Silver AJ, et al. Clonal hematopoiesis and risk of atherosclerotic cardiovascular disease. N Engl J Med 2017;377(2):111–21.

[8] Steensma DP, Bejar R, Jaiswal S, et al. Clonal hematopoiesis of indeterminate potential and its distinction from myelodysplastic syndromes. Blood 2015;126(1):9–16.

[9] Papaemmanuil E, Gerstung M, Bullinger L, et al. Genomic classification and prognosis in acute myeloid leukemia. N Engl J Med 2016;374(23):2209–21.

[10] Papaemmanuil E, Gerstung M, Malcovati L, et al. Clinical and biological implications of driver mutations in myelodysplastic syndromes. Blood 2013;122(22):3616–27 [quiz: 3699].

[11] Gelsi-Boyer V, Brecqueville M, Devillier R, et al. Mutations in ASXL1 are associated with poor prognosis across the spectrum of malignant myeloid diseases. J Hematol Oncol 2012;5:12.

[12] Smith ZD, Meissner A. DNA methylation: roles in mammalian development. Nat Rev Genet 2013;14(3):204–20.

[13] Valent P, Orazi A, Steensma DP, et al. Proposed minimal diagnostic criteria for myelodysplastic syndromes (MDS) and potential pre-MDS conditions. Oncotarget 2017;8(43):73483–500.

[14] Welch JS, Ley TJ, Link DC, et al. The origin and evolution of mutations in acute myeloid leukemia. Cell 2012;150(2):264–78.

[15] Cargo CA, Rowbotham N, Evans P, et al. Targeted sequencing identifies patients with preclinical MDS at high risk of disease progression. Blood 2015;126(21):2362–5.

[16] Font P, Loscertales J, Benavente C, et al. Inter-observer variance with the diagnosis of myelodysplastic syndromes (MDS) following the 2008 WHO classification. Ann Hematol 2013;92(1):19–24.

[17] Font P, Loscertales J, Soto C, et al. Interobserver variance in myelodysplastic syndromes with less than 5 % bone marrow blasts: unilineage vs. multilineage dysplasia and reproducibility of the threshold of 2 % blasts. Ann Hematol 2015;94(4):565–73.

[18] Steensma DP. Dysplasia has A differential diagnosis: distinguishing genuine myelodysplastic syndromes (MDS) from mimics, imitators, copycats and impostors. Curr Hematol Malig Rep 2012;7(4):310–20.

[19] Cazzola M, Della Porta MG, Malcovati L. The genetic basis of myelodysplasia and its clinical relevance. Blood 2013;122(25):4021–34.

[20] Kwok B, Hall JM, Witte JS, et al. MDS-associated somatic mutations and clonal hematopoiesis are common in idiopathic cytopenias of undetermined significance. Blood 2015;126(21):2355–61.

[21] Malcovati L, Karimi M, Papaemmanuil E, et al. SF3B1 mutation identifies a distinct subset of myelodysplastic syndrome with ring sideroblasts. Blood 2015;126(2): 233–41.

[22] Malcovati L, Gallì A, Travaglino E, et al. Clinical significance of somatic mutation in unexplained blood cytopenia. Blood 2017;129(25):3371–8.

[23] Bowman RL, Busque L, Levine RL. Clonal hematopoiesis and evolution to hematopoietic malignancies. Cell Stem Cell 2018;22(2):157–70.

[24] Patel JL, Schumacher JA, Frizzell K, et al. Coexisting and cooperating mutations in NPM1-mutated acute myeloid leukemia. Leuk Res 2017;56:7–12.

[25] Ivey A, Hills RK, Simpson MA, et al. Assessment of minimal residual disease in standard-risk AML. N Engl J Med 2016;374(5):422–33.

[26] Jongen-Lavrencic M, Grob T, Hanekamp D, et al. Molecular minimal residual disease in acute myeloid leukemia. N Engl J Med 2018;378(13):1189–99.

[27] Bejar R, Stevenson K, Abdel-Wahab O, et al. Clinical effect of point mutations in myelodysplastic syndromes. N Engl J Med 2011;364(26):2496–506.

[28] Bejar R. Clinical and genetic predictors of prognosis in myelodysplastic syndromes. Haematologica 2014; 99(6):956–64.

[29] Arber DA, Orazi A, Hasserjian R, et al. The 2016 revision to the World Health Organization classification of myeloid neoplasms and acute leukemia. Blood 2016; 127(20):2391–405.

[30] Greenberg PL, Tuechler H, Schanz J, et al. Revised international prognostic scoring system for myelodysplastic syndromes. Blood 2012;120(12):2454–65.

[31] Schanz J, Tüchler H, Solé F, et al. New comprehensive cytogenetic scoring system for primary myelodysplastic syndromes (MDS) and oligoblastic acute myeloid leukemia after MDS derived from an international database merge. J Clin Oncol 2012;30(8): 820–9.

Advances in Molecular Pathology 1 (2018) 43–50
ADVANCES IN MOLECULAR PATHOLOGY

Comprehensive Monitoring of Patients with Chronic Myeloid Leukemia

Ranjana Arora, MD, MPH
Hematology Molecular Clinical Services, Clinical Molecular and Genomics Laboratory, Department of Pathology and Laboratory Medicine, University of Kentucky, 800 Rose Street, Lexington, KY 40536, USA

KEYWORDS
• Chronic myeloid leukemia • CML • International scale • Molecular monitoring • Tyrosine kinase inhibitors • TKI

KEY POINTS

- Molecular methodologies enable precise and deep level monitoring for minimal residual disease in chronic myeloid leukemia (CML).
- The International Scale offers standardization of molecular testing for CML across laboratories.
- Mutations in BCR-ABL1 kinase domain may confer resistance requiring switching of TKIs.
- Successful treatment-free remission is a possibility for a subset of patients, and there is optimism for others with newer therapies and future research.

INTRODUCTION

Chronic myeloid leukemia (CML) is a myeloproliferative disorder characterized by chromosomal translocation t(9;22)(q34.1; q11.2) that results in the formation of the pathognomonic Philadelphia chromosome (Ph) containing the BCR-ABL1 fusion gene. This BCR-ABL1 fusion gene leads to constitutive activation of tyrosine kinase required for initiation and propagation of CML in patients [1]. The approach of treating CML saw a dramatic change following the results of phase 3 of the International Randomized Study of Interferon STI571 (IRIS) clinical trial and subsequent US Food and Drug Administration (FDA) approval of imatinib mesylate (also known as ST1571; Gleevec) in 2001. The current primary treatment of CML includes imatinib as the first-generation tyrosine kinase inhibitor (TKI), whereas the second-line therapy includes several more potent TKIs, such as bosutinib, dasatinib, nilotinib, ponatinib, and omacetaxine [2–4]. These changes in treatment of CML have led to an evolution in diagnosis and follow-up. From being solely based on morphologic and cytogenetic response (CyR) criteria, the reliance is on molecular methodologies that include quantitative reverse transcriptase polymerase chain reaction (qRT-PCR), digital PCR, and next-generation sequencing (NGS) for monitoring of BCR-ABL1 transcripts. These methods are much more sensitive for assessment of molecular response to monitor TKI treatment [5,6].

The indicators measured to monitor response to therapy include complete hematologic response, CyR, molecular response, and relapse.[3] Hematologic response refers to complete normalization of peripheral blood counts (leukocyte count $<10 \times 10^9$/L and platelet count $<450 \times 10^9$/L) with no immature cells or blasts in blood and disappearance of palpable splenomegaly. Complete cytogenetic response (CCyR) is the absence of Ph^+ metaphases. Once CCyR is achieved in these patients, only molecular methods make it possible to monitor minimal residual disease (MRD) for follow-up of treatment response. The revised 2016 World Health

Disclosure Statement: The author has nothing to disclose.

E-mail address: Ranjana.arora@uky.edu

https://doi.org/10.1016/j.yamp.2018.07.006
2589-4080/18/

Organization (WHO) diagnostic guidelines have included a "provisional" response to TKI for defining accelerated phase of CML in addition to hematological and cytogenetic criteria, which will require additional clinical trials data for validation [7].

Using the International Scale (IS) for standardized reporting, the molecular response is monitored as Early Molecular Response ([EMR]; BCR-ABL1 [IS] ≤10% at 3 and 6 months) or Major Molecular Response ([MMR]; BCR-ABL1 [IS] ≤0.1% or ≥3-log reduction in BCR-ABL1 messenger RNA (mRNA) from the standardized baseline, if quantitative PCR (qPCR) (IS) is not available) [3]. The terminology used to define deeper molecular response refers to the assay's level of sensitivity, for example, MR^4 (BCR-ABL1 [IS] ≤0.01%; ≥4-log reduction from IRIS baseline), $MR^{4.5}$ (BCR-ABL1 [IS] ≤0.0032%; 4.5-log reduction from IRIS baseline), and MR^5 (BCR-ABL1 [IS] ≤0.001%; 5-log reduction from IRIS baseline) [8]. Any loss to response (hematologic or cytogenetic relapse) or 1-log increase in BCR-ABL1 transcript levels (ie, loss of MMR) requires a prompt evaluation. In such a scenario, a bone marrow biopsy for disease progression to accelerated or blast phase, and BCR-ABL1 kinase domain mutation analysis for resistance to TKI therapy is indicated. These patients are evaluated for alternative TKI therapy/clinical trials or allogenic hematopoietic stem cell transplantation.

SIGNIFICANCE

It has been more than a decade of experience with TKI therapy in CML, and molecular monitoring has rapidly become the new norm. Against the backdrop of newer updated guidelines for clinical practice guidelines, this article attempts to discuss the present and future of comprehensive monitoring of CML.

The current National Comprehensive Cancer Network (NCCN) and European LeukemiaNet (ELN) recommendations advocate regular monitoring of TKI therapy in CML patients for BCR-ABL1 transcript levels standardized to the IS. MMR was defined in the IRIS trial as a 3-log reduction in BCR-ABL1 transcript levels from a standardized baseline (defined as ≤0.1% BCR-ABL on the IS). The qRT-PCR analysis for this trial was standardized across 3 laboratories using separate laboratory procedures and different control genes [9]. The standardization became essential because these differences, such as the use of varied control genes (which include ABL1, GUSB, G6PD, beta-2-microglobulin), risk introduction of disparity in reporting of quantitative assays. Several studies have explored this issue, and although ABL1 is the most commonly used reference gene across the United States, different testing laboratories have their own preferred choice. Whereas one study [10] established the ABL1 gene as the most stable reference gene, another study [11] showed significantly skewed ABL1 gene expression under differing cellular conditions during treatment with TKIs. This study proposed GUSB to be the most suitable control gene for accurate quantitative estimation of BCR-ABL1 [11,12]. Although at low levels the performance is reported to be equally good for the commonly used genes, GUSB has the advantage over ABL1 in terms of lack of distortion at high levels of disease. Whether that is clinically important in today's day and age of low-level precise quantitative monitoring is debatable. Furthermore, considering that much of the available published data is ABL1 related, it remains the most popular choice for testing.

The treatment guidelines for CML patients require serial molecular analysis of these values and reporting standardized MRD levels to achieve consistent treatment decisions. The need for reporting standardized levels underscores the importance of achieving comparability for the interpretation of data derived from different laboratories using a global scale [13]. Unfortunately, there can be a large amount of heterogeneity in BCR-ABL1 measurement because of a slew of factors, including variability in methodology, equipment, reagents, and reporting of results. These factors played a key role in establishing a standardized IS for measuring of BCR-ABL1 transcripts. The IS scale was designed to allow comparability and equivalency between values reported by different laboratories, a key factor to ensure quality clinical care as well as validity of research and inform regulatory decisions [13].

The testing laboratories offering or contemplating the same require in-house validation of their methodology from start to finish. The in-house validation translates to starting from specimen selection to nucleic acid extraction and all the way to report generation and interpretation. For the analytical stage, there are 2 key words: calibration and conversion factor (CF). The calibration of the BCR-ABL to IS can be done by exchanging a series of samples [14–24] with a reference laboratory that is already calibrated on IS. The CF is generated by comparing the data generated by the field method and reference laboratory. It is derived using linear regression and calculating the bias, which is based on the tendency of the field data to deviate from the reference data [2,13]. This CF is the antilog of the mean bias between the data from the 2 laboratories. Therefore, importantly, the CF will be determined by factors specific and unique to each testing laboratory. Once the CF has been calibrated, a second set of validation using sample exchange with the reference laboratory is done to validate the CF. The BCR-ABL1 value that is generated by the testing laboratory can then be converted to the IS by multiplying the BCR-ABL1 value with the CF [2,13].

The WHO recently established an International Genetic Reference Panel for BCR-ABL1 testing that consists of 4 dilutions of lyophilized cell lines with fixed BCR-ABL1 (IS) of ~0.01%, 0.1%, 1%, and 10% on the IS. This material can be used as reference material for laboratories working on calibrating to IS [25]. However, this material is available in only limited quantities. Consequently, several laboratories use commercially available secondary reference material, which is calibrated to the WHO primary reference standards. Increasing use of the secondary reference material is anticipated especially with a move toward obtaining US FDA approval by commercial testing platform manufacturers.

There have been ongoing efforts to address the challenges for BCR-ABL1 standardization and reproducibility. The European Treatment and Outcome Study group has developed a network of laboratories standardized to IS and has published detailed technical specifications and recommendations that would impact the accuracy, limit of detection, and precision of molecular monitoring [26]. The College of American Pathologists (CAP) has also developed guidelines for development and validation of laboratory-developed qRT-PCR for quantitative detection of BCR-ABL1 transcripts [27]. Most of the laboratories that offer BCR-ABL1 (IS) quantitative assays participate in CAP-offered semiannual proficiency testing. Although there has been a significant and optimistic increase in adoption of IS by laboratories across the United States [1], adoption to IS has not yet achieved 100%, which is required for universal standardization of molecular monitoring of TKI therapy.

For molecular monitoring, qRT-PCR should be carried out on blood or bone marrow RNA specimens for initial workup to establish the presence of quantifiable BCR-ABL1 mRNA transcripts at baseline. Most patients with CML express the transcripts e14a2 (also known as b3a2) or e13a2 (also known as b2a2), which result from rearrangement of the major breakpoint cluster regions (M-BCR) generating a 210-kDa fusion protein. Rarely, the breakpoints occur in the μ-BCR generating a larger fusion protein of 230 kDa; or in the minor breakpoint region, m-BCR, generating a short fusion protein of 190 kDa [28]. The baseline evaluation of these transcripts is important from a clinical point of view because conversion to IS from this value is used for any future comparisons for trend or monitoring the response to treatment. Although interpreting the baseline levels, one should be cognizant of the fact that both the major and the minor BCR-ABL1 transcripts have been reported in normal healthy individuals. Although the levels in normal healthy individuals tend to be at a much lower level ($1-10/10^8$ white blood cells), the incidence of finding these low-level transcripts increases with advancing age [29,30].

NCCN guidelines recommend risk scoring in patients with chronic phase CML before initiation of TKI therapy using either the Sokal or the Hasford scoring system [3]. This system stratifies patients into low-, intermediate-, and high-risk groups [14,15]. Both NCCN and ELN recommend monitoring for BCR-ABL1 (IS) every 3 months for all patients after initiating TKI therapy to monitor the response milestones at 3, 6, and 12 months (Table 1). NCCN guidelines consider BCR-ABL1 (IS) ≤10% at 3 and 6 months, BCR-ABL1 (IS) ≤1% at 12 months, and BCR-ABL1

TABLE 1
Goals for Molecular Response to First-Line Tyrosine Kinase Inhibitors Therapy

	NCCN Guidelines Response Milestone (RM) Time Point (mo)				ELN Guidelines RM Time Point (mo)		
BCR-ABL (IS)	3	6	12	>12	3	6	12
>10%	RM (B)	RM (C)	RM (C)	RM (C)	RM (D)		
>1–10%	RM (A)	RM (A)	RM (B)	RM (C)		RM (E)	
>0.1%–1%	RM (A)	RM (A)	RM (A)	RM (B)			RM (F)
≤0.1%	RM (A)	RM (A)	RM (A)	RM (A)			

Data from NCCN clinical practice guidelines in oncology: chronic myeloid leukemia. Version 4.2018. 2018. Available at: http://www.nccn.org. Accessed March 15, 2018; and Baccarani M, Deininger M, Rosti G, et al. European LeukemiaNet recommendations for the management of chronic myeloid leukemia. Blood 2013;122:872–84.

(IS) ≤0.1% at ≥12 months (see Table 1; Table 2) as adequate response. ELN recommendations consider BCR-ABL1 (IS) >10% at 3 months to be a warning response warranting frequent monitoring (see Tables 1 and 2) [3,4]. If these response milestones are not achieved, the results would be grounds for a switch in therapy. Deep molecular response should be monitored every 3 months after CCyR has been achieved, for 2 years and every 3 to 6 months thereafter.

Secondary drug resistance in CML patients occurs most commonly as point mutations in the BCR-ABL1 kinase domain. These mutations are associated with variable degrees of imatinib resistance [16,17] and are associated with poor prognosis and disease progression [18,19]. Although many kinase domain mutations have been described, not all patients show clinical response to switched TKI therapy. The wide spectrum of mutations underscores the importance of identification of specific mutations that would impact management strategy [1]. There have been several studies that predict kinase domain mutation in patients with an increase in BCR-ABL RNA; because of a lack of consensus, there are no specific guidelines for mutational screening. Most of the laboratories advocate a 2- to 3-fold range of increase in BCR-ABL1 transcripts [20,21]. Because the precise increase in the levels of transcripts depends on the performance characteristics of the qPCR [21], NCCN guidelines advocate clinical judgment in deciding when and in whom to screen for these mutations based on change in the level of molecular response.

TABLE 2
Recommendations for Response Milestones

Response Milestones (RM)	Clinical Considerations and Treatment Options
RM (A): NCCN	Continue monitoring response and continue same TKI
RM (B):NCCN	Evaluate for patient compliance, drug interactions, and mutational analysis. Follow-up options include continue same TKI, dose escalation of imatinib (to maximum of 800 mg), switch to alternate TKI, and evaluate for HCT
RM (C): NCCN	Evaluate patient compliance, drug interactions, and mutational analysis. Switch to alternate TKI and evaluate for HCT
RM (D): ELN	Warning response. More frequent monitoring to allow for timely change in therapy in case of treatment failure Treatment failure is lack of complete hematologic response and/or >95% Ph+ metaphases. No designation for molecular response for treatment failure at 3 mo
RM (E): ELN	Warning response >10% BCR-ABL1 (IS) at 6 mo is treatment failure
RM (F): ELN	Warning response >1% BCR-ABL1 (IS) at 12 mo is treatment failure

The spectrum of resistance for different mutations is varied. Although being able to confer resistance across several TKIs, they may spare one or more of the others. NCCN guidelines suggest switching to nilotinib for F317L/V/I/C, T315A, or V299L, dasatinib for Y253H, E255K/V, or F359V/C/I, and switching to bosutinib for E255K/V, F317L/V/I/C, F359V/C/I, T315A, and Y253H (Fig. 1). The presence of T315I mutation is associated with resistance to imatinib, dasatinib, nilotinib, and bosutinib [22], and switching to Ponatinib could be effective [23]. In addition to T315I mutation, Ponatinib is also active against E255V, Y253H, and F359V mutations [24]. The variation in resistance spectrum highlights the importance of understanding the resistance profile of each mutation to determine which treatment to switch to in the scenario of resistance.

PRESENT RELEVANCE AND FUTURE AVENUES TO CONSIDER OR TO INVESTIGATE

There has been increasing evidence from clinical trials showing better outcome in patients with chronic phase CML who are treated with dasatinib or nilotinib in comparison with imatinib (Table 3). More patients achieved MMR or $MR^{4.5}$ with dasatinib (DASISION trial) or nilotinib (ENESTnd study) than imatinib (IRIS trial) [31,32]. Long-term follow-up of selected cohorts from all these clinical trials showed fewer transformations to accelerated phase-CML or blast phase–CML [31–34].

Recently, there is active research in identification of molecular markers that predict response to TKI therapy [5]. Several clinical trials have demonstrated that achievement of EMR is an indicator of successful response to treatment and good prognosis, underscoring the importance of accurate and precise

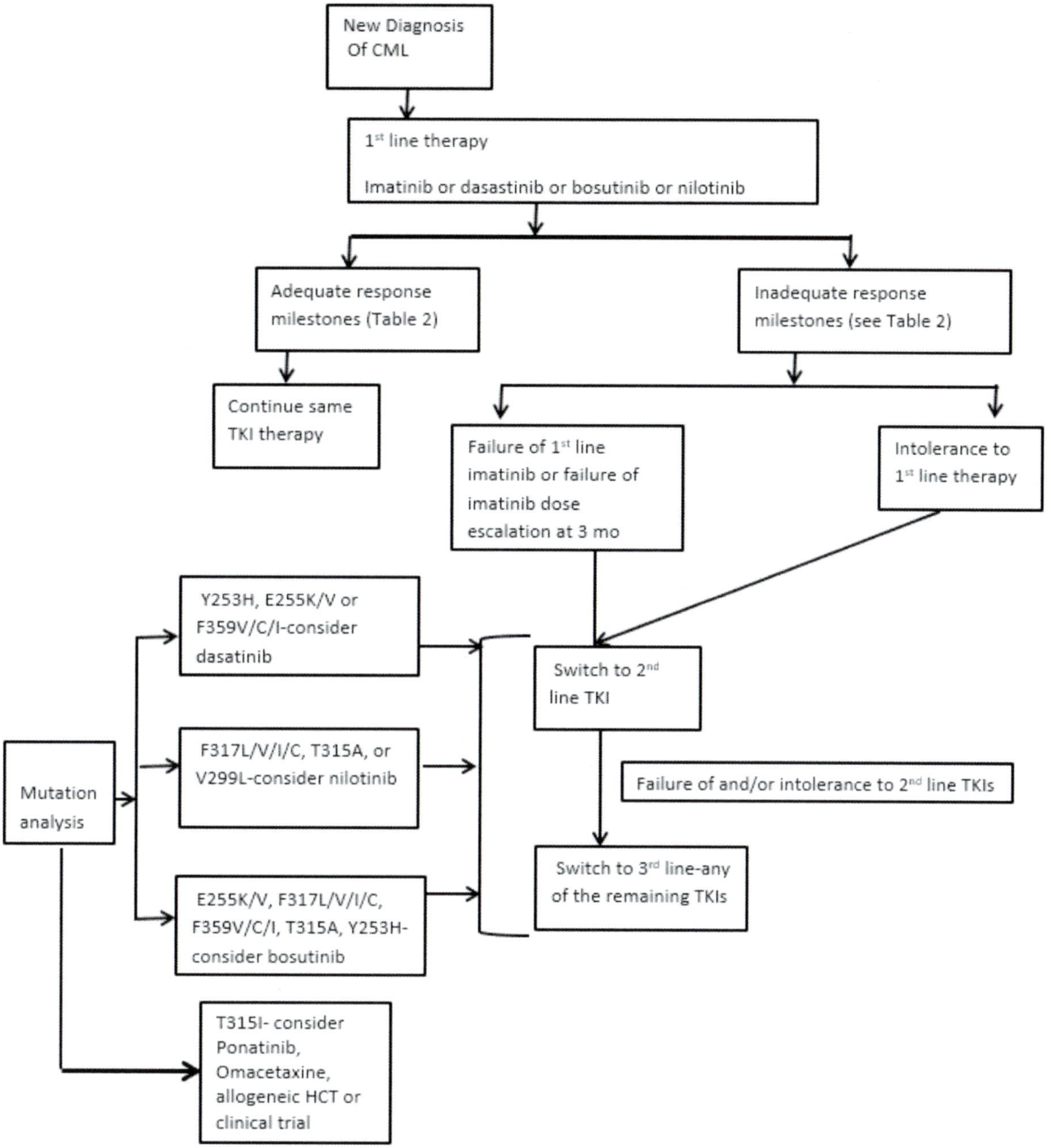

FIG. 1 Treatment algorithm suggested for chronic phase CML patients. HCT, hematopoietic stem cell transplantation. (*Data from* Refs. [3,22,41])

quantification of BCR-ABL1 on the IS [2]. Current research is directed toward either modification of conventional qRT-PCRs assays to improve quality of total mRNA [35] or in the form of additional assay development. A cartridge-based technique (GeneXpert, Sunnyvale, CA, USA) is an easy and inexpensive technology but has not been validated to levels below MR^4 [5]. In comparison to RNA-based assays, DNA-

TABLE 3
Long-Term Follow-up Comparative Data of Deep Molecular Monitoring for Different Tyrosine Kinase Inhibitors Used to Treat Chronic Phase Chronic Myeloid Leukemia

	IRIS Study [34] (n = 1106)	DASISION Study [31] (n = 519)	ENESTnd Study [32] (n = ~281)	BFORE Study [33] (n = 536)
Drugs	Imatinib	Dasatinib vs imatinib	Nilotinib vs imatinib	Bosutinib vs imatinib
Study duration	10 y (n = 123)	5 y	5 y	12 mo
Molecular response	MMR (imatinib): 93% (3 log reduction in BCR-ABL1 from baseline)	MMR (dasatinib): 76% MMR (imatinib): 64% P = .002 $MR^{4.5}$ (dasatinib): 42% $MR^{4.5}$ (imatinib): 33% P = .025	MMR (nilotinib 300 & 400 mg): 77% MMR (imatinib): 60% P<.001 $MR^{4.5}$ (nilotinib 300 mg): 54% $MR^{4.5}$ (nilotinib 400 mg): 52% $MR^{4.5}$ (imatinib): 31% P<.001)	MMR (bosutinib): 47% MMR (imatinib): 37% P = .02

based qPCRs would have numerous benefits for residual disease detection in CML because DNA is more stable and easier to extract than RNA. The major obstacle in adopting this technique is the difficulty in mapping the genomic breakpoints of translocation that occur over widespread intronic sequences. These limitations are being overcome using targeted DNA based digital PCR [6].

The importance of kinase domain resistance mutations in patients undergoing TKI therapy cannot be overstated. Ability to detect compound mutations, which are emerging as potential acquired driver mutations using NGS methods, is being investigated actively [36,37]. The efficient ability of NGS technology over routine Sanger sequencing to distinguish between true compound mutations and *in trans* (on separate alleles) mutations is being explored and could guide clinical decisions in the future [5,38].

Discontinuation of TKI therapy was investigated in The Stop Imatinib trial in 100 patients on imatinib with complete molecular remission for more than 2 years who then stopped treatment [39,40]. The median follow-up after discontinuation of treatment on these patients was for 77 months; recurrence-free survival was 43% at 6 months and 38% at 60 months [40]. Molecular relapse was seen in 61% of the patients, with most of the events occurring within 6 months of cessation of treatment [39].

Successful treatment-free remission is a possibility in some patients, and long-term discontinuation of TKI would produce substantial economic impact. However, treatment discontinuation should be considered in patients with high-quality and close monitoring. TKI treatment for at least 5 years, achievement of $MR^{4.5}$, and maintenance of a stable deep molecular response ($\geq MR^4$) for at least 2 years are significant determining variables for patient selection [3,41]. The patients should have access to reliable and sensitive qPCR with at least $MR^{4.5}$ (BCR-ABL1 $\leq$ 0.0032% IS) sensitivity level and provides results within 2 weeks for frequent molecular monitoring. The NCCN guidelines version 4.2018 for CML recommendation updated January 24, 2018 has modified the monitoring guidelines for discontinuation. In place of earlier recommendation to monitor monthly during the first half year, 6 weekly during the second half-year followed by 3 monthly monitoring later, now it recommends monthly monitoring for 1 year, then every 6 weeks for the second year, and every 12 weeks thereafter (indefinitely) in patients who remain in MMR after discontinuation of TKI therapy [3,42,43]. Furthermore, for patients with loss of MMR after discontinuation, the recommendation is to promptly resume TKI within 4 weeks with molecular monitoring every 4 weeks until MMR is reestablished and then every 12 weeks thereafter indefinitely for such patients. If resumption of TKI therapy does not result in MMR, BCR-ABL1 kinase domain mutation testing is recommended along with continuation of monthly molecular monitoring for another 6 months. Long-term monitoring of patients with discontinuation of therapy or failure to achieve MMR, as well as further research toward the scope and impact of mutations, would generate additional data leading to treatment-free remission for a larger subset of patients.

SUMMARY

Treatment of CML has evolved rapidly with the availability of newer TKIs. With this has come the necessity to accurately and precisely monitor the response to therapy. Deep molecular monitoring based on qRT-PCR, digital PCR, and NGS is enabling measurements at levels previously not possible with cytogenetic or hematologic monitoring. The higher sensitivity of molecular tests exposes them to the risk of lack of comparability and reproducibility. These risks can be mitigated to a considerable extent by adopting standardization to the IS by collaboration between new and reference laboratories for calibration and validation of BCR-ABL1 testing. Updated clinical practice guidelines emphasize the need for continuous monitoring during and after discontinuation of treatment. Failure to respond or loss of MMR is a likely predictor of resistance warranting change of therapy. Future investigations into more stable (eg, DNA based) testing methodologies and further research into understanding of mutations will contribute to better utilization of newer therapies and successful treatment-free remission for patients.

REFERENCES

[1] Press RD, Kamel-Reid S, Ang D. BCR-ABL1 Rt-qPCR for monitoring the molecular response to tyrosine kinase inhibitors in chronic myeloid leukemia. J Mol Diagn 2013; 15:565–76.

[2] Arora R, Press RD. Measurement of BCR-ABL1 transcripts on the International Scale in the United States: current status and best practices. Leuk Lymphoma 2017;58(1):8–16.

[3] NCCN clinical practice guidelines in oncology: chronic myeloid leukemia. Version 4.2018. 2018. Available at: http://www.nccn.org. Accessed March 15, 2018.

[4] Baccarani M, Deininger M, Rosti G, et al. European LeukemiaNet recommendations for the management of chronic myeloid leukemia. Blood 2013;122:872–84.

[5] Marum JE, Branford S. Current developments in molecular monitoring in chronic myeloid leukemia. Ther Adv Hematol 2016;7(5):237–51.

[6] Alikian M, Ellery P, Forbes M, et al. Next-generation sequencing-assisted DNA-based digital PCR for a personalized approach to the detection and quantification of residual disease in chronic myeloid leukemia patients. J Mol Diagn 2016;18:176–89.

[7] Arber DA, Orazi A, Hasserjian R, et al. The 2016 revision to the World Health Organization classification of myeloid neoplasms and acute leukemia. Blood 2016; 127:2391–405.

[8] Cross NCP, White HE, Colomer D, et al. Laboratory recommendations for scoring deep molecular response following treatment for chronic myeloid leukemia. Leukemia 2015;29:999–1003.

[9] Hughes TP, Kaeda J, Branford S, et al. Frequency of major molecular responses to imatinib or interferon alfa plus cytarabine in newly diagnosed chronic myeloid leukemia. N Engl J Med 2003;349:1423–32.

[10] Beillard E, Pallisgaard N, van der Velden VH, et al. Evaluation of candidate control genes for diagnosis and residual disease detection in leukemic patients using 'real-time' quantitative reverse-transcriptase polymerase chain reaction (RQ-PCR) – a Europe against cancer program. Leukemia 2003;17:2474–86.

[11] Lee JW, Chen Q, Knowles DM, et al. beta- Glucuronidase is an optimal normalization control gene for molecular monitoring of chronic myelogenous leukemia. J Mol Diagn 2006;8:385–9.

[12] Zhang T, Grenier S, Nwachukwu B, et al. Inter-laboratory comparison of chronic myeloid leukemia minimal residual disease monitoring: summary and recommendations. J Mol Diagn 2007;9:421–30.

[13] Branford S, Fletcher L, Cross NC, et al. Desirable performance characteristics for BCR-ABL measurement on an international reporting scale to allow consistent interpretation of individual patient response and comparison of response rates between clinical trials. Blood 2008; 112(8):3330–8.

[14] Sokal J, Cox E, Baccarani M, et al. Prognostic discrimination in "good-risk" chronic granulocytic leukemia. Blood 1984;63(4):789–99.

[15] Hasford J, Pfirrmann M, Hehlmann R, et al. A new prognostic score for survival of patients with chronic myeloid leukemia treated with interferon alfa. Writing Committee for the Collaborative CML Prognostic Factors Project Group. J Natl Cancer Inst 1998;90:850–8.

[16] Apperley JF. Part I: mechanisms of resistance to imatinib in chronic myeloid leukaemia. Lancet Oncol 2007;8(11): 1018–29.

[17] O'Hare T, Eide CA, Deininger MW. Bcr-Abl kinase domain mutations, drug resistance and the road to a cure of chronic myeloid leukemia. Blood 2007;110(7): 2242–9.

[18] White DL, Saunders VA, Dang P, et al. OCT-1–mediated influx is a key determinant of the intracellular uptake of imatinib but not nilotinib (AMN107): reduced OCT-1 activity is the cause of low in vitro sensitivity to imatinib. Blood 2006;108(2):697–704.

[19] Soverini S, Martinelli G, Rosti G, et al. ABL mutations in late chronic phase chronic myeloid leukemia patients with up-front cytogenetic resistance to imatinib are associated with a greater likelihood of progression to blast crisis and shorter survival: a study by the GIMEMA working party on chronic myeloid leukemia. J Clin Oncol 2005;23(18):4100–9.

[20] Branford S, Rudzki Z, Parkinson I, et al. Real-time quantitative PCR analysis can be used as a primary screen to

identify patients with CML treated with imatinib who have BCR-ABL kinase domain mutations. Blood 2004; 104(9):2926–32.

[21] Press RD, Willis SG, Laudadio J, et al. Determining the rise in BCR-ABL RNA that optimally predicts a kinase domain mutation in patients with chronic myeloid leukemia on imatinib. Blood 2009;114(13): 2598–605.

[22] Jabbour E, Kantarjian H, Jones D, et al. Characteristics and outcomes of patients with chronic myeloid leukemia and T315I mutation following failure of imatinib mesylate therapy. Blood 2008;112(1):53–5.

[23] Cortes JE, Kantarjian H, Shah NP, et al. Ponatinib in refractory Philadelphia chromosome-positive leukemias. N Engl J Med 2012;367:2075–88.

[24] Cortes JE, Kim D-W, Pinill-Ibarz J, et al. A phase 2 trial of Ponatinib in Philadelphia chromosome-positive leukemias. N Engl J Med 2013;369:1783–96.

[25] White HE, Matejtschuk P, Rigsby P, et al. Establishment of the first World Health Organization International Genetic Reference Panel for quantitation of BCR-ABL mRNA. Blood 2010;116:e111–7.

[26] Muller MC, Cross NC, Erben P, et al. Harmonization of molecular monitoring of CML therapy in Europe. Leukemia 2009;23:1957–63.

[27] Jennings LJ, Smith FA, Halling KC, et al. Design and analytic validation of *BCR-ABL1* quantitative reverse transcription polymerase chain reaction assay for monitoring minimal residual disease. Arch Pathol Lab Med 2012;136:33–40.

[28] Chasseriau J, Rivet J, Bilan F, et al. Characterization of the different *BCR-ABL* transcripts with a single multiplex RT-PCR. J Mol Diagn 2004;6(4):343–7.

[29] Bose S, Deininger M, Gora-Tybor J, et al. The presence of typical and atypical BCR-ABL fusion genes in leukocytes of normal individuals: biologic significance and implications for the assessment of minimal residual disease. Blood 1998;92(9):3362–7.

[30] Biernaux C, Loos M, Sels A, et al. Detection of major bcr-abl gene expression at a very low level in blood cells of some healthy individuals. Blood 1995;86(8): 3118–22.

[31] Cortes JE, Saglio G, Kantarjian HM, et al. Final 5-year study results of DASISION: the dasatinib versus imatinib study in treatment-naïve chronic myeloid leukemia patients trial. J Clin Oncol 2016;34(20): 2333–40.

[32] Hochhaus A, Saglio G, Hughes TP, et al. Long-term benefits and risks of frontline nilotinib vs imatinib for chronic myeloid leukemia in chronic phase: 5-year update of the randomized ENESTnd trial. Leukemia 2016; 30(5):1044–54.

[33] Cortes JE, Gambacorti-Passerini C, Deininger MW, et al. Bosutinib versus Imatinib for newly diagnosed chronic myeloid leukemia: results from the randomized BFORE trial. J Clin Oncol 2017;28:231–7.

[34] Hochhaus A, Larson RA, Guilhot F, et al. Long-term outcomes of imatinib treatment for chronic myeloid leukemia. N Engl J Med 2017;376:917–27.

[35] Yeung D, Parker W, Phillis, et al. BCR-ABL assay sensitivity of MR4.5 achieved in >90%, and MR5 in >75% of samples, through mRNA selection before qRT-PCR. Blood 2015;126:2777.

[36] Khorashad J, Kelley T, Szankasi P, et al. BCR-ABL1compound mutations in tyrosine kinase inhibitor resistant CML: frequency and clonal relationships. Blood 2013; 121:489–98.

[37] Shah N, Skaggs B, Branford S, et al. Sequential ABL kinase inhibitor therapy selects for compound drug resistant BCR-ABL mutations with altered oncogenic potency. J Clin Invest 2007;117:2562–9.

[38] Parker W, Phillis S, Yeung D, et al. Detection of BCR-ABL1 compound and polyclonal mutants in chronic myeloid leukemia patients using a novel next generation sequencing approach that minimises PCR and sequencing errors. Blood 2014;124:399.

[39] Mahon FX, Réa D, Guilhot J. Discontinuation of imatinib in patients with chronic myeloid leukaemia who have maintained complete molecular remission for at least 2 years: the prospective, multicentre Stop Imatinib (STIM) trial. Lancet Oncol 2010;11(11):1029–35.

[40] Etienne G, Guilhot J, Rea D, et al. Long-term follow-up of the french stop imatinib (STIM1) study in patients with chronic myeloid leukemia. J Clin Oncol 2017; 35(3):298–305.

[41] Hochhaus A, Saussele S, Rosti G, et al. Chronic myeloid leukemia: ESMO clinical practice guidelines for diagnosis, treatment and follow-up. Ann Oncol 2017;28(4):iv41–51.

[42] SauBele S, Richter J, Hochhaus A, et al. The concept of treatment free remission in chronic myeloid leukemia. Leukemia 2016;30:1638–47.

[43] Hughes TP, Ross DM. Moving treatment-free remission into mainstream clinical practice in CML. Blood 2016; 128:17–23.

Advances in Molecular Pathology 1 (2018) 51–64
ADVANCES IN MOLECULAR PATHOLOGY

Genomic Biomarkers in Pathogenesis and Clinical Care of Chronic Lymphocytic Leukemia

Kalpana S. Reddy, MD[a], Keyur P. Patel, MD, PhD[b,*]

[a]Department of Pathology and Laboratory Medicine, Division of Hematopathology, Zucker School of Medicine at Hofstra/Northwell, 6 Ohio Drive, Suite 202, Lake Success, NY 11042, USA; [b]Department of Hematopathology, The University of Texas MD Anderson Cancer Center, 6565 MD Anderson Boulevard Unit 1062, Houston, TX 77030, USA

KEYWORDS

• CLL • IGHV mutation • CLL genomics • CLL mutations • TP53 mutation • Resistance mutation • Hereditary CLL

KEY POINTS

- Genetic heterogeneity underlies the heterogeneity observed in the clinical presentation and the clinical course of chronic lymphocytic leukemia.
- Novel and clinically significant clonal mutations in genes such as *ATM, NOTCH1*, *SF3B1*, *XPO1*, *BIRC3*, and *FBXW7* provide useful prognostic information for clinical decision making.
- Subclonal mutations are common in chronic lymphocytic leukemia and are associated with poor prognosis.
- Molecular biomarkers can predict poor response to chemoimmunotherapy (*TP53*) and allow detection of emerging resistance to targeted therapy (*BTK*, *PLCG2*).
- Although most cases are acquired, it is important to recognize inherited form of chronic lymphocytic leukemia, which accounts for less than 10% of chronic lymphocytic leukemia cases, for obvious treatment and familial implications.

INTRODUCTION

Chronic lymphocytic leukemia (CLL)/small lymphocytic lymphoma is the most common adult leukemia in the Western world accounting for approximately 25% of total cases. The age adjusted incidence of CLL in the US United States is 5.7 per 100,000 per year [1], and the median age at diagnosis is 68 years. The 5-year relative survival has increased from 67.5% in 1975 to 83.2% in 2014. Details for diagnosis, initial workup, specific indications for treatment as well as response assessment to therapy and supportive management are described in the current revised 2018 version of the International Workshop on Chronic Lymphocytic Leukemia guidelines [2]. Based on the presence or absence of peripheral blood lymphocytosis and extramedullary involvement, cases with clonal CLL or CLL-like cells are classified as chronic lymphocytic leukemia (CLL), small lymphocytic lymphoma (SLL) or monoclonal B-cell lymphocytosis (MBL). Transformation to Richter syndrome (RS), either diffuse large B-cell lymphoma (DLBCL) or classical Hodgkin lymphoma (CHL), occurs in approximately 2% to 8% and 1% of patients with CLL, respectively. Although earlier CLL prognostication relied on clinical and hematologic

Disclosure: The authors have nothing to disclose.

*Corresponding author, *E-mail address:* kppatel@mdanderson.org

https://doi.org/10.1016/j.yamp.2018.06.001
2589-4080/18/

findings, *TP53* and *IGHV* mutation status now constitute 2 of the 5 parameters in the International Prognostic Index for CLL [3].

GENOMIC BIOMARKERS IN CHRONIC LYMPHOCYTIC LEUKEMIA

Genomic studies have provided critical insights into the underlying pathobiology of CLL, which aids in clinical decision making (Fig. 1). Comprehensive genomic analyses indicate a model of sequential genetic evolution in CLL, which is initiated by chromosomal aberrations. Additional acquired mutations may alter the course of the disease, rendering it more aggressive and refractory to therapy. Early drivers commonly include deletion of chromosome 13q (del13q) in 55% of cases and 10% of cases with deletion of chromosome 11q (del11q) as well as 10% to 20% cases showing trisomy 12 [4]. Also, del13q leads to loss of microRNAs [5], whereas del11q causes *ATM* gene loss [6]. Deletion of chromosome 17p (del17p), occurring in 5% to 8% of cases, is typically acquired at later stages and deletes tumor suppressor gene *TP53*. More than 50% of these cases also carry mutations in the remaining *TP53* allele, altering the pathway [7]. Mutations in *BIRC3*, *FBXW7*, *KRAS*, and *MGA* also act as late drivers [4]. Somatic gene mutations such as *POT1* and *SF3B1* [8] that behave as intermediate drivers have been identified. *XPOL1*, *KLHL6*, and *MYD88* are examples of some other recurrent somatic gene mutations seen.

Chromosomal Changes in Chronic Lymphocytic Leukemia

Cytogenetic and fluorescence in situ hybridization studies (FISH) for recurrent abnormalities are well-established components of CLL workup and are covered only briefly in this review. More than 80% of patients with CLL have acquired chromosomal abnormalities, most often deletions of 13q14, 17p13, 11q22-23, and trisomy 12 [9]. An isolated abnormality such as del13q has a better outcome and has been described as an early event in CLL, whereas del11q, del17p as well as 2p gain are associated with progression and relapse [10]. Statistically significant associations between cytogenetic abnormalities exist, as in (i) del11q and 2p gain and (ii) trisomy 12 with trisomies 18 and 19, 14q deletion, and translocations involving *BCL2*, *BCL3*, and *MYC* [11]. A complex karyotype (≥3 abnormalities) is associated with an unfavorable prognosis and a poor response to therapy, as well as a shorter

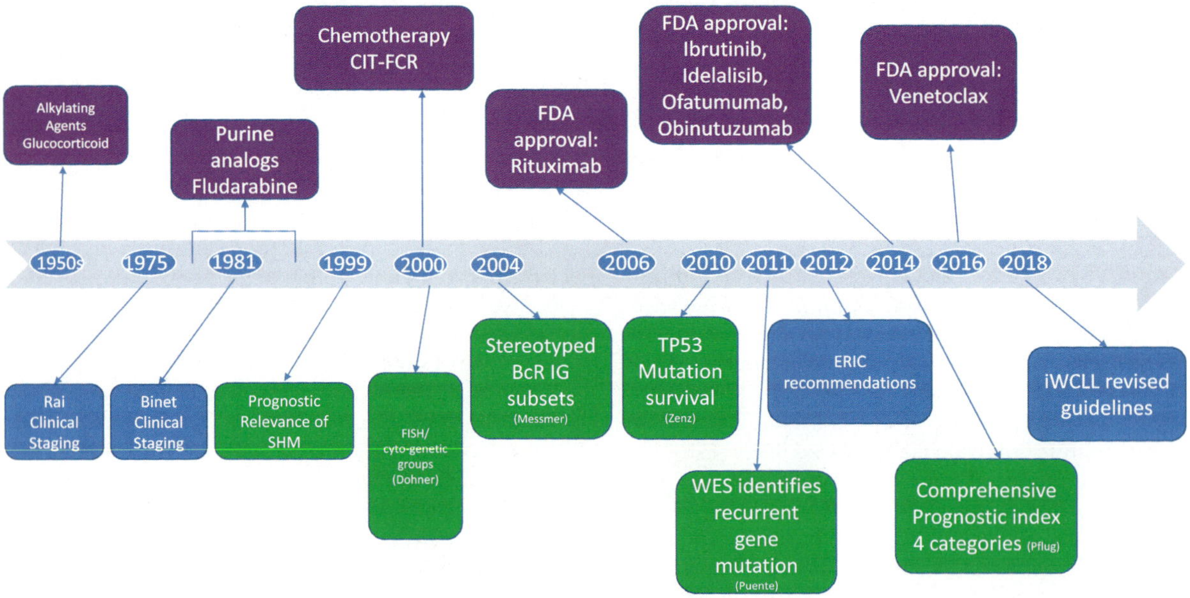

FIG. 1 Timeline of landmark genomic discoveries and treatments in chronic lymphocytic leukemia (CLL). CIT-FCR, chemoimmunotherapy–fludarabine, cyclophosphamide and rituximab; ERIC, European Research Initiative on Chronic Lymphocytic Leukemia; FDA, US Food and Drug Administration; FISH, fluorescence in situ hybridization; iWCLL, International Workshop on Chronic Lymphocytic Leukemia; SHM, somatic hypermutation; WES, whole-exome sequencing.

time to first treatment (TTFT) [12,13]. It is also an independent and powerful predictor of poor response to ibrutinib therapy [14,15]. Several reports have indicated that a higher FISH percentage of abnormalities is also associated with increased risk in del 17p [16] and del11q [17].

TP53 mutation or deletion is associated with advanced stage, rapidly progressive disease, and RS, in addition to being an independent predictor of overall survival (OS) after RS transformation [18]. *TP53* mutations not only predict for shorter OS, progression-free survival (PFS), time to treatment, but are also associated with refractoriness to fludarabine-containing regimens independent of del17p cooccurrence [19].

Immunoglobulin heavy chain rearrangements

Immunoglobulin heavy chain gene variable region sequence (*IGHV*) mutation status is a well-established prognostic factor in CLL [20]. The degree of somatic hypermutation (SHM) with a cutoff of 2% deviation or 98% sequence identity to germline VH gene sequence is currently used to subdivide patients with CLL into good mutated (M-CLL) and bad unmutated (U-CLL) groups [21]. However, other studies have used various IGHV percentage cutoff points (1%–5%). Also, results from the ibrutinib trial [22] indicated that separating patients into M-CLL and U-CLL may no longer be useful. A relatively recent study identified IGHV% as a continuous variable with higher levels being incrementally associated with favorable PFS and OS in patients with CLL treated with fludarabine, cyclophosphamide, and rituximab. This concept may also be a more relevant prognostic indicator in patients treated with ibrutinib and venetoclax [14]. Another recent study [23] showed that, while $IgHV^{unmut}$ CLL mainly displays coding mutations in driver genes and an aging signature, $IgHV^{mut}$ CLL has a high incidence of promoter and enhancer mutations secondary to aberrant activation-induced cytidine deaminase activity.

Currently, there is recognition of specific variant chain usage in disease pathogenesis and clinical behavior. CLL clones show a preferential usage of certain V regions, with *VH4-34* often seen in cases with hypermutation and *VH1-69* and *VH4-39* seen in unmutated cases. In addition, 30% of patients with CLL show highly similar heavy chain complementary determining region (HCDR3) amino acid sequences in their B-cell receptors, referred to as *stereotyped receptors*. These findings suggest that antigen stimulation by autoantigens [24] and superantigens [25] including *Staphylococcus aureus* protein A and cytomegalovirus phosphoprotein pUL32 is likely involved in CLL pathogenesis. Furthermore, specific use of *VH3-21* and stereotyped "subset 2" is an adverse prognostic marker that is independent of *IGHV* mutation status. Also, *VH4-39* gene use and stereotyped "subset 8" are polyreactive to various antigens in patients with CLL with predisposition to increased risk of RS [26]. As of now, although assessment of BcR IG stereotypes is not a part of routine CLL prognostic workup [2], studies have shown clear associations summarized and are summarized here [27].

- Subset #1 (2.4%): U-CLL; very aggressive TTFT 1.9 years.
- Subset #2 (2.8%): U-CLL and M-CLL; very aggressive TTFT 1.6 years. Aberrant spliceosomes, increased *SF3B1*, and low frequency of *TP53* mutations seen.
- Subset # 8 (0.5%): primarily women; U-CLL; highest risk for RT and very aggressive TTFT 1.5 years. Promiscuous antigen binding reactivity. High frequency of trisomy 12, *NOTCH1* mutations noted.
- Subset #4 (1%): M-CLL very indolent TTFT 11 years. B-cell anergy, only a few gene mutations, mainly del13q14. Intraclonal diversification owing to ongoing somatic hypermutation (SHM); also seen IG gene.

Recurrent Gene Mutations in Chronic Lymphocytic Leukemia

Whole-genome sequencing [28,29] and whole-exome sequencing [8] have provided a comprehensive picture of the complex mutational landscape in CLL that are helpful in diagnosis, prognosis, and treatment. An important finding was that specific recurrent mutations were identified in M-CLL (*MYD88*, *CHD2*, and *KLHL6*) and U-CLL (*NOTCH1*, *TP53*, *SF3B1*, *POT1*, and *XPO1*). Mutations that are shown to have an adverse prognostic impact include *TP53*, *NOTCH1*, and *SF3B1*. Numerous recurrent acquired mutations in the coding regions of *TP53*, *SF3B1*, *NOTCH1*, *BIRC3*, *ATM*, *RPS15*, *POT1*, and *SAMHD1* have been associated with chemorefractoriness, advanced disease, poor prognosis, and/or transformation [30]. In addition to increasing numbers of somatic gene mutations being identified in coding regions, a study [31] for the first time pointed to the significance of noncoding mutations in CLL, by characterizing a kataegis region affecting an enhancer site 300 kb upstream of the *PAX5* gene [23].

Mutations predictably affect several key cellular pathways involving RNA metabolism, DNA damage, cell cycle control, apoptosis, NOTCH1 signaling, genome/chromatin modification, inflammatory pathway, and B-cell signaling [4,30,31].

RNA splicing and processing pathways

The incidence of *SF3B1* mutation in patients with CLL is about 5% to 15% at diagnosis, increasing to 20% in those with advanced disease. These somatic mutations are composed of missense nucleotide alterations (mutation hotspots at codons 662, 666, and 700) clustered in specific HEAT repeats of the SF3B1 protein. They are associated with inferior response to chemoimmunotherapy [32], aggressive disease and shorter TTFT and OS, as well as unmutated *IGHV*, but are not seen in RS. *SF3B1* mutations are associated with specific variant chain usage, typically in *IGHV3-21*, possibly *IGHV1-69*, and are mutually exclusive of *IGHV1-2*. These mutations are more common in patients with normal karyotype or del11q, but are not seen in patients with trisomy 12 [33].

XPO1, a gene located on 2p15, is most frequently mutated in exon 15 codon 571 (p.E571K), resulting in overexpression of exportin-1 and drug resistance [34]. Mutations are seen primarily in patients with CLL with unmutated IGHV (approximately 5%). Selinexor (KPT-330 or KPT8602), a selective inhibitor of nuclear export, synergizes with ibrutinib ex vivo and has also been shown to disrupt B-cell receptor signaling by suppressing *BTK* gene expression [30].

Low-frequency mutated gene *DDX3X*, a member of the DEAD-box RNA helicase family, is involved in many steps of RNA metabolism [35] and occurs in 2% of cases. A recent analysis suggested that CLL *DDX3X* mutations were associated with unmutated *IGHV* and poor outcome, associated with worse PFS [36].

DNA repair and cell cycle control

TP53, a tumor suppressor gene localized at 17p, is inactivated by deletions and mutations in CLL [9,37]. *TP53* mutations and del17p are associated with poor survival (median 5-year OS) and resistance to chemotherapy [38]. In addition, *TP53* inactivation is associated with disease progression to aggressive DLBCL, being noted in 40% of patients with RS and predicts OS after transformation [18,32].

More than 95% of *TP53* mutations in CLL occur in exons 5 to 8, encoding the DNA binding domain [38]. The overexpression of MDM2, a TP53-specific ubiquitin ligase that mediates its degradation, can also inactivate TP53. Lower levels of miR34A are seen in TP53-inactivated CLL cells and correspond with more aggressive disease [39,40]. Activated TP53 induces miR34A expression, which activates TP53 by inhibiting SIRT1. Small molecules targeting the MDM2–TP53 interaction induce apoptosis in patients with CLL by overcoming ATM-mediated resistance to fludarabine [41,42]. Furthermore, ibrutinib was shown to synergize with MDM2 inhibitors in the induction of apoptosis in CLL cells independent of the TP53 status [43]. A novel MDM2 inhibitor (RG7112) is under evaluation in clinical trials [44].

ATM, a tumor suppressor gene, encodes a cell cycle checkpoint kinase linking DNA damage with cell cycle/DNA repair and also controls many other cellular functions, including metabolism and chromatin structure. Clonal *ATM* mutations are associated with a shorter PFS and OS after first-line treatment, but this does not apply to subclonal *ATM* mutations [45,46]. Targeted treatments of ATM-mutant CLL cells were investigated in preclinical studies. ATM-deficient cells rely on alternate DNA damage response pathways for DNA double strand breaks repair. Hence, poly(ADP-ribose) polymerase 1 and protein kinase DNA-PKcs inhibitors might display selective toxicity against ATM-defective cells [47]. A recent study [48] reported that AZD6738, a selective inhibitor of ATR (ATM and Rad3-related protein), led to synthetic lethality in primary CLL with *ATM* or *TP53* deficiency in vitro owing to accumulation of unrepaired DNA damage, resulting in cell death by mitotic catastrophe.

SAMHD1 encodes the sterile a motif and histidine-aspartic domain containing protein 1. It is a deoxynucleoside triphosphate triphosphohydrolase that is required for DNA synthesis and maintenance [49]. *SAMHD1* loss of function results in increased deoxynucleoside triphosphate cellular levels, DNA synthesis, and cell cycle progression, leading to cell proliferation and survival. About 3% to 5% of patients with CLL have acquired mutations in *SAMHD1* at diagnosis and this increases to 9% to 11% in relapsed/refractory CLL without associated poor risk factors, such as del11q or unmutated *IGHV* [49]. Standard CLL therapies may select preexisting clones carrying *SAMHD1* mutations. Some studies suggest that *SAMHD1* mediates cytarabine (Ara-C) resistance by decreasing intracellular Ara-CTP. Conversely, *SAMHD1* inactivation increases sensitivity to Ara-C and, to a lesser extent, fludarabine [50].

NOTCH signaling

NOTCH1 mutations are found in about 10% of patients with newly diagnosed CLL, increasing to 20% in more advanced disease and 30% in RS. These mutations are mainly confined to exon 34, with 80% to 90% comprising the c.7541_7542delCT variant causing early termination of the PEST domain, resulting in a degradation-resistant protein. This process in turn leads to sustained NOTCH signaling, increased cell survival, and resistance to apoptosis [28]. A large-scale study identified a novel biological mechanism that also leads to the removal of NOTCH1 PEST domain [31]. Noncoding splice-site mutations in *NOTCH1*, have also been identified in 3% of cases [31] and are correlated with clinical outcome, but were found to be mutually exclusive to *NOTCH1* coding variants [51]. *NOTCH1* mutations are rare in del13q [33], but are enriched in trisomy 12 [31] and associated with unmutated *IGHV*, more aggressive disease, poor response to anti-CD20 monoclonal antibodies, and fludarabine resistance, as well as predisposition to RT; correlating with shorter TTFS and adverse outcome [52].

Mutations in additional genes, whose products participate in Notch pathway control, have been noted at a lower frequency. Inactivating mutations of *SPEN* gene were also detected in 1% of patients with CLL [31]. It is noted that SPEN functions as a co-repressor of RBPJ (Recombination signal Binding Protein for immunoglobulin kappa J region), the nuclear effector of the Notch pathway.

Dysregulated NOTCH1 signaling is of particular interest, because this may provide a target for therapy. The gamma-secretase inhibitor PF-03084014 showed inhibition of NOTCH1 signaling and enhances cytotoxic effect of fludarabine [53]. Using gene expression-based screening, a calcium channel modulator bepridil was recently identified as a new NOTCH1 pathway inhibitor [54].

FBXW7 encodes an E3 ubiquitin ligase that in turn regulates the stability of several proteins, including NOTCH1, MYC, MTOR, and MCL1, by targeting them for ubiquitination and degradation. About 2.5% patients with CLL displayed inactivating mutations of *FBXW7* [33].

MED12 (the mediator complex subunit 12) gene encodes a subunit kinase module that is associated with the 26-subunit mediator core complex that regulates different transcriptional programs important in tumorigenesis. Missense *MED12* mutations noted in 2% to 5% patients with CLL, lie within exon 2, target G44, and potentially lead to an increase in NOTCH1 signaling. They are associated with known poor prognostic markers such as U-*IGHV* [55,56].

Nuclear factor-κB signaling/Toll-like receptor signaling

NFKBIE (nuclear factor [NF]-κB inhibitor I-kappa-B-epsilon) gene encodes a negative regulator of NF-κB signaling that traps cytoplasmic REL protein; it also involves B-cell receptor and Toll-like receptor signaling. Recurrent 4-bp truncating and rare point mutations of *NFKBIE* occur in 5% to 10% of CLLs, are enriched in advanced disease, and carry a poor prognosis [57,58]. In CLL, *NFKBIE* deletions were associated with shorter TTFT similar to IGHV-unmutated or 17p-deleted patients.

The *BIRC3* (baculoviral inhibitor of apoptosis protein repeat containing 3) gene encodes a member of the inhibitor of apoptosis protein family involved in the negative regulation of MAP3K14 via cooperation with TRAF3 and TRAF2. In CLL, inactivating *BIRC3* mutations lead to constitutive activation of the noncanonical NF-κB signaling [59]; rare mutations in TRAF2 and TRAF3 are also described. *BIRC3* mutations are strongly associated with unmutated *IGHV*, *ATM* mutations, del11q, and shorter TTFT [60], occurring in 3% to 8% at the time of diagnosis. However, these mutations may continue to emerge over time [31,59–61] and the frequency of *BIRC3* disruptions may increase to 24% among fludarabine-refractory patients, being mutually exclusive with TP53 abnormalities [59,61] and may be associated with refractoriness to the BTK inhibitor ibrutinib [59,61]. *BIRC3* mutations constitute high-risk CLL in the integrated model.

MYD88 is an adaptor protein for interleukin 1 and Toll-like receptor signaling. Mutations in *MYD88* consisting mainly of p.L265P substitution are found in 2% to 4% of Caucasian patients with CLL [33], although a higher rate of 8% is reported in Asia [62]. These mutations lead to downstream activation of NF-κB and JAK2 pathways. Initial studies reported that most patients with *MYD88* mutations were younger at diagnosis, belonging to *IGHV*-mutated group [28,63] with longer time to treatment and OS than those with wild-type *MYD88*. However, this conclusion was controversial [60]. A more recent study [64] did not observe a preferable *IGHV* 3-23 gene usage in *MYD88*-mutated cases and suggested that these mutations may in fact predict unfavorable prognosis within the *IGHV*-mutated CLL subgroup.

RAS/MAPK signaling

Mutations in this pathway, which lies downstream of B-cell receptor signaling [12], have been reported in patients with CLL. Mutated *BRAF* (3%–10%) was identified as an independent prognostic driver for shorter TTF [31] and dismal prognosis. *BRAF* mutations in CLL, can involve exon 11 in addition to codon V600 (exon 15) and represent a subclonal population [65]. They may be less susceptible to the inhibitor vemurafenib.

KRAS mutations occur in 2% to 6% of patients with CLL and correlated with a poor response to chemoimmunotherapy [12]. *NRAS* and *MAPK1* mutations each account for about 3% of patients with CLL.

Telomere maintenance/stability

POT1 mutations are present in 3% to 5% of patients with clinically aggressive CLL [66] causing telomere dysfunction, disruption of DNA maintenance, and in turn control of chromatin structure and splicing regulation [67]. They were also reported to occur at greater frequency in RS [18]. Germline *POT1* mutations are also associated with familial CLL [68]. A prospective clinical trial [12] recently reported that complex karyotypes and *POT1* mutations are significant prognostic factors for an unfavorable survival independent of IGHV mutation status, Binet stage, and serum beta-2-microglobulin. Thus, monitoring of *POT1* mutation seems to be warranted.

Ribosomal proteins

All *RPS15* mutations lie within a hotspot region in exon 4 and target a 7 amino acid evolutionary conserved region. *RPS15* is recurrently mutated in CLL (approximately 5%) and associated with a shorter PFS; an aggressive, relapsing form of CLL; and resistance to fludarabine-based chemotherapy [4,69]. *RPS15* mutations are frequently associated with *TP53* mutations. Mutant RPS15 p.G132A experimentally increased TP53 degradation through increased ubiquitination, as compared with wild-type RPS15 [69].

Transcription factors

Mutations in *EGR2* gene encoding transcription factor controlling B-cell biology are heterozygous missense mutations that are localized in the DNA-binding sites of the 3 zinc-finger domains predominantly affecting the codons E356, H384, and D411. *EGR2* mutations are significantly enriched in patients with CLL with aggressive disease and, in particular, treatment-refractory cases [69,70].

About 2% of patients with CLL display heterozygous missense mutations (L116R/P) in the DNA-binding domain of the *IRF4* gene, with the majority also carrying trisomy 12 [71] In CLL, *IKZF3* is affected by a recurrent missense mutation p.L162R substitution that resides in the second zinc finger domain [4].

Recurrent somatic intergenic mutations were identified in genomic regions within chromosome 9p13 and the region was identified as a distant PAX5 transcription regulatory element [31,58]. The *PAX5* mutation was shown to be associated with *MYD88*, *ATM*, *NOTCH1*, *SF3B1*, and *ZMYM3* mutations in CLL [58].

Chromatin modification

CHD2 gene, a chromatin remodeler displays somatic mutations in 5% of CLL and 7% in MBL cases. Most mutations are truncating or target functional domains in turn impacting *CHD2* association with active chromatin, leading to altered nuclear distributions [72].

SETD2 is a histone methyltransferase responsible for the trimethylation of lysine 36 on histone 3 (H3K36me3), an epigenetic marker involved in transcriptional elongation [73]. In human cells, *SETD2* interacts with RNA pol II and plays a role in alternative splicing and DNA repair. *SETD2* loss results in a dysfunctional mitotic spindle and abnormalities in cytokinesis leading to genomic instability [74] secondary to its role in methylation of α-tubulin. Somatic *SETD2* mutations occur in up to 4% of patients with CLL and affect 1 copy with no evidence of inactivation of the other [4,31,75]. In CLL, *SETD2* mutations are identified as early loss-of-function events and are linked to aggressive disease [75].

Other genes encoding proteins involved in the control of chromatin modification, including *ASXL1*, *KMT2D*, *ZMYM3*, *ARID1A*, and *HIST1H1B*, are recurrently mutated at low frequency [4,31].

MicroRNAs

MicroRNAs are a class of small, highly conserved noncoding RNA molecules that act as negative regulators of gene expression by RNA silencing (owing to messenger RNA degradation and/or inhibits messenger RNA translation). In addition to being useful biomarkers, miR profiling in CLL has provided an understanding of disease biology. Many additional studies have followed the pivotal identification of the miR-15a and miR-16-1 cluster being located within a 30-kb deletion between exons 2-5 of the *DLEU2* gene in chromosome 13q14-deletions. In 2005 it was discovered that miR-15/16 function as tumor suppressors by directly targeting *BCL2*, one of the most important oncogenes that inhibits apoptosis [76]. Thus, the main cause for BCL2 overexpression, a hallmark of CLL, is loss of the negative regulators miR15/16. More recently, the US Food and Drug Administration has approved a specific BCL2 inhibitor ABT-199 (venetoclax) for CLL treatment [76]. However, this drug fails to eradicate MRD in most patients. Other studies have found that deletion of miR-15/16 may lead to overexpression of *ROR1*, a receptor for Wnt5a, which may in turn promote cell proliferation, and can be targeted by cirmtuzumab, a humanized anti-ROR1 monoclonal antibody [77]. Thus, combining agents that target different oncogenes may possibly result in an additive effect to more effectively treat patients.

Recently, novel miR-155-5p involved in regulating salient transcription factors such as E2F2, FOXO3333, and HIF1 seems to be a promising independent and unfavorably prognostic molecular biomarker. It has been shown that miR-155 expression progressively increases from normal controls to those with MBL to patients with CLL [78], but its role in overt CLL development is not understood fully.

Subclonal mutations and clonal evolution

CLL displays extremely high interpatient and intrapatient genomic heterogeneity that makes it vulnerable to clonal evolution owing to differing responses to varying stressors such as microenvironment and therapy [79,80]. A temporal ordering of events also exists. Several studies have demonstrated that there is either no clonal evolution or 2 other types of clonal evolution can occur: (1) linear evolution, wherein there is a founder clone with successive new mutations associated with Richter transformation and (2) branched or parallel evolution of multiple clones associated with rapid disease progression and poor prognosis [30,58]. Prior studies [81] showed that convergent mutational evolution (>1 mutation in the same gene) is a common phenomenon in CLL. Studies showed that subclonal driver mutations of *TP53* and *SF3B1* expand over time [29]. Previously unrecognized driver genes *RPS15* and *IKZF3* as well as recurrent *RPS15* mutations occur in relapsed cases [69]. In absence of any intervening therapy, these subclones are typically stable. A recent study [46] of 28 CLL driver genes showed that small subclones are more common than clonal mutations (55% vs 45%). Also, although copy number alterations tend to be stable, gene mutations are continually acquired. The total number of gene alterations or mutational complexity (*SF3B1*, *BRAF*, *ATM*, *NOTCH1*, and *MGA*) gradually shortened TTFT independent of IGHV status and Binet stage. However, decreased OS was associated with increasing subclonal diversity (*FBXW7*, *NOTCH1*, *SF3B1*, and *TP53*) and was not independent of age, IGHV, and *TP53* status.

CLINICAL APPLICATIONS OF GENOMIC BIOMARKERS IN CHRONIC LYMPHOCYTIC LEUKEMIA

Current Status of Genomic Biomarkers in Chronic Lymphocytic Leukemia Treatment Decisions

The treatment for CLL is as heterogeneous as the disease itself and a detailed description is beyond the scope of this review. Briefly, low-risk patients may be kept under observation with no intervention or may be treated based on their comorbidities. The initiation of treatment is generally guided by several characteristics—clinical, hematology, clinical chemistry, and genomic findings (unmutated *IGHV*, specific chromosomal lesions). The poorest outcome CLL patient groups include those carrying a del17p (including *TP53*), del11q, and UM-*IGHV*. Thus, currently, the biomarkers most critical for decision making in CLL are *TP53* gene defects, including chromosomal aberrations of 17p13 (deletions of *TP53* locus) and *TP53* mutations, that are associated with chemoimmunotherapy resistance and poor clinical outcomes. The current 2018 guidelines from National Cancer Center Network and the European Research Initiative on Chronic Lymphocytic Leukemia recommend that *TP53* gene mutation assessments should be performed before the initiation of the first and every subsequent line of treatment [82]. Thus, all patients with de novo CLL, outside clinical trial patients eligible for an allogeneic stem cell transplantation or other intensive therapies, as well as in previously treated patients with wild-type TP53 at the initial diagnosis if further therapy is required fall under this category [65]. By using multivariate analysis in CLL 8 trail, the presence of del17p, *TP53* mutations, and U-CLL was shown to have a negative prognostic impact on PFS and OS [83]. Patients with a mutated IgVH obtained 80% remission to reach minimal residual disease (MRD), whereas those with unmutated IgVH relapsed despite reaching MRD [84].

Newer therapeutic agents that target a specific signaling pathway or molecule are rapidly being adopted into clinical practice. These include ibrutinib (an inhibitor of BTK signaling), idelalisib (a potent and highly selective inhibitor of the phosphatidylinositol 3-kinase [PI3K]), ABT199 (venetoclax, a Bcl-2 inhibitor, which has been approved by the US Food and Drug Administration for relapsed or refractory CLL), gefitinib (a tyrosine kinase inhibitor), fostamatinib (a competitive inhibitor of SYK), selinexor (a selective inhibitor of nuclear export exportin-1 [CRM1/XPO1]), anti-microRNAs, and chimeric antigen receptor T cells. Molecular biomarkers play an important role as therapeutic targets (*SYK*, *XPO1*) or markers of treatment resistance (*BTK*, *PLCG2*).

Diagnostic

Although rarely needed in current practice owing to the availability of flow cytometry, clonal *IGHV* rearrangements may provide clonality assessment in challenging cases to establish the diagnosis. None of the molecular biomarkers have been shown to be specific to CLL; however, specific association of recurrent mutations with clinically significant presentations have been noted. Mutations most commonly associated with unmutated *IGHV* and poor prognosis include *ATM1*, *BIRC3*, *TP53*, *SF3B1*, and *NOTCH1*.

Although the distinction between MBL and CLL is made based primarily on the blood counts, high count MBL ($\geq 0.5 \times 10^9$/L) is similar to low stage CLL (Rai stage 0), but with a greater proportion of *IGHV* mutation and progress to frank CLL requiring therapy at a rate of 1% to 2% per year [85,86]. High count MBL and Rai stage 0 CLL have a similar distribution of *SF3B1* and *NOTCH1* mutations, CD38 and ZAP70 positivity, cytogenetic abnormalities, IGHV family use, and frequency of stereotyped *IGHV* gene sequences. MBL patients had longer PFS possibly a reflection of lower tumor burden rather than biological differences [87]. Thus, high count MBL can potentially be considered with CLL and followed clinically for progression.

Prognostic

The evidence for the prognostic usefulness of individual biomarkers continues to develop, but currently no consensus exists on the list of genes to be included in the prognostic workup for CLL. Fig. 2 shows clinical correlates of molecular biomarkers at different stages of care [55,81].

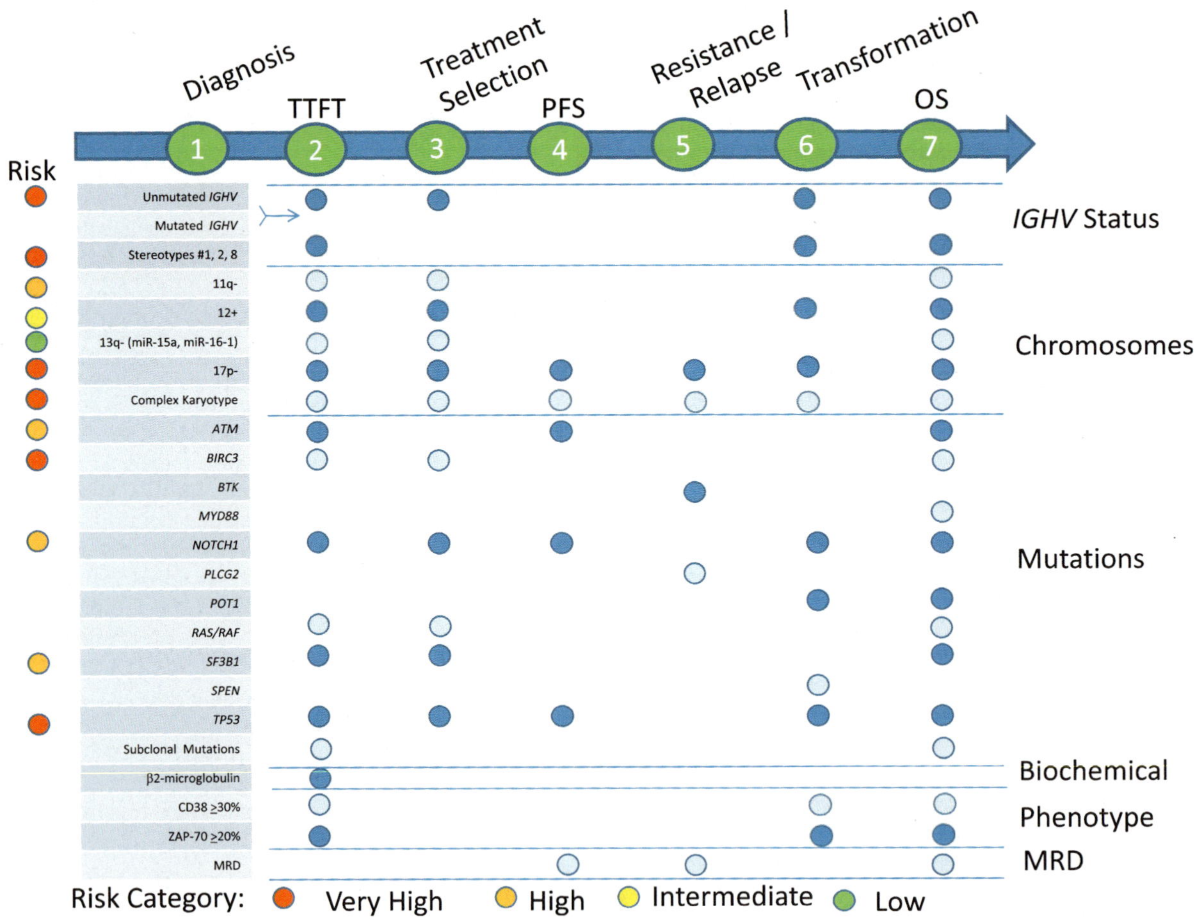

FIG. 2 Clinical usefulness of genomic biomarkers during each stage of clinical care in chronic lymphocytic leukemia (CLL). Genomic biomarkers are represented in alternating light and dark rows with matching circles in columns corresponding to specific clinical end-point. Overall risk category associated with each biomarker is shown using colored circles to the left of each biomarker. OS, overall-survival; PFS, progression-free survival; TTFT, time to first treatment; MRD, minimal residual disease.

Predictive

The association of *TP53* loss with resistance to fludarabine, cyclophosphamide, and rituximab therapy was detailed elsewhere in this article. In comparison, mutations in *BTK* and *PLCG2* are typically noted in patients treated with targeted B-cell receptor signaling inhibitor drugs like ibrutinib (BTK inhibitor) or idelalisib (PI3K delta inhibitor). Mutations in *BTK* can change the binding site of the inhibitor such as C481S [88] or occur in the SH2 domain (T316A) [89]. A gain-of-function mutation activating PLCγ2 may also exist. In addition, *PLCG2* mutations occurring in exon19, exon 20, and exon 24 cause deletion of S707 and A708 [90]. Other potential resistance mechanisms such as del8p can occur with additional mutations [91]. Patients with CLL with acquired ibrutinib resistance displayed subclonal *BTK* and *PLCG2* mutations arising concurrently in different cells or on different alleles [90]. Resistance mechanisms to idelalisib have not yet been fully elucidated.

Venetoclax (a selective inhibitor of BCL2) resistance may be mediated by upregulation of MCL1, BCL-XL, or constitutive activation of AKT [92,93]. More recently, *BTG1* mutations and homozygous deletions of CDKN2A/B were detected as recurrent events during venetoclax relapse [94]. *BTG1* is regulated by BCL2 and seems to be the underlying event. *BRAF* mutations and a high level focal amplification of *CD274* (PD-L1) were also identified, and may offer areas that can be exploited for further therapeutic intervention (vemurafenib and PD-L1 inhibitors).

Progression and Transformation

Both germline and somatic mutations can predispose an individual with CLL to develop RT. Germline mutations conferring modestly increased risk of RT single nucleotide polymorphisms in *CD38*, *LRP4*, and *BCL-2* genes [95]. There seem to be 2 main, mutually exclusive genetic pathways that lead to RS-DLBCL. The first pathway occurring in 50% of cases involves the acquisition of mutations in *TP53* or *CDKN2A*. The oncogene *C-MYC* is activated in a subset of patients with *TP53* aberration. The second pathway noted in 30% of RS cases involves the activation of the *NOTCH1* pathway through somatic mutations, most frequently in patients with trisomy 12. The remaining 20% of patients have heterogeneous genomic aberrations. RS genomic profiling is intermediate between CLL and de novo DLBCL and *CDKN2A* inactivation is the most frequently acquired lesion at the time of transformation [91,96]. Some other molecular features associated with RT include stereotyped B-cell receptor, unmutated *IGHV* status, and del11q; CD38 expression and Zap70 positivity are also considered risk factors [91,97].

Biologically transformed DLBCL can be clonally related, arising from linear evolution of the original clone [98]. This type is the most common, with a very poor prognosis, and it is seen in *IGVH* unmutated cases. However, approximately 20% of the DLBCL-type RS and approximately 50% of Hodgkin lymphoma-type RS have IGHV-DJ rearrangements that differ from that of the original CLL clone. Clonally unrelated DLBCL is more often seen in *IGHV* mutated cases and shows a prognosis identical to de novo DLBCL in the setting of immune dysregulation. Rarely, Epstein-Barr virus–associated large B-cell lymphoma occurs, often after alemtuzumab treatment [99].

The majority of heavily pretreated patients (median number of 3 prior therapies) had high-risk features such as del17p. This finding suggests that aggressive subclones are present before treatment, then most likely emerge under selective pressure of therapy, and that RT is not induced by therapies. In the setting of relapsed/refractory disease, RT is a frequent event in patients receiving novel agents. The incidence of RT was 16% in a phase I study of relapsed/refractory CLL/small lymphocytic lymphoma patients receiving venetoclax [100], whereas it was 5% in previously treated patients receiving ibrutinib. With the use of novel agents in previously treated CLL, transformation occurred within 12 to 18 months of treatment initiation, although the risk of RT subsequently plateaued.

Studies have attempted to identify the mechanisms underlying transformation to RT in ibrutinib-treated patients, but they remain unclear. Several studies [90,101] found *BTK* C481S and *BTK* C481Y mutations, as well as activating mutations in *PLCG2*, in the majority of patients with progressive CLL during ibrutinib therapy, but these mutations were lacking or infrequent in RT. Studies also suggested a branched evolution pattern [96]. The only recurrent new abnormality noted in RT but not in original CLL cells was gain on chromosome 8q. There is no published information on the molecular drivers of RT in idelalisib- or venetoclax-treated patients [102].

Minimal Residual Disease Monitoring

MRD assessment can be done using sensitive multicolor flow cytometry and remains the mainstay for majority of the clinical laboratories. Recently, next-generation sequencing–based approaches for IGH clonality have shown comparable sensitivities, but such assays are not widely available for routine clinical care [2]. In addition, next-generation sequencing–based MRD determination requires a high amount of input DNA and the analysis of multiple replicates to achieve a high degree of sensitivity and specificity.

Familial Chronic Lymphocytic Leukemia

Although CLL is considered a multifactorial disease, genetic susceptibility is a well-established risk factor. About 5% to 10% of patients with CLL display evidence of familial predisposition. First-degree relatives have an increased incidence of MBL as well as an overall increased risk of developing CLL that is 8.5-fold higher [103]. Significant linkage has been noted at the 2q21.2-containing *CXCR4* gene, and rare coding mutations have been identified [104]. About 19% of familial risk of CLL seems to be associated with 32 single nucleotide polymorphisms from 28 loci, including genes such as *BAK1*, *BCL2*, *BCL2L11*, *BMF*, *CASP8/CASP10*, *FAS*, *PMAIP1* (apoptosis), *HLA-DQA1*, *IRF3* (B-cell receptor activation), *POT1*, *TERT*, *TERC* (telomere function), *LEF1*, *IRF8*, *PRKD3*, and *SP140* (transcription factors in B-cell differentiation) [103]. Germline loss of function in shelterin (a telomere specific protein complex) encoded by *POT1*, *ACD*, *TERF2IP*, *TERF1*, *TERF2*, and *TINF2* leads to telomere dysregulation that seems to be strategic in CLL development [68]. Mapping of the 15q15.1 CLL risk locus identified the single nucleotide polymorphism rs539846 located in a *BMF* intron leading to disruption of RELA transcription factor-binding site and reduced expression of BMF [105]. However, there is currently no recommendation to screen for germline mutations in CLL.

Future Directions

The increased use and accessibility of massively parallel DNA and RNA sequencing has further advanced our understanding of genomes and transcriptomes. However, this information does not tell the full story in CLL that is now viewed as a dynamic disease. Genomic studies do not predict posttranslational modifications, which can directly impact protein function. Therefore, to more completely understand its biology, the proteomics of the CLL cells should also be probed and the information analyzed in concert with the genomic and transcriptomic data [106].

Further studies incorporating newer methods/tools such as iTRAQ and SWATH MS with more comprehensive protein databases may enable the development of predictive biomarkers and new targeted therapies to allow patients to receive optimal treatment [106]. Considering the escape mechanisms of tumor cells, the search for new drugs and new potential therapeutic targets should be constant, while considering the specificity and toxicity of each drug.

Genomic studies have identified mutations and deletions in numerous key molecular drivers in CLL, such as *NOTCH1*, *SF3B1*, *BIRC3*, *NF-κB*, and *BCL2* [107]. The development of evidence-based clinical molecular diagnostic tests will be required to translate genomic discoveries into bedside tools that improve patient outcomes. Given the high degree of genomic heterogeneity, test platforms that can interrogate all possible genomic alterations in a cost-effective manner will need to be developed.

REFERENCES

[1] Chronic lymphocytic leukemia. National Cancer Institute, NIH. Bethesda (MD): SEER Cancer Stat Facts; 2018. Available at: https://seer.cancer.gov/statfacts/html/cllsll.html.

[2] Hallek M, Cheson BD, Catovsky D, et al. iwCLL guidelines for diagnosis, indications for treatment, response assessment and supportive management of CLL. Blood 2018;131(25):2745–60.

[3] International CLL-IPI Working Group. An international prognostic index for patients with chronic lymphocytic leukaemia (CLL-IPI): a meta-analysis of individual patient data. Lancet Oncol 2016;17(6):779–90.

[4] Landau DA, Tausch E, Taylor-Weiner AN, et al. Mutations driving CLL and their evolution in progression and relapse. Nature 2015;526(7574):525–30.

[5] Klein U, Dalla-Favera R. New insights into the pathogenesis of chronic lymphocytic leukemia. Semin Cancer Biol 2010;20(6):377–83.

[6] Schaffner C, Stilgenbauer S, Rappold GA, et al. Somatic ATM mutations indicate a pathogenic role of ATM in B-cell chronic lymphocytic leukemia. Blood 1999;94(2):748–53.

[7] Zenz T, Krober A, Scherer K, et al. Monoallelic TP53 inactivation is associated with poor prognosis in chronic lymphocytic leukemia: results from a detailed genetic characterization with long-term follow-up. Blood 2008;112(8):3322–9.

[8] Quesada V, Conde L, Villamor N, et al. Exome sequencing identifies recurrent mutations of the splicing factor SF3B1 gene in chronic lymphocytic leukemia. Nat Genet 2011;44(1):47–52.

[9] Dohner H, Stilgenbauer S, Benner A, et al. Genomic aberrations and survival in chronic lymphocytic leukemia. N Engl J Med 2000;343(26):1910–6.

[10] Ouillette P, Saiya-Cork K, Seymour E, et al. Clonal evolution, genomic drivers, and effects of therapy in chronic lymphocytic leukemia. Clin Cancer Res 2013;19(11):2893–904.

[11] Ibbotson R, Athanasiadou A, Sutton LA, et al. Coexistence of trisomies of chromosomes 12 and 19 in chronic lymphocytic leukemia occurs exclusively in the rare IgG-positive variant. Leukemia 2012;26(1):170–2.

[12] Herling CD, Klaumunzer M, Rocha CK, et al. Complex karyotypes and KRAS and POT1 mutations impact outcome in CLL after chlorambucil-based

chemotherapy or chemoimmunotherapy. Blood 2016; 128(3):395–404.
[13] Puiggros A, Collado R, Calasanz MJ, et al. Patients with chronic lymphocytic leukemia and complex karyotype show an adverse outcome even in absence of TP53/ATM FISH deletions. Oncotarget 2017;8(33): 54297–303.
[14] Jain P, Keating M, Wierda W, et al. Outcomes of patients with chronic lymphocytic leukemia after discontinuing ibrutinib. Blood 2015;125(13):2062–7.
[15] Thompson PA, O'Brien SM, Wierda WG, et al. Complex karyotype is a stronger predictor than del(17p) for an inferior outcome in relapsed or refractory chronic lymphocytic leukemia patients treated with ibrutinib-based regimens. Cancer 2015;121(20):3612–21.
[16] Tam CS, Shanafelt TD, Wierda WG, et al. De novo deletion 17p13.1 chronic lymphocytic leukemia shows significant clinical heterogeneity: the M. D. Anderson and Mayo Clinic experience. Blood 2009;114(5):957–64.
[17] Van Dyke DL, Werner L, Rassenti LZ, et al. The Dohner fluorescence in situ hybridization prognostic classification of chronic lymphocytic leukaemia (CLL): the CLL Research Consortium experience. Br J Haematol 2016; 173(1):105–13.
[18] Fabbri G, Khiabanian H, Holmes AB, et al. Genetic lesions associated with chronic lymphocytic leukemia transformation to Richter syndrome. J Exp Med 2013; 210(11):2273–88.
[19] Chiaretti S, Marinelli M, Del Giudice I, et al. NOTCH1, SF3B1, BIRC3 and TP53 mutations in patients with chronic lymphocytic leukemia undergoing first-line treatment: correlation with biological parameters and response to treatment. Leuk Lymphoma 2014;55(12): 2785–92.
[20] Hamblin TJ, Davis ZA, Oscier DG. Determination of how many immunoglobulin variable region heavy chain mutations are allowable in unmutated chronic lymphocytic leukaemia - long-term follow up of patients with different percentages of mutations. Br J Haematol 2008;140(3):320–3.
[21] Chiorazzi N. Implications of new prognostic markers in chronic lymphocytic leukemia. Hematology Am Soc Hematol Educ Program 2012;2012:76–87.
[22] O'Brien S, Jones JA, Coutre SE, et al. Ibrutinib for patients with relapsed or refractory chronic lymphocytic leukaemia with 17p deletion (RESONATE-17): a phase 2, open-label, multicentre study. Lancet Oncol 2016; 17(10):1409–18.
[23] Burns A, Alsolami R, Becq J, et al. Whole-genome sequencing of chronic lymphocytic leukaemia reveals distinct differences in the mutational landscape between IgHV(mut) and IgHV(unmut) subgroups. Leukemia 2018;32(2):573.
[24] Schweighofer CD, Huh YO, Luthra R, et al. The B cell antigen receptor in atypical chronic lymphocytic leukemia with t(14;19)(q32;q13) demonstrates remarkable stereotypy. Int J Cancer 2011;128(11):2759–64.
[25] Dal-Bo M, Del Giudice I, Bomben R, et al. B-cell receptor, clinical course and prognosis in chronic lymphocytic leukaemia: the growing saga of the IGHV3 subgroup gene usage. Br J Haematol 2011;153(1):3–14.
[26] Gounari M, Ntoufa S, Apollonio B, et al. Excessive antigen reactivity may underlie the clinical aggressiveness of chronic lymphocytic leukemia stereotyped subset #8. Blood 2015;125(23):3580–7.
[27] Stamatopoulos K, Agathangelidis A, Rosenquist R, et al. Antigen receptor stereotypy in chronic lymphocytic leukemia. Leukemia 2017;31(2):282–91.
[28] Puente XS, Pinyol M, Quesada V, et al. Whole-genome sequencing identifies recurrent mutations in chronic lymphocytic leukaemia. Nature 2011;475(7354): 101–5.
[29] Landau DA, Wu CJ. Chronic lymphocytic leukemia: molecular heterogeneity revealed by high-throughput genomics. Genome Med 2013;5(5):47.
[30] Ghamlouch H, Nguyen-Khac F, Bernard OA. Chronic lymphocytic leukaemia genomics and the precision medicine era. Br J Haematol 2017;178(6):852–70.
[31] Puente XS, Bea S, Valdes-Mas R, et al. Non-coding recurrent mutations in chronic lymphocytic leukaemia. Nature 2015;526(7574):519–24.
[32] Rossi D, Bruscaggin A, Spina V, et al. Mutations of the SF3B1 splicing factor in chronic lymphocytic leukemia: association with progression and fludarabine-refractoriness. Blood 2011;118(26):6904–8.
[33] Jeromin S, Weissmann S, Haferlach C, et al. SF3B1 mutations correlated to cytogenetics and mutations in NOTCH1, FBXW7, MYD88, XPO1 and TP53 in 1160 untreated CLL patients. Leukemia 2014;28(1): 108–17.
[34] Cosson A, Chapiro E, Bougacha N, et al. Gain in the short arm of chromosome 2 (2p+) induces gene overexpression and drug resistance in chronic lymphocytic leukemia: analysis of the central role of XPO1. Leukemia 2017;31(7):1625–9.
[35] Montpetit B, Thomsen ND, Helmke KJ, et al. A conserved mechanism of DEAD-box ATPase activation by nucleoporins and InsP6 in mRNA export. Nature 2011;472(7342):238–42.
[36] Ojha J, Secreto CR, Rabe KG, et al. Identification of recurrent truncated DDX3X mutations in chronic lymphocytic leukaemia. Br J Haematol 2015;169(3):445–8.
[37] Zenz T, Mertens D, Kuppers R, et al. From pathogenesis to treatment of chronic lymphocytic leukaemia. Nat Rev Cancer 2010;10(1):37–50.
[38] Rossi D, Cerri M, Deambrogi C, et al. The prognostic value of TP53 mutations in chronic lymphocytic leukemia is independent of Del17p13: implications for overall survival and chemorefractoriness. Clin Cancer Res 2009;15(3):995–1004.
[39] Zenz T, Habe S, Denzel T, et al. Detailed analysis of p53 pathway defects in fludarabine-refractory chronic lymphocytic leukemia (CLL): dissecting the contribution of 17p deletion, TP53 mutation, p53-p21 dysfunction,

and miR34a in a prospective clinical trial. Blood 2009; 114(13):2589–97.

[40] Asslaber D, Pinon JD, Seyfried I, et al. microRNA-34a expression correlates with MDM2 SNP309 polymorphism and treatment-free survival in chronic lymphocytic leukemia. Blood 2010;115(21):4191–7.

[41] Kojima K, Konopleva M, McQueen T, et al. Mdm2 inhibitor Nutlin-3a induces p53-mediated apoptosis by transcription-dependent and transcription-independent mechanisms and may overcome Atm-mediated resistance to fludarabine in chronic lymphocytic leukemia. Blood 2006;108(3):993–1000.

[42] Bixby D, Kujawski L, Wang S, et al. The pre-clinical development of MDM2 inhibitors in chronic lymphocytic leukemia uncovers a central role for p53 status in sensitivity to MDM2 inhibitor-mediated apoptosis. Cell Cycle 2008;7(8):971–9.

[43] Voltan R, Rimondi E, Melloni E, et al. Ibrutinib synergizes with MDM-2 inhibitors in promoting cytotoxicity in B chronic lymphocytic leukemia. Oncotarget 2016; 7(43):70623–38.

[44] Andreeff M, Kelly KR, Yee K, et al. Results of the phase I trial of RG7112, a small-molecule MDM2 antagonist in leukemia. Clin Cancer Res 2016;22(4):868–76.

[45] Skowronska A, Parker A, Ahmed G, et al. Biallelic ATM inactivation significantly reduces survival in patients treated on the United Kingdom Leukemia Research Fund Chronic Lymphocytic Leukemia 4 trial. J Clin Oncol 2012;30(36):4524–32.

[46] Nadeu F, Clot G, Delgado J, et al. Clinical impact of the subclonal architecture and mutational complexity in chronic lymphocytic leukemia. Leukemia 2018;32(3): 645–53.

[47] Knittel G, Liedgens P, Reinhardt HC. Targeting ATM-deficient CLL through interference with DNA repair pathways. Front Genet 2015;6:207.

[48] Kwok M, Davies N, Agathanggelou A, et al. ATR inhibition induces synthetic lethality and overcomes chemoresistance in TP53- or ATM-defective chronic lymphocytic leukemia cells. Blood 2016;127(5):582–95.

[49] Clifford R, Louis T, Robbe P, et al. SAMHD1 is mutated recurrently in chronic lymphocytic leukemia and is involved in response to DNA damage. Blood 2014; 123(7):1021–31.

[50] Schneider C, Oellerich T, Baldauf HM, et al. SAMHD1 is a biomarker for cytarabine response and a therapeutic target in acute myeloid leukemia. Nat Med 2017; 23(2):250–5.

[51] Larrayoz M, Rose-Zerilli MJ, Kadalayil L, et al. Non-coding NOTCH1 mutations in chronic lymphocytic leukemia; their clinical impact in the UK CLL4 trial. Leukemia 2017;31(2):510–4.

[52] Villamor N, Conde L, Martinez-Trillos A, et al. NOTCH1 mutations identify a genetic subgroup of chronic lymphocytic leukemia patients with high risk of transformation and poor outcome. Leukemia 2013; 27(5):1100–6.

[53] Lopez-Guerra M, Xargay-Torrent S, Rosich L, et al. The gamma-secretase inhibitor PF-03084014 combined with fludarabine antagonizes migration, invasion and angiogenesis in NOTCH1-mutated CLL cells. Leukemia 2015;29(1):96–106.

[54] Baldoni S, Del Papa B, Dorillo E, et al. Bepridil exhibits anti-leukemic activity associated with NOTCH1 pathway inhibition in chronic lymphocytic leukemia. Int J Cancer 2018;143(4):958–70.

[55] Guieze R, Wu CJ. Genomic and epigenomic heterogeneity in chronic lymphocytic leukemia. Blood 2015; 126(4):445–53.

[56] Kampjarvi K, Jarvinen TM, Heikkinen T, et al. Somatic MED12 mutations are associated with poor prognosis markers in chronic lymphocytic leukemia. Oncotarget 2015;6(3):1884–8.

[57] Damm F, Mylonas E, Cosson A, et al. Acquired initiating mutations in early hematopoietic cells of CLL patients. Cancer Discov 2014;4(9):1088–101.

[58] Rose-Zerilli MJ, Gibson J, Wang J, et al. Longitudinal copy number, whole exome and targeted deep sequencing of 'good risk' IGHV-mutated CLL patients with progressive disease. Leukemia 2016;30(6):1301–10.

[59] Rossi D, Fangazio M, Rasi S, et al. Disruption of BIRC3 associates with fludarabine chemorefractoriness in TP53 wild-type chronic lymphocytic leukemia. Blood 2012;119(12):2854–62.

[60] Baliakas P, Hadzidimitriou A, Sutton LA, et al. Recurrent mutations refine prognosis in chronic lymphocytic leukemia. Leukemia 2015;29(2):329–36.

[61] Cortese D, Sutton LA, Cahill N, et al. On the way towards a 'CLL prognostic index': focus on TP53, BIRC3, SF3B1, NOTCH1 and MYD88 in a population-based cohort. Leukemia 2014;28(3):710–3.

[62] Xia Y, Fan L, Wang L, et al. Frequencies of SF3B1, NOTCH1, MYD88, BIRC3 and IGHV mutations and TP53 disruptions in Chinese with chronic lymphocytic leukemia: disparities with Europeans. Oncotarget 2015;6(7):5426–34.

[63] Martinez-Trillos A, Pinyol M, Navarro A, et al. Mutations in TLR/MYD88 pathway identify a subset of young chronic lymphocytic leukemia patients with favorable outcome. Blood 2014;123(24):3790–6.

[64] Qin SC, Xia Y, Miao Y, et al. MYD88 mutations predict unfavorable prognosis in chronic lymphocytic leukemia patients with mutated IGHV gene. Blood Cancer J 2017; 7(12):651.

[65] Onaindia A, Medeiros LJ, Patel KP. Clinical utility of recently identified diagnostic, prognostic, and predictive molecular biomarkers in mature B-cell neoplasms. Mod Pathol 2017;30(10):1338–66.

[66] Ramsay AG. Identifying CLL antigens for future combinational therapy. Blood 2013;122(19):3241–2.

[67] Colla S, Ong DS, Ogoti Y, et al. Telomere dysfunction drives aberrant hematopoietic differentiation and myelodysplastic syndrome. Cancer Cell 2015;27(5): 644–57.

[68] Speedy HE, Kinnersley B, Chubb D, et al. Germ line mutations in shelterin complex genes are associated with familial chronic lymphocytic leukemia. Blood 2016;128(19):2319–26.
[69] Ljungstrom V, Cortese D, Young E, et al. Whole-exome sequencing in relapsing chronic lymphocytic leukemia: clinical impact of recurrent RPS15 mutations. Blood 2016;127(8):1007–16.
[70] Young E, Noerenberg D, Mansouri L, et al. EGR2 mutations define a new clinically aggressive subgroup of chronic lymphocytic leukemia. Leukemia 2017;31(7): 1547–54.
[71] Shukla V, Ma S, Hardy RR, et al. A role for IRF4 in the development of CLL. Blood 2013;122(16):2848–55.
[72] Rodriguez D, Bretones G, Quesada V, et al. Mutations in CHD2 cause defective association with active chromatin in chronic lymphocytic leukemia. Blood 2015; 126(2):195–202.
[73] Li J, Duns G, Westers H, et al. SETD2: an epigenetic modifier with tumor suppressor functionality. Oncotarget 2016;7(31):50719–34.
[74] Park IY, Powell RT, Tripathi DN, et al. Dual chromatin and cytoskeletal remodeling by SETD2. Cell 2016; 166(4):950–62.
[75] Parker H, Rose-Zerilli MJ, Larrayoz M, et al. Genomic disruption of the histone methyltransferase SETD2 in chronic lymphocytic leukaemia. Leukemia 2016; 30(11):2179–86.
[76] Pekarsky Y, Balatti V, Croce CM. BCL2 and miR-15/16: from gene discovery to treatment. Cell Death Differ 2018;25(1):21–6.
[77] Rassenti LZ, Balatti V, Ghia EM, et al. MicroRNA dysregulation to identify therapeutic target combinations for chronic lymphocytic leukemia. Proc Natl Acad Sci U S A 2017;114(40):10731–6.
[78] Furtado FM, Scheucher PS, Santana BA, et al. Comparison of microRNA expression in high-count monoclonal B-cell lymphocytosis and Binet A chronic lymphocytic leukemia. Rev Bras Hematol Hemoter 2017;39(3):237–43.
[79] Malcikova J, Stano-Kozubik K, Tichy B, et al. Detailed analysis of therapy-driven clonal evolution of TP53 mutations in chronic lymphocytic leukemia. Leukemia 2015;29(4):877–85.
[80] Rossi D, Gaidano G. Lymphocytosis and ibrutinib treatment of CLL. Blood 2014;123(12):1772–4.
[81] Jethwa A, Hullein J, Stolz T, et al. Targeted resequencing for analysis of clonal composition of recurrent gene mutations in chronic lymphocytic leukaemia. Br J Haematol 2013;163(4):496–500.
[82] Pospisilova S, Gonzalez D, Malcikova J, et al. ERIC recommendations on TP53 mutation analysis in chronic lymphocytic leukemia. Leukemia 2012;26(7):1458–61.
[83] Fischer K, Bahlo J, Fink AM, et al. Long-term remissions after FCR chemoimmunotherapy in previously untreated patients with CLL: updated results of the CLL8 trial. Blood 2016;127(2):208–15.
[84] Thompson PA, Wierda WG. Eliminating minimal residual disease as a therapeutic end point: working toward cure for patients with CLL. Blood 2016;127(3): 279–86.
[85] Rawstron AC, Shingles J, de Tute R, et al. Chronic lymphocytic leukaemia (CLL) and CLL-type monoclonal B-cell lymphocytosis (MBL) show differential expression of molecules involved in lymphoid tissue homing. Cytometry B Clin Cytom 2010;78(Suppl 1):S42–6.
[86] Vardi A, Dagklis A, Scarfo L, et al. Immunogenetics shows that not all MBL are equal: the larger the clone, the more similar to CLL. Blood 2013;121(22):4521–8.
[87] Morabito F, Cutrona G, Gentile M, et al. Prognostic relevance of in vitro response to cell stimulation via surface IgD in Binet stage a CLL. Br J Haematol 2010; 149(1):160–3.
[88] Woyach JA, Bojnik E, Ruppert AS, et al. Bruton's tyrosine kinase (BTK) function is important to the development and expansion of chronic lymphocytic leukemia (CLL). Blood 2014;123(8):1207–13.
[89] Sharma S, Galanina N, Guo A, et al. Identification of a structurally novel BTK mutation that drives ibrutinib resistance in CLL. Oncotarget 2016;7(42):68833–41.
[90] Ahn IE, Underbayev C, Albitar A, et al. Clonal evolution leading to ibrutinib resistance in chronic lymphocytic leukemia. Blood 2017;129(11):1469–79.
[91] Burger JA, Landau DA, Taylor-Weiner A, et al. Clonal evolution in patients with chronic lymphocytic leukaemia developing resistance to BTK inhibition. Nat Commun 2016;7:11589.
[92] Choudhary GS, Al-Harbi S, Mazumder S, et al. MCL-1 and BCL-xL-dependent resistance to the BCL-2 inhibitor ABT-199 can be overcome by preventing PI3K/AKT/ mTOR activation in lymphoid malignancies. Cell Death Dis 2015;6:e1593.
[93] Oppermann S, Ylanko J, Shi Y, et al. High-content screening identifies kinase inhibitors that overcome venetoclax resistance in activated CLL cells. Blood 2016;128(7):934–47.
[94] Herling CD, Abedpour N, Weiss J, et al. Clonal dynamics towards the development of venetoclax resistance in chronic lymphocytic leukemia. Nat Commun 2018;9(1):727.
[95] Parikh SA, Shanafelt TD. Risk factors for Richter syndrome in chronic lymphocytic leukemia. Curr Hematol Malig Rep 2014;9(3):294–9.
[96] Chigrinova E, Rinaldi A, Kwee I, et al. Two main genetic pathways lead to the transformation of chronic lymphocytic leukemia to Richter syndrome. Blood 2013; 122(15):2673–82.
[97] Parikh SA, Rabe KG, Call TG, et al. Diffuse large B-cell lymphoma (Richter syndrome) in patients with chronic lymphocytic leukaemia (CLL): a cohort study of newly diagnosed patients. Br J Haematol 2013;162(6): 774–82.
[98] Rossi D. Venetoclax: a new weapon to treat high-risk CLL. Lancet Oncol 2016;17(6):690–1.

[99] Lepretre S, Aurran T, Mahe B, et al. Excess mortality after treatment with fludarabine and cyclophosphamide in combination with alemtuzumab in previously untreated patients with chronic lymphocytic leukemia in a randomized phase 3 trial. Blood 2012;119(22):5104–10.

[100] Roberts AW, Davids MS, Pagel JM, et al. Targeting BCL2 with venetoclax in relapsed chronic lymphocytic leukemia. N Engl J Med 2016;374(4):311–22.

[101] Kadri S, Lee J, Fitzpatrick C, et al. Clonal evolution underlying leukemia progression and Richter transformation in patients with ibrutinib-relapsed CLL. Blood Adv 2017;1(12):715–27.

[102] Khan M, Siddiqi R, Thompson PA. Approach to Richter transformation of chronic lymphocytic leukemia in the era of novel therapies. Ann Hematol 2018;97(1):1–15.

[103] Cerhan JR, Slager SL. Familial predisposition and genetic risk factors for lymphoma. Blood 2015;126(20):2265–73.

[104] Crowther-Swanepoel D, Qureshi M, Dyer MJ, et al. Genetic variation in CXCR4 and risk of chronic lymphocytic leukemia. Blood 2009;114(23):4843–6.

[105] Kandaswamy R, Sava GP, Speedy HE, et al. Genetic predisposition to chronic lymphocytic leukemia is mediated by a BMF super-enhancer polymorphism. Cell Rep 2016;16(8):2061–7.

[106] Thurgood LA, Chataway TK, Lower KM, et al. From genome to proteome: looking beyond DNA and RNA in chronic lymphocytic leukemia. J Proteomics 2017;155:73–84.

[107] Alsagaby SA, Brennan P, Pepper C. Key molecular drivers of chronic lymphocytic leukemia. Clin Lymphoma Myeloma Leuk 2016;16(11):593–606.

Infectious Disease

Advances in Molecular Pathology 1 (2018) 65–80
ADVANCES IN MOLECULAR PATHOLOGY

Molecular Monitoring of Viral Infections

Esther Babady, PhD[a,b,*]
[a]Clinical Microbiology Service, Department of Laboratory Medicine, Memorial Sloan Kettering Cancer Center, 327 East 64th Street CLM 522, New York, NY 10065, USA; [b]Infectious Disease Service, Department of Medicine, Memorial Sloan Kettering Cancer Center, 327 East 64th Street CLM 522, New York, NY 10065, USA

KEYWORDS
• Viral load • Nucleic acids amplification test
• Solid-organ transplant (SOT) and hematopoietic stem cell transplant (HSCT) • Standardization • International units

KEY POINTS
- Viral load monitoring is accomplished using nucleic acid amplification tests.
- Recommendations for viral load monitoring vary with viruses and patient population.
- Standardization of viral load assays impact the establishment of threshold for clinical management.

INTRODUCTION

Viral infections are responsible for significant mortality and morbidity in transplant patients including solid organ transplantation (SOT) and hematopoietic stem cell transplant (HSCT) recipients. Molecular tests are well-established for the rapid diagnosis of viral infections and are now considered the gold standard for both diagnosis and monitoring. The first molecular tests introduced in clinical virology were cumbersome and required a high level of expertise to design and perform and, hence, were limited largely to references laboratories. Today, several commercial options are available, from research use only (RUO) kits and analyte-specific reagents (ASR) that facilitate the development of laboratory-developed tests (LDT) to assays cleared by the US Food and Drug Administration (FDA) for diagnosing and monitoring viral infections in various transplant populations.

The first available in vitro diagnostic nucleic acids amplification tests (NAT) targeted the detection and monitoring of bloodborne viral pathogens including human immunodeficiency virus (HIV), hepatitis B virus (HBV), and hepatitis C virus (HCV). These NATs have significantly evolved since their introduction on the market, with increased analytical sensitivity, improved and simplified workflows, and decreased costs. Furthermore, all commercial assays for bloodborne viral pathogens are calibrated to the World Health Organization (WHO) international standards, making comparison across laboratories seamless. This is not necessarily the case for double-stranded DNA viruses of significance to transplant patients including cytomegalovirus (CMV), Epstein-Barr virus (EBV), BK polyoma virus (BKV), and adenoviruses (ADV), where in vitro diagnostic tests are lacking, or have only been recently introduced, and standardization remains a challenge.

This article provides an update on the use of molecular tests for the monitoring of bloodborne viral

Disclosure: This work was supported in part through the National Institute of Heath/National Cancer Institute Cancer Center Support [Grant P30 CA008748].

*Clinical Microbiology Service, Department of Laboratory Medicine, Memorial Sloan Kettering Cancer Center, 327 East 64th Street CLM 522, New York, NY 10044. *E-mail address:* babadyn@mskcc.org

https://doi.org/10.1016/j.yamp.2018.06.006
2589-4080/18/

pathogens (HIV, HBV, and HCV), herpesviruses (CMV and EBV), BKV, and ADV.

BLOODBORNE VIRAL PATHOGENS

Human Immunodeficiency Virus

HIV is an enveloped, positive sense, single-stranded RNA *Lentivirus* in the *Retroviridae* family. HIV-1, the most common HIV species, is found worldwide and is divided into 4 groups (M, N, O, and P), 9 subtypes (A–D, F–H, J, and K), and an increasing number of circulating recombinant forms [1]. In the Western hemisphere, including Europe and North America, HIV-1, group M, subtype B, is the most common species, whereas HIV-1, subtype C, predominates in Africa and South-East Asia [1,2]. HIV-2 is restricted to West Africa and is divided into 9 groups, with 2 circulating groups (A and B), 7 noncirculating groups (E–I), and a few subtypes and circulating recombinant forms [3].

The diversity of HIV sequences has a significant impact on the design and interpretation of molecular assays for viral load measurements. Most commercial assays are designed to target only HIV-1 with an emphasis on group M. The HIV genome is a 9.7-kb segmented genome containing 9 to 10 proteins encoded primarily by 3 genes that are used as target for monitoring and resistance testing molecular assays: the *gag* core gene, encoding the p24 capsid protein, the p12 protease, and the p66/p51 reverse transcriptase; the *pol* gene encoding the integrase proteins; and the *env* gene encoding the envelope proteins, gp 120 and gp 41 [1].

HIV is transmitted through several routes with sexual transmission being the most common. Other less common routes of transmission include percutaneous transmission through sharing of infected needles, perinatal transmission from infected mother to child, and through transfusion and organ transplantation, with the latter 2 routes occurring rarely given the current screening regulations for blood and organ donor screening [1].

Laboratory diagnosis of HIV infection has significantly improved in the last few years owing in part to the increased sensitivity of both immunoassays and nucleic acids amplifications tests. The most recent testing recommendations from the Centers for Diseases Control and Prevention (CDC) and the Association of Public Health Laboratories (APHL) were issued in 2014 and aimed at more accurately identifying cases of acute HIV. The CDC/APHL recommendations start with screening using fourth-generation immunoassays, which detect both the p24 antigen and HIV-1/2 IgM and IgG antibodies, a combination that shortens the diagnosis of acute HIV by 5 days when compared with previous, third-generation immunoassays. A reactive screening assay is followed up by a supplemental serologic test to distinguish between HIV-1 antibody, HIV-2 antibody, and p24 antigen. If the supplemental test is negative or indeterminate, further testing using a qualitative NAT test (Aptima HIV-1 RNA; Aptima, Inc, Woburn, MA) is performed. The CDC/APHL algorithm has been widely adopted across laboratories, with 0.1% of laboratories using the algorithm in 2011 compared with 64% in 2015, resulting in a significant increase in the percentage of diagnosed patients linked to care within 30 days of the HIV diagnosis [4].

Once an HIV diagnosis has been established, additional testing including measurement of the CD4 T-cell counts and baseline HIV viral loads is performed. Several FDA-cleared quantitative HIV NATs are commercially available to measure HIV-1 viral loads and are generally optimized for group M subtypes (Table 1). The lower limit of detection (LOD) and the lower limit of quantification (LLOQ) of these assays range between 20 and 175 copies/mL. The newer, real-time reverse transcriptase polymerase chain reaction (RT-PCR) assays have a lower analytical sensitivity and simpler, automated extraction and amplification workflows that have significantly decrease the labor and turnaround time to results. Several studies have compared the performance characteristics of several of the newer HIV-1 viral loads, showing an overall high correlation between various methods, but with some differences observed at the threshold that may be important for clinical decisions [5–10].

Given the importance of viral monitoring in establishing successful response to antiretroviral therapy, comparison of viral load assays focuses primarily on the performance at the lower end of the analytical range. Virologic blips (isolated' detectable HIV RNA level that is followed by a return to virologic suppression) and low-level viremia (detectable HIV RNA of <200 copies/mL) may be early indicators of virologic failure (the inability to achieve or maintain suppression of viral replication to an HIV RNA level of <200 copies/mL) [11]. Amendola and colleagues [10] compared the performance of the Abbott RealTime HIV-1 (Abbott, Abbott Park, IL) with the Roche CAP/CT HIV-1 v.2.0 (Roche Diagnostics, Indianapolis, IN) on residual clinical plasma samples with viral loads of less than 1000 copies/mL and National Institute and Biological Standards and Control (NIBSC) HIV-1 RNA reagent diluted to a concentration of less than 1000

TABLE 1
Select FDA-Cleared Molecular Monitoring Tests

Manufacturer	Test Name	Method	Sample Type	Linear Range	Indication
Abbott Molecular	Real*time* CMV	PCR	Plasma	50–1.56 × 10^8 IU/mL	HSCT
	Real*time* HBV	PCR	Plasma/serum	1.0 × 10^1-1.0 × 10^9 IU/mL 1.5 × 10^1-1.0 × 10^9 IU/mL	Chronic HBV
	Real*time* HCV	RT-PCR	Plasma/serum	1.2 × 10^1-1.0 × 10^8 IU/mL	HCV infection
	Real*time* HIV-1	RT-PCR	Plasma	4.0 × 10^1-1.0 × 10^7 cp/mL	HIV infection
Hologic Inc.	Aptima HBV Quant Dx	TMA	Plasma/serum	1.0 × 10^1-1.0 × 10^9 IU/mL	Chronic HBV
	Aptima HCV Quant Dx	TMA	Plasma/serum	1.0 × 10^1-1.0 × 10^8 IU/mL	HCV infection
	Aptima HIV Quant Dx	TMA	Plasma	3.0 × 10^1-1.0 × 10^7 cp/mL	HIV infection
Qiagen, Inc.	ARTUS CMV RGQ MDX KIT	PCR	Plasma	1.59 × 10^2-7.94 × 10^7 IU/mL	SOT
Roche Molecular	Cobas CMV	PCR	Plasma	1.5 × 10^1-1.0 × 10^8 IU/mL	SOT HSCT
	CAP/CTM quantitative CMV, v2.0.	PCR	Plasma	1.37 × 10^2-9.1 × 10^6 IU/mL	SOT
	Cobas HBV	PCR	Plasma/serum	1.0 × 10^1-1.0 × 10^9 IU/mL	Chronic HBV
	CAP/CTM quantitative HBV, v2.0.	PCR	Plasma/serum	2.0 × 10^1-1.7 × 10^7 IU/mL	Chronic HBV
	COBAS TaqMan HBV Test For Use With The High Pure System	PCR	Plasma/serum	2.9 × 10^1-1.1 × 10^8 IU/mL	Chronic HBV
	CAP/CTM quantitative HCV v.2.0	RT-PCR	Plasma/serum	1.5 × 10^1-1.0 × 10^8 IU/mL	HCV infection
	Cobas HCV	RT-PCR	Plasma/serum	1.5 × 10^1-1.0 × 10^8 IU/mL	HCV infection
	COBAS TaqMan HCV Test For Use With The High Pure System	RT-PCR	Plasma/serum	2.5 × 10^1- 3.0 × 10^8 IU/mL	HCV infection
	CAP/CTM quantitative HIV-1 v.2.0	RT-PCR	Plasma	2.0 × 10^1 – 1.0 × 10^7 cp/mL	HIV infection
	Cobas HIV	RT-PCR	Plasma Serum	2.0 × 10^1 – 1.0 × 10^7 cp/mL 6.0 × 10^1 – 1.0 × 10^7 cp/mL	HIV infection
Siemens	VERSANT HCV 3.0	bDNA	Plasma/serum	6.15 × 10^2-7.69 × 10^6 IU/mL	HCV infection

Abbreviations: bDNA, branched DNA signal amplification; CAP/CTM, cobas ampliprep/cobas TaqMan; CMV, cytomegalovirus; cp: copies; HBV, hepatitis B virus; HCV, hepatitis C virus; HIV, human immunodeficiency virus; HSCT, hematopoietic stem cell transplant; PCR, polymerase chain reaction; RT-PCR, reverse transcriptase PCR; SOT, solid organ transplant; TMA, transcription-mediated amplification.

copies/mL. The investigators showed that, although the qualitative agreement between the 2 methods were substantial (κ = 0.762), the quantitative agreement was low, with a mean difference between the 2 methods of 0.193 log copies/mL, and the Roche assay being more sensitivity while the Abbott assay being more accurate. Discrepant viral loads were similarly observed in approximately 14% of samples tested in a study that compared the bioMérieux NucliSENS EasyQ HIV-1 v2.0 (bioMérieux, Marcy-l'Étoile, France) versus the Roche Cobas CAP/CTM v2.0 and Abbott RealTime HIV-1 assays [8]. A comparison of the new Hologic Aptima (Hologic, Marlborough, MA) with the CAP/CTM and Abbott RealTime showed that on average, the HIV-1 viral loads measured by Aptima were higher than those measured by the Roche CAP/CTM and the Abbott RealTime tests by 0.21 and 0.30 log, respectively, and that the Aptima test had a higher sensitivity, with the potential to detect more positive samples near the LOD of the assay [9]. Therefore, although HIV viral loads measured between various in vitro diagnostic platforms correlate well, the monitoring of patients on antiretroviral therapy should preferably be done using a single assay.

Hepatitis C Virus

HCV is a single-stranded, positive-sense, linear RNA virus belonging to the *Flaviviridae* family and the sole member of the *Hepacivirus* genus. Its genome is approximately 9.6 kb in length, encoding structural proteins (a core protein, transmembrane protein, and 2 glycoproteins), nonstructural proteins (NS2, NS3, NS4A, NS4B, NS5A, and NS5B) and flanked by 5′ and 3′ untranslated regions. HCV is divided into 7 major genotypes and more than 80 subtypes, with genotypes having less than 60% sequence identity in the overall genome, and subtypes having more than 75% to 85% identity in their core/E1 and NS5B sequences [12,13]. The frequency of HCV genotypes varies with geographic locations with the following distribution: genotypes 1 and 3 worldwide; genotype 1 in Western countries; genotype 2 in North Africa, Mediterranean countries, and the Far East; genotype 3 in Europe; genotype 4 in the Middle East; and genotype 5 in South Africa and genotype 6 in Asia [14]. In the United States, genotype 1 is the most frequently recovered HCV genotype (75.4%), followed by genotype 2 (12.6%) and genotype 3 (10.2%) [15]. Information on HCV genotype and subtype is essential for clinical management and treatment strategies, particularly since the introduction of new therapies including direct-acting antiviral agents (DAA) [16].

HCV is responsible for more than 177.5 million infections worldwide [14]. In the United States, an increase in the number of acute HCV infections has been observed over the last several years (an average of 16,500 new cases in 2011 compared with an average of 39,000 new cases in 2015) with an estimated 2.7 to 3.9 million cases of chronic HCV [17]. HCV infection is acquired by contact with infected blood, tissues, organs, and needles; through sexual intercourse; and perinatally during child delivery. Acute HCV hepatitis may be asymptomatic or may produce nonspecific symptoms such as malaise, nausea, dark urine, and jaundice. The incubation period varies between 0 and 6 months and infection may resolve without any treatment. If not cleared, infection progresses to chronic HCV in 50% to 85% of acute hepatitis cases and without management can cause hepatic fibrosis, cirrhosis, end-stage liver diseases, and hepatocellular carcinoma [18].

The diagnosis of HCV infections include serology to detect total HCV antibodies and molecular methods to detect HCV RNA [19]. Screening immunoassays have high sensitivity. However, in low prevalence populations, specificity may only be moderate and, as such, confirmation of positive results is required. The current CDC algorithm for diagnosis of HCV recommends confirmation using a qualitative HCV RNA NAT.

Quantitative NAT for HCV are used for monitoring treatment response. Most quantitative HCV NATs target the NS regions of HCV with linear ranges varying between 12 IU/mL and 10^9 IU/mL (see Table 1). Monitoring of HCV viral loads is recommended at baseline, after 4 weeks of treatment, and 12 weeks after completion of treatment. In addition, viral loads may be measured at the end of treatment and 24 weeks or longer after completion of treatment. Measurement of viral loads at 6 weeks is recommended if HCV RNA is detectable at week 4 and treatment should be discontinued if viral load increases by greater than 10-fold (>1 $\log_{10}$ IU/mL) on repeat testing [20]. Patients treated with standard treatment regimen of pegylated interferon alpha and ribavirin achieved a sustained virologic response (SVR) in 55% to 60% of cases, whereas new treatment regimens, including DAA drugs such as protease inhibitors (eg, telaprevir and boceprevir) or polymerase inhibitors (eg, lediprivir) have the potential to cure HCV with reported SVR of 80% or greater and a decrease in mortality and morbidity. However, these new treatment regimens are currently targeted primarily at HCV genotype 1 [21].

Several commercial methods are available for HCV quantitation (see Table 1). The most recently approved test is the Aptima HCV Quant Dx assay. This method is based on transcription-mediated amplification and performed on both plasma and serum samples. Nucleic acid extraction, amplification, detection, and quantitation are automated on the Panther system (Hologic). The Aptima HCV assay is validated for genotypes 1 to 6 with the LLOQ of 10 IU/mL and LOD of 3.9 IU/mL for plasma and 3.4 IU/mL for serum. Of note, the LOD of the assay is lowest for genotype 5 in serum (2.1 IU/mL) and lowest for genotype 4 (2.3 IU/mL) in plasma.

Other FDA-cleared quantitative HCV NAT are based on real-time RT-PCRs (see Table 1). The Cobas HCV is performed on both plasma and serum samples with automated nucleic acids extraction, detection, and quantitation performed on the new Cobas 6800 System and Cobas 8800 System. The assay uses dual probes to detect amplified RNA and a non-HCV armored RNA quantitation standard in each sample that serves both as an internal control and a quantification standard. Genotypes 1 to 6 are detected and quantified with an overall LLOQ of 15 IU/mL and a LOD of 12 IU/mL in plasma and 13.7 IU/mL in serum samples depending on the platform used. The CAP/CTM HCV test has similar chemistry to the Cobas HCV test, but is performed on the Cobas AmpliPrep and Cobas TaqMan 48. The overall LLOQ of the CAP/CTM HCV v.2 assay is 15 IU/mL, lower than the first version of the assay which had an LLOQ of 43 IU/mL, a value that was not adequate for monitoring SVR for patients on therapy [22].

The Abbott RealTime HCV assay also uses real-time RT-PCR to amplify HCV RNA from genotypes 1 to 6 and integrates nucleic acids extraction and amplification on the Abbott m2000sp and m2000rt and is performed on both serum or plasma samples. Fluorescent probes are used to detect the amplified complementary DNA and the cycle threshold value for each sample is converted into a concentration using a stored calibration curve generated using 2 levels of calibrators (3.00 and 7.00 log IU/mL). The overall LLOQ is 12 IU/mL and a LOD of 10.5 IU/mL in plasma and 7.2 IU/mL in serum samples.

One important characteristic of quantitative HCV NAT used for monitoring of HCV infection is the LLOQ, because the establishment of SVR or cure depends on a laboratory report of "undetectable" HCV RNA. Therefore, an adequate HCV quantitative assay should have an LLOQ of at least 25 IU/mL with a LOD of 15 IU/mL. Several studies have been published that compares that performance characteristics of quantitative HCV RNA tests with overall conclusions that the viral load obtained using the various FDA-approved assays were comparable, meaning that they were mostly within $\pm 0.5\ \log_{10}$ IU/mL [5,23,24]. Differences in viral loads are particularly pronounced at the lower end of the linear ranges. In one study, the overall agreement for samples with viral loads 25 IU/mL or less was 89% between the Aptima and Roche CAP/CTM HCV assay [23], whereas another study reported lower viral load values at the lower end of the linear range on the Cobas 6800 compared with the CAP/CTM and Abbott HCV assays, particularly compared with the Abbott HCV tests [5]. In another study, the viral loads obtained by the Abbott HCV were significantly lower than those obtained by the CAP/CTM for values between 25 and 3500 IU/mL [24]. Therefore, although results correlate well over the linear range of FDA-cleared methods, the monitoring of patients should ideally be done using a single assay.

Hepatitis B Virus

HBV is a small, circular, and partially double-stranded DNA virus from the *Hepadnaviridae* family, in the *Orthohepadnavirus* genus. Up to 10 HBV genotypes (genotypes A–H, I, and J) and more than 30 subtypes have been described to date. HBV genotypes differ by greater than 8% in their genome sequences and the subtypes differ by 4% to 8% [25]. HBV has a worldwide distribution with genotypes showing great geographic variation. The 2 new genotypes, I and J, were identified in Vietnam/Laos and in the Ryukyu Islands, respectively [25]. In the United States, genotypes A, B, and C are the most prevalent with reported rates of 35%, 22%, and 31%, respectively [26].

Approximately 257 million people are infected with HBV worldwide and in 2015,887,000 people died from complications of HBV [27]. In high prevalence regions (ie, >8% hepatitis B surface antigen prevalence), transmission of HBV most often occurs perinatally, from infected mothers to babies during delivery. In low endemicity regions, transmission occurs primarily through percutaneous and sexual routes or from close contacts [28]. In 2015, approximately 3300 cases of acute hepatitis B and 14,400 case of chronic HBV cases were identified in the United States [17]. For most infected patients, acute HBV infection is self-limited and does not progress to chronic HBV. Only a small group of patients develops chronic HBV, with the host immune state and the age of exposure to the virus being identified as risk factors [28,29]. Complications of chronic HBV infections include liver cirrhosis and hepatocellular carcinomas, which carry high morbidity and mortality rates [30].

The incubation period after exposure to HBV ranges from 6 weeks to 6 months. While immunoassays are used for screening and diagnosis of acute and chronic HBV infections, quantitative HBV DNA NATs are essential for the management of chronic HBV being used for to establish pretreatment baseline and to monitor response to treatment [31]. Patients with viral loads of at least 2,000 IU/mL (if hepatitis B e antigen is negative) or 20,000 IU/mL (if hepatitis B e antigen is positive) and elevated liver enzymes qualify for antiviral treatment [29].

There are currently several FDA-cleared quantitative molecular tests for HBV (see Table 1). HBV quantitative NAT are run on the same platforms used for both HIV and HCV quantitative NAT. The most recently approved test is the Aptima HBV Quant Dx assay (Hologic) and is performed on both plasma and serum samples. The Aptima HBV assay is validated for genotypes A to H with the LLOQ of 10 IU/mL and a LOD of 4.8 IU/mL for plasma and 5.9 IU/mL for serum. The LOD of the assay is lowest for genotype B in serum (3.9 IU/mL) and lowest for genotype G (2.8 IU/mL) in plasma.

Other FDA-cleared quantitative HBV NAT are based on real-time RT-PCRs and include 3 Roche tests—the Cobas HBV, the CAP/CTM HBV test v.2, and the CTM HBV test—and 1 Abbott test—the RealTime HBV test (see Table 1). The assay principle is the same for all 3 tests. The CTM HBV test was the first molecular assay available for monitoring of HBV DNA in both serum and plasma samples. The assay is semiautomated, requiring a manual extraction with the High Pure Viral Nucleic Acid kits before amplification on the COBAS TaqMan 48. The manual extraction is a disadvantage of this method and many laboratories using this method modified it to include an automated extraction step. The CTM HBV test has a LLOQ of 29 IU/mL with an LOD of 10 IU/mL. The Cobas HBV is the newest Roche product with automated nucleic acids extraction, detection, and quantitation performed on the Cobas 6800 System and Cobas 8800 System. The assay is approved for testing of both plasma and serum samples. A single probe is used to detect amplified HBV DNA for genotypes A to H. A DNA quantitation standard is added to each sample and serves both as an internal control and a quantification standard. The overall LLOQ is 10 IU/mL with a LOD of 6.6 IU/mL in plasma and 3.5 IU/mL in serum samples. The overall LLOQ of the CAP/CTM HCV v.2 assay is 20 IU/mL and the assay similarly detects HBV genotypes A to H. Thus, the newer Roche tests have increased sensitivity and wider quantification range compared to the CTM HBV.

The Abbott RealTime HBV assay amplifies the surface gene of HBV genotypes A to H from both plasma and serum samples. The cycle threshold value for each sample is converted into a concentration using a stored calibration curve generated using 2 levels of calibrators (3.00 and 7.00 log IU/mL). The overall LLOQ and LOD vary depending on the input volume (0.5 mL vs 0.2 mL) and range from 10 to 15 IU/mL for LLOQ and 6.4 to 10.66 IU/mL for LOD.

One recent multicenter, international study compared the performance characteristics of the 4 generations of HBV Roche quantitative assays, the Cobas 6800/8800 HBV, the CAP/CTM HBV v2.0, the CTM HBV, and the Cobas 4800 HBV test (not available in the United States) [32]. The evaluation was performed using the 7-member WHO HBV standard panels for LOD and linear range comparisons and clinical samples for accuracy studies, with a focus around the clinical decision points of 2,000 to 20,000 copies/mL. The authors showed high concordance, ranging from 91.7% to 96.3% across all paired comparisons for the range of concentration tested including the 2,000 IU/mL threshold. However, they did observe greater variability (59.6%–78.9%) when analyzing a subset of samples closer to the 2000 IU/mL threshold, highlighting that, although the assays had high commutability, careful interpretation of assay results at that threshold is necessary when testing is performed using different platforms.

Yeh and colleagues [33] compared the Abbott RealTime HBV assay with the Roche CAP/CTM HBV DNA using 220 HBV serum samples. The correlation between the 2 assays was excellent (R^2 = 0.961) with a mean difference between viral loads of 0.31 $\log_{10}$ IU/mL, well within the 0.5 $\log_{10}$ IU/mL difference considered significant. Correlation at low level viremia (<3 $\log_{10}$ IU/mL) was lower with differences of greater than 1 $\log_{10}$ IU/mL observed. Using the CAP/CTM HBV DNA as the reference method, the sensitivity and specificity of the Abbott RealTime HBV was 98.2% and 100%, respectively.

The new Aptima HBV Dx was evaluated against the CAP/CTM HBV test v2.0 and the Abbott Realtime HBV on plasma samples from untreated patients infected with HBV genotypes A through F [34]. The performance of the 3 methods was comparable, although the HBV DNA viral loads were slightly lower for the Aptima HBV compared with both the CAP/CTM HBV and Abbott Realtime HBV for all genotypes. All differences were lower than 0.5 $\log_{10}$ IU/mL, except for genotype F, where the difference in viral loads between the 2 specimens tested was 0.84 log IU/mL between the Aptima HBV and the CAP/CTM HBV.

DOUBLE-STRANDED DNA VIRUSES

Human Cytomegalovirus

Human CMV belongs to the *Herpesviridae* family in the *Betaherpesvirinae* subfamily. CMV is a double-stranded DNA virus with a genome size of approximately 240 kb and over 200 open reading frames, encoding approximately 164 proteins [35]. CMV is one of the most common infections worldwide, with an estimated age-adjusted seroprevalence of 50.4% in the United States [36]. CMV is transmitted through several routes including vertical transmission from mother to child in utero or perinatally at birth, horizontal transmission through close contact with infected body fluids and through blood transfusion or organ transplantations. CMV has wide cell tropism resulting in a range of syndromes from asymptomatic infections to severe meningitis. Like other herpesviruses, CMV establishes lifelong latency in various cells after primary infections and can reactivate after immune trauma, such as inflammation or immunosuppression [37].

CMV infection (the presence of detectable CMV DNA/RNA or antigens without clinical symptoms) and CMV disease (CMV infections with clinical symptoms) are significant causes of morbidity and mortality in SOT and HSCT recipients [38,39]. Results of donor (D) and recipient (R) CMV serologies play a significant role in assessing risk of developing CMV infection or CMV disease after transplantation [40,41]. The lowest risk of infection is seen in donor/recipient negative (D^-/R^-) pair while the highest risk of infections is seen for donor positive/recipient negative (D^+/R^-) pair [41,42]. Factors associated with increased risk of infections include the type of organ transplanted and the type and degree of immunosuppression.

In addition to predicting risk for CMV infection or disease after transplantation, the donor and recipient CMV serostatus are used to establish the frequency of viral load monitoring [41]. Current management strategies to prevent CMV infection or disease in transplant patients include 2 approaches: antiviral prophylaxis and preemptive therapy. With antiviral prophylaxis, low-dose antiviral drugs (eg, acyclovir, ganciclovir) are administered to prevent the development of CMV infections or disease. Given the increased risk of drug-related toxicity with prolonged therapy, many centers have abandoned this prevention strategy, except for special situation such as patients with a high risk of CMV infections, including recipients of mismatched or T-cell–depleted allografts [43]. With preemptive therapy, treatment depends on the detection of CMV DNA or pp 65 antigen in blood or plasma samples [41,44]. To ensure early detection of CMV reactivation, most transplant centers have developed a viral load monitoring schedule based on risk factors for CMV infection and disease. Given that CMV viremia occurs frequently in transplant patients before the development of CMV disease, monitoring of CMV viremia to prevent disease is a preferred approach and has been shown to prevent end-organ disease [45].

Viral load thresholds for initiation of therapy are not universal and vary depending on the center, the type of transplant, the risk factors, the type of assays used for monitoring, and the initial viral loads. Antiviral prophylaxis and preemptive therapy have decreased the rate of CMV diseases [41]. However, late CMV disease still occurs in many transplant groups. The most serious CMV disease manifestation in HSCT recipient is CMV pneumonia, which has a significantly high mortality rate, even with the current antiviral management approaches [46,47]. In a single-center retrospective study, the all-cause mortality of HSCT patients after the onset of CMV pneumonia was still high, with only 30% survival at 6 months [46]. Similarly, a retrospective study of lung transplant recipients showed a high rate of CMV infections and disease despite use of extended antiviral prophylaxis [48]. These studies illustrate the continued challenge of accurately diagnosing CMV disease.

Routine monitoring is recommended for patients at high risk for CMV disease [49,50]. Although a few centers may still be using the detection of CMV pp65 antigen, a 65-kD phosphoprotein found in infected leukocytes and endothelial cells [51], to monitor CMV in blood, most centers have converted to molecular tests for rapid and more sensitive detection of CMV infection. CMV quantitative assays are an integral part of the clinical management of transplant patients. Until recently, there were no FDA-cleared assays and most laboratories used LDT for CMV quantitative NATs. A high degree of variability across centers exist when comparing results of LDT CMV quantitative NATs. This variability is due in part to differences in genes targeted for amplification, samples types used, nucleic acids extraction and amplification methodologies, and units used to express results [52]. Testing of CMV in whole blood and plasma using the same assay has shown that viral loads in whole blood tend to be higher than in plasma samples, although low level viremia can be detected most frequently in plasma samples than in whole blood samples [53,54]. The introduction of the first WHO CMV international standards has allowed for the standardization of viral loads obtained with

LDTs. However, some variability remains even with the use of WHO standards [55,56].

Four molecular assays are FDA cleared for the quantitation of CMV DNA (see Table 1). All FDA-cleared assays have traceability to the first WHO International Standard for Human Cytomegalovirus. The CAP/CTM CMV assay was the first FDA-cleared test. Automated extraction on the Cobas Ampliprep is followed by real-time PCR on the Cobas TaqMan 48 and detection occurs using a dual-labeled probe. A standard is included and processed with each sample, serving both as an internal control and a quantitation standard. The CAP/CTM assay is approved for performance on plasma samples of SOT recipients and has a LOD of 91 IU/mL and an LLOQ of 137 IU/mL. The Cobas CMV is the most recent test from Roche, with automated nucleic acids extraction, detection, and quantitation performed on the Cobas 6800 System and Cobas 8800 System. The LOD and LLOQ of the Cobas CMV test is 34.5 IU/mL on plasma samples of both SOT and HSCT recipients. In a multicenter, international study, the Roche CAP/CTM CMV quantitative assay was shown to perform consistently well across laboratories when testing was performed on a standardized CMV panel. However, some variability between LDTs from each center and the Roche assay remained when tested on a set of plasma samples from immunosuppressed patients [57].

The artus CMV RGQ MDx Kit (Qiagen Inc., Hilden, Germany) combines automated extraction on the EZ1 Advanced or EZ1 Advanced XL instruments and real-time PCR on the Rotor-Gene Q instruments to measure CMV viral loads in plasma samples of SOT recipients. Quantitation is performed using a standard curve and concentrations calculated by the instrument software to convert Ct values to copies per milliliter as well as international units per milliliter. The artus CMV assay has a LOD of 77 IU/mL and an LLOQ of 159 IU/mL. One study compared the Artus CMV assay to the CAP/CTM CMV assay on a small number of HSCT patients and found good correlation ($r = 0.80$) for 98% of samples tested [58].

The Abbott RealTime CMV assay detects amplified CMV DNA from plasma samples of HSCT recipients. The LOD and LLOQ are 31.2 IU/mL and 50 IU/mL respectively. Tsai and colleagues [59] compared the performance of the Abbott RealTime CMV with that of the CAP/CTM assay. As expected, given the claimed LOD of each assay, the Abbott CMV test had higher sensitivity than the CAP/CTM CMV test but correlation between the viral loads obtained by both methods was high ($R^2 = 0.94$). However, the viral loads measured by the Abbott CMV were generally higher than those measured by the CAP/CTM CMV test [59].

Given that institutional guidelines for initiating therapy rely on specific numerical values generated by the laboratory, a clear understanding of the test performance characteristics, including the specimen type used, the LOD, the limit of quantification, the linear range and the reproducibility of the assay, is necessary for accurate interpretation of the CMV viral loads and establishment of clinically significant thresholds.

Epstein-Barr Virus

EBV belongs to the *Herpesviridae* family in the *Gammaherpesvirinae* subfamily. EBV is a double-stranded DNA virus with a genome size of approximately 170 kb and about 90 coding genes [60]. Transmission of EBV occurs after contact with oral secretions, blood products, or transplanted cells and/or organs. Exposure to EBV occurs early in life and similar to other herpesviruses, EBV establishes latency in various cells, including B lymphocytes [61]. Infections with EBV may be asymptomatic or cause mild illness including infectious mononucleosis in immunocompetent hots. In immunosuppressed hosts (eg, SOT and HSCT recipients), after the loss of T-cell functions, EBV reactivation can result in posttransplant lymphoproliferative disorders (PTLD) [62]. PTLD is the most significant EBV-associated syndrome in SOT and HSCT recipients [63]. In SOT recipients, the incidence of PTLD ranges from 1% to 20%, with a lower incidence in renal and liver transplant recipients and highest incidence in intestinal and multivisceral transplants. In allogeneic HSCT recipients, rates of PTLD range from 0.45% to 29.0% occurring primarily in the postengraftment and late phase posttransplant. Incidence rates depends on several factors including the type of transplants and the conditioning regimens and generally occurs in the postengraftment and late phases after transplantation [60,62]. Although PTLD is loosely defined as lymphoproliferation after transplant, the syndrome represents a large group of histopathologically heterogenous presentations, from early lesions (eg, mononucleosis-like lesions), to polymorphic PTLD (polyclonal or monoclonal) and monomorphic PTLD (eg, lymphoma) [63]. Manifestations of PTLD vary from benign to severe diseases related to the oncogenic properties of EBV with EBV associated lymphomas (eg, Burkitt's lymphoma) and carcinomas (eg, nasopharyngeal carcinoma) representing the high end of the spectrum [60,62,63].

Given the high mortality associated with EBV-related PTLD, routine monitoring of EBV DNA is performed at most transplant centers. Molecular assays are used for monitoring of EBV reactivation in blood samples (whole blood, serum, plasma or peripheral blood monocyte) of high-risk SOT and HSCT recipients [64]. The most recent guidelines from the American Society of Transplantation recommends routine monitoring of EBV DNA only in high risk SOT patients, EBV seropositive donor/seronegative recipient (D^+/R^-) and patients receiving antilymphocyte globulin [65]. A recent European survey, however, showed that routine monitoring of EBV was frequently done in both low-risk and high-risk patients, despite limited evidence on the usefulness of routine monitoring in low-risk patients [66]. EBV may reactivate without resulting in active disease and viral thresholds to distinguish between background EBV viral loads and clinically significant viral loads are established by individual centers. Because viral loads may be high in patients without PTLD, a general rule, based on knowledge of EBV replication kinetics is that a change of viral load of greater than 0.5 log copies/mL between consecutive samples is considered significant more so than the viral load itself.

To date, there are no FDA-cleared molecular tests for detection and quantitation of EBV viral loads. Therefore, monitoring of EBV viral loads is accomplished exclusively using LDT based on a variety of reagents (Table 2). The variability in viral loads obtained across laboratories using LDT has been established [52,56]. For EBV, factors contributing to variability included commercial reagents, calibrators, nucleic acid extraction methods, viral gene target, and a pipetting method [52]. In 2011, the first WHO International standards for EBV became available for calibration of secondary reference materials to international units. A recent report showed that conversion of viral loads from copies per milliliter to international units per milliliter resulted in lower EBV values and reduced variability in viral load measurements, which may ultimately result in more standardized viral loads across centers, and the potential to establish universally clinically significant, EBV viral load thresholds [56].

Human Herpesvirus-6

Human herpesvirus-6 (HHV-6) belongs to the *Herpesviridae* family in the *Betaherpesvirinae* subfamily. HHV-6 is a double-stranded DNA virus with a genome size of approximately 170 kb and about 100 coding genes. Although HHV-6 was traditionally considered one virus with 2 variants, HHV-6A and HHV-6B, recently these 2 viruses were established as 2 separate species [67]. Collectively, HHV-6A and HHV-6B infect more than 90% of individuals before the age of 2 to 5. Primary infections result in roseola infantum (sixth disease), a self-limited disease characterized by high fever for 2 to 5 days and the presence of a maculopapular rash on the neck and torso, which resolves within a couple of days [68]. After resolution of primary infection, HHV-6 establishes latency mainly in mononuclear cells and has the unique ability to integrate the host chromosomes [69].

In SOT recipients, the incidence of HHV-6 infections ranges from 10% to 60% and occurs within the first month after transplantation [70]. Although most infections are asymptomatic, end-organ diseases including hepatitis, encephalitis, and pneumonitis, occurs in less than 1% of SOT recipients, with most cases caused by HHV-6B [70,71]. In HSCT recipients and patients with hematologic malignancies, HHV-6 reactivation occurs in 50% to 95% of HSCT recipients after immunosuppression or chemotherapy, with higher reactivation rates seen in cord blood transplants [72]. The clinical impact of HHV-6 reactivation in HSCT recipients varies, with some studies reporting that early reactivation of HHV6 posttransplantation may be associated with delayed neutrophils and platelets engraftment, increased mortality, and the development of acute graft-versus-host disease [73,74], whereas other studies showed no impact from HHV-6 reactivation [75]. These differences in outcomes may be due in part to differences in the type of transplants (eg, cord blood vs HSCT). A complication associated with reactivation of HHV-6 is posttransplant acute limbic encephalitis (PALE) in allogeneic HSCT recipients [76]. In the study by Seeley and colleagues [76], PALE was identified only in HSCT recipient positive for HHV-6 in the cerebral spinal fluid, but other studies have shown some overlap in viral loads for HHV-6 of HSCT patients with or without PALE [77]. Risk factors for development of HHV-6 disease are not well-defined and studies evaluating the utility of preemptive therapy or antiviral prophylaxis to present PALE or HHV-6 disease have been inconclusive [78–80].

Other complications associated with HHV-6 infections includes graft rejection, graft-versus-host disease and an increased all-cause mortality [81]. Although subclinical, asymptomatic infections do not require treatment, HHV-6 diseases are usually treated using foscarnet, cidofovir, and ganciclovir, but the efficacy of these therapies has not been fully evaluated in clinical trials [81].

TABLE 2
Select Commercial Reagents for Molecular Assays

Manufacturer	Name	Status	Methodology
Altona	RealStar Adenovirus PCR kit	RUO	Hydrolysis probes
	RealStar BKV PCR	RUO	Hydrolysis probes
	RealStar EBV PCR	RUO	Hydrolysis probes
	RealStar HHV-6 PCR Kit	RUO	Hydrolysis probes
bioMérieux	Adenovirus R-Gene	RUO	Hydrolysis probes
	BK Virus R-Gene	RUO	Hydrolysis probes
	EBV R-Gene	RUO	Hydrolysis probes
	HHV6,7,8 R-Gene	RUO	Hydrolysis probes
ELITechGroup	MGB Alert Adenovirus Primer Mix MGB Alert Adenovirus Probe Mix	ASR	Minor groove binder probes
	MGB Alert BKV Primer Mix MGB Alert BKV Probe Mix	ASR	Minor groove binder probes
	MGB Alert EBV Primer Mix MGB Alert EBV Probe Mix	ASR	Minor groove binder probes
	MGB Alert HHV6 2.0 Primer Mix MGB Alert HHV6 2.0 Probe Mix	ASR	Minor groove binder probes
Luminex	MultiCode Adenovirus Primers	ASR	Labeled primers
	MultiCode BK Virus Primers	ASR	Labeled primers
	MultiCode EBV Primers	ASR	Labeled primers
Qiagen	Artus BK Virus RG PCR	RUO	TaqMan probes
	BK virus Primers BK virus Probes	ASR	TaqMan probes
	EBV Primers EBV Probes	ASR	TaqMan probes
Roche	EBV Primer Pair EBV Probes 1 and 2	ASR	HybProbes

Abbreviations: ASR, analyte-specific reagents; EBV, Epstein–Barr virus; HHV, human herpesvirus; PCR, polymerase chain reaction; RUO, research use only.

Although the benefit of routine monitoring of HHV-6 viral loads has not been completely demonstrated and not supported by the most recent guidelines, many transplant centers include HHV-6 screening as part of their routine screen after transplantation [75,82,83]. Quantitative molecular diagnostics assays are the primary methods for the detection and monitoring of HHV-6 infections. There are currently no FDA-cleared molecular tests for HHV-6 quantitation. Several commercial ASR are available for LDTs (see Table 2). To date, no WHO international standards are available for standardization of HHV-6 viral loads assays, and as such, comparisons of viral loads obtained from different laboratories are not comparable [56,84]. Additionally, unique to HHV-6, viral loads testing alone cannot accurately differentiate between actively replicating HHV-6 and chromosomally integrated HHV-6 (ciHHV-6), which is present in approximately 1% of the population. HHV-6 can be detected in whole blood or plasma samples and high viral loads (eg, $>10^6$ in whole blood or $>10^4$ copies/mL in plasma) may indicate ciHHV-6. Sedlak and colleagues [85] developed a digital PCR to distinguish between ciHHV-6 and cell free HHV-6 using the ratio of HHV-6 to total cell counts of approximately 1 to indicate ciHHV-6.

Human Adenovirus

Human ADV belong to the *Adenoviridae* family, in the *Mastadenovirus* genus. ADV are double-stranded, nonenveloped DNA viruses responsible for a wide spectrum of clinical manifestations including upper respiratory tract infections, pneumonia, nephritis, hemorrhagic cystitis, hepatitis and colitis [86]. Based on serologic and sequencing methods, up to 7 species (A-G) and more than 70 types of ADV have been characterized to date, with many of the ADV showing specific tissue-tropism [86].

Clinical presentations vary between different patient populations and ranges from asymptomatic, self-limited infections to severe and life-threatening disseminated disease [87]. After primary infections, ADV establishes long-term latency in the lymphoid cells of various tissues [86]. In immunosuppressed hosts, including SOT and HSCT recipients, ADV infections can results from reactivation of latent viruses or from de novo infections. End-organ diseases includes hepatitis, pneumonitis, encephalitis, colitis, and hemorrhagic cystitis and are associated with significant morbidity and mortality [86,88].

Adenovirus infections rates in HSCT recipients range from 5% to 15%, with rates and outcomes varying with the type of transplant and the level of immunosuppression [82,89–91]. Lee and colleagues [92] reported an attributable adenovirus mortality rate of 22% in a cohort of HSCT recipients transplanted with $CD34^+$ selected stem cells, and mortality rates were significantly lower in a cohort of patients with an alemtuzumab-based allogeneic stem cell transplantation [91]. Of note, adenovirus viremia is associated with mortality rates as high as 44% in some studies [92–94]. In a recent study, ADV viremia in allogeneic HSCT recipients occurred at a median of 14 days before end-organ disease and in the context of persistent viremia [95]. In SOT recipients, the incidence of adenovirus ranges from 3.5% to 57.0% in pediatric SOT recipients, with the highest rate seen in intestinal and multivisceral transplants, much higher than in adult SOT patients were the rates range from 4.1% to 7.2% [88].

Routine surveillance for ADV is suggested for patients at highest risk of developing infections and end-organ diseases. The most recent guidelines for HSCT recipients suggest weekly adenovirus viral loads monitoring in the first 6 months after transplant using quantitative PCR. However, no standardized threshold values have been established for initiation of therapy or withdrawal of immunosuppression when possible [82,96]. Therapy options for adenovirus infections are limited and include cidofovir or ribavirin for preemptive antiviral therapy in selected high-risk HCT patients, although data on efficacy is limited. Unlike in HSCT recipients, routine surveillance for adenovirus infections in SOT recipients is not recommended given the low frequency of end-organ disease.

Quantitative adenovirus PCR tests are the method of choice for monitoring of adenovirus viremia. Most quantitative PCRs are performed on plasma or whole blood samples at predetermined intervals posttransplant. In addition to plasma or blood samples, active surveillance for adenovirus using stool samples has also been proposed [97,98]. Although adenovirus gastroenteritis is caused primarily by serotypes 40/41, in immunocompromised patients, many other serotypes have been associated with gastroenteritis [99]. There are currently no FDA-cleared molecular methods for adenovirus monitoring and most centers rely on LDTs (see Table 2). Given the large number of adenovirus serotypes, ASR or other reagents for LDTs should be carefully selected and evaluated for maximum inclusivity. WHO international standards are not yet available and quantitative PCR tests are not standardized, making establishment of valid, actionable threshold challenging.

BK Polyoma Virus

BKV is a small, nonenveloped, circular, double-stranded DNA viruses that belongs to the *Polyomaviridae* family, in the *Betapolyomavirus* genus [100]. The BKV genome is approximately 5 kB in length and divided into 3 regions; the early region, coding for the tumor antigen genes, a noncoding control region, and a late region, coding for structural viral proteins. BKV are divided in 4 genotypes, I to IV, and several subgroups with BKV genotype I responsible for most infections worldwide [101]. Transmission of BKV is thought to occur through the respiratory or oral routes. Primary infection occurs early in life and results in mostly asymptomatic infections with the virus establishing latency in the epithelial cells of the urinary tract system [102].

Immunocompetent hosts can intermittently shed high levels of BKV in urine without symptoms. Two BKV syndromes are associated with immunosuppressed states including polyomavirus associated nephropathy (PyVAN) in kidney transplant recipients and polyomavirus associated hemorrhagic cystitis in HSCT recipients [103]. In kidney transplants, PyVAN occurs in 1% to 10% of cases and can arise from primary infections or from reactivation of latent infections. The specific risk factors for development of PyVAN have not been clearly defined with some studies suggesting increased risks being associated with a positive donor BKV serostatus, the recipient immune system, the source of the organs, donor–recipient HLA mismatch, recipient age, and the type of immunosuppressants used [103,104]. In HSCT recipients, hemorrhagic cystitis occurs in 5% to 15% of patients within 3 to 6 weeks posttransplant [82]. Similar to renal transplant patients, the risk factors for hemorrhagic cystitis in HSCT recipients are not well defined but a few risk factors, including male gender, conditioning regimen (eg, cyclophosphamide), and an unrelated donor, have been identified in a few studies [105,106].

In kidney transplant recipients, BKV viremia precedes the development of PyVAN and, as such, routine screening is recommended by the American Society of transplantation. Various, center-specific recommendations based on BK virus incidence exist, including screening every 3 months for the first 2 years posttransplant then annually until year 5 [103]. Options for screening includes molecular viral load testing of urine samples, with BKV viruria of greater than 10^7 copies/mL as a threshold for further testing including BKV viremia followed by allograft biopsy if BKV viremia is $>10^4$ copies/mL [103].

BKV viruria is present in 60% to 80% of HSCT recipients with viral loads as high as 10^7 copies/mL but less than 20% of patients developing hemorrhagic cystitis [107]. In HSCT recipients, diagnosis of hemorrhagic cystitis is further complicated by overlapping symptomologies with other viral etiologies including adenovirus and CMV [46]. In some studies, high viral loads of greater than 10^7 copies/mL were associated with risk of developing hemorrhagic cystitis, although significant overlap occurred between control and patient cohorts [106,107]. There are no recommendations for routine monitoring of BKV in HSCT patients, but testing of symptomatic patients may be warranted [82,107]. Although fluoroquinolones and cidofovir are used for treatment of BKV infections, there is no evidence to support their use as prophylaxis or in preemptive therapy of asymptomatic patients and although a decrease in immunosuppression is an option in kidney transplant recipients, the risk for further complications including graft-versus-host disease in HSCT recipients excludes it as an option.

There are currently no FDA-cleared molecular methods for BKV monitoring and most centers rely on real-time PCR LDTs. LDTs are based on amplification of the viral proteins or tumor antigen genes of BKV but the design of BKV LDTs is challenged by high homology with other polyomaviruses [108–110]. Several kits and reagents are commercially available to facilitate BKV detection and quantitation (see Table 2). Standardization of LDTs is still lacking, which results in high variability in viral loads across centers and challenging the feasibility of establishing clinical decision viral thresholds that are consistent across transplant centers [56,109,110]. Variability in viral loads generated by LDTs may be due to differences in standards used for quantitation as well as differences in commercial reagents used (see Table 2). Most recently, the first WHO international standard for BK virus became recently available [111]. In one study, calibration of LDTs using the WHO BKV standards changed the viral load of 10,000 copies/mL, which used as a threshold for intervention, in one assay to 2500 IU/mL in another assay [112]. Such changes in the numeric value of the viral loads will need to be closely assessed given their impact on monitoring of BK viremia or BK viruria.

SUMMARY

Monitoring of bloodborne viruses and double-stranded DNA viruses continues to play a significant role in the clinical management of a variety of patients including HSCT and SOT recipients. As standardization continues to improve and more quantitative molecular assays gain FDA clearance, viral loads obtained across centers worldwide will become more consistent. This will in turn facilitate the development and implementation of more accurate thresholds to define cure, predict disease and administer appropriate therapy in a timely manner to prevent poor outcomes.

REFERENCES

[1] Maartens G, Celum C, Lewin SR. HIV infection: epidemiology, pathogenesis, treatment, and prevention. Lancet 2014;384(9939):258–71.

[2] McCutchan FE. Global epidemiology of HIV. J Med Virol 2006;78(Suppl 1):S7–12.

[3] Visseaux B, Damond F, Matheron S, et al. Hiv-2 molecular epidemiology. Infect Genet Evol 2016;46:233–40.

[4] Peruski AH, Dong X, Selik RM. Trends in testing algorithms used to diagnose HIV infection, 2011-2015, United States and 6 dependent areas. J Clin Virol 2018;103:19–24.

[5] Wirden M, Larrouy L, Mahjoub N, et al. Multicenter comparison of the new Cobas 6800 system with Cobas Ampliprep/Cobas TaqMan and Abbott RealTime for the quantification of HIV, HBV and HCV viral load. J Clin Virol 2017;96:49–53.

[6] Braun P, Delgado R, Drago M, et al. A European multicenter study on the comparison of HIV-1 viral loads between VERIS HIV-1 Assay and Roche COBAS(R) TAQMAN(R) HIV-1 test, Abbott RealTime HIV-1 Assay, and Siemens VERSANT HIV-1 assay. J Clin Virol 2017; 92:75–82.

[7] Schonning K, Johansen K, Landt B, et al. Comparison of the Hologic Aptima HIV-1 Quant Dx assay to the Roche COBAS Ampliprep/COBAS TaqMan HIV-1 test v2.0 for the quantification of HIV-1 RNA in plasma samples. J Clin Virol 2017;92:14–9.

[8] Mourez T, Delaugerre C, Vray M, et al. Comparison of the bioMerieux NucliSENS EasyQ HIV-1 v2.0-HIV-1 RNA quantification assay versus Abbott Real-Time HIV-1 and Roche Cobas TaqMan HIV-1 v2.0 on current epidemic HIV-1 variants. J Clin Virol 2015;71:76–81.

[9] Manak MM, Hack HR, Nair SV, et al. Evaluation of Hologic Aptima HIV-1 Quant Dx assay on the panther system on HIV subtypes. J Clin Microbiol 2016;54(10): 2575–81.

[10] Amendola A, Marsella P, Bloisi M, et al. Ability of two commercially available assays (Abbott RealTime HIV-1 and Roche Cobas AmpliPrep/Cobas TaqMan HIV-1 Version 2.0) to quantify low HIV-1 RNA Levels (<1,000 copies/milliliter): comparison with clinical samples and NIBSC working reagent for nucleic acid testing assays. J Clin Microbiol 2014;52(6):2019–26.

[11] Department of Health and Human Services. Panel on antiretroviral guidelines for adults and adolescents. Guidelines for the use of antiretroviral agents in adults and adolescents living with HIV. Department of Health and Human Services; 2017. Available at: http://aidsinfo.nih.gov/contentfiles/lvguidelines/AdultandAdolescentGL.pdf. Accessed April 7, 2018.

[12] Smith DB, Bukh J, Kuiken C, et al. Expanded classification of hepatitis C virus into 7 genotypes and 67 subtypes: updated criteria and genotype assignment web resource. Hepatology 2014;59(1):318–27.

[13] IC TV Online (ICTV). HCV classification. 2018. Available at: https://talk.ictvonline.org/ictv_wikis/flaviviridae/w/sg_flavi/56/hcv-classification. Accessed April 8, 2018.

[14] Petruzziello A, Marigliano S, Loquercio G, et al. Global epidemiology of hepatitis C virus infection: an up-date of the distribution and circulation of hepatitis C virus genotypes. World J Gastroenterol 2016;22(34): 7824–40.

[15] Gordon SC, Trudeau S, Li J, et al. Race, age, and geography impact hepatitis C genotype distribution in the United States. J Clin Gastroenterol 2017. [Epub ahead of print].

[16] Ghany MG, Liang TJ. Current and future therapies for hepatitis C virus infection. N Engl J Med 2013;369(7): 679–80.

[17] Centers for Disease Control and Prevention. Surveillance for Viral Hepatitis – United States, 2015. 2015. Available at: https://www.cdc.gov/hepatitis/statistics/2015surveillance/pdfs/2015HepSurveillanceRpt.pdf. Accessed April 8, 2018.

[18] Ghany MG, Strader DB, Thomas DL, et al, American Association for the Study of Liver Diseases. Diagnosis, management, and treatment of hepatitis C: an update. Hepatology 2009;49(4):1335–74.

[19] Centers for Disease Control and Prevention (CDC). Testing for HCV infection: an update of guidance for clinicians and laboratorians. MMWR Morb Mortal Wkly Rep 2013;62(18):362–5.

[20] AASLD-IDSA. Recommendations for testing, managing, and treating hepatitis C. 2017. Available at: http://hcvguidelines.org/. Accessed April 8, 2018.

[21] Liang TJ, Ghany MG. Current and future therapies for hepatitis C virus infection. N Engl J Med 2013; 368(20):1907–17.

[22] Colucci G. Molecular diagnostic and predictive tests in the evolution of chronic hepatitis C anti-viral therapies. BMC Infect Dis 2012;12(Suppl 2):S8.

[23] Worlock A, Blair D, Hunsicker M, et al. Analytical characteristics and comparative evaluation of Aptima HCV quant Dx assay with the Abbott RealTime HCV assay and Roche COBAS AmpliPrep/COBAS TaqMan HCV quantitative test v2.0. Virol J 2017; 14(1):66.

[24] Kessler HH, Cobb BR, Wedemeyer H, et al. Evaluation of the COBAS (R) AmpliPrep/COBAS (R) TaqMan (R) HCV Test, v2.0 and comparison to assays used in routine clinical practice in an international multicenter clinical trial: the ExPECT study. J Clin Virol 2015;67: 67–72.

[25] Sunbul M. Hepatitis B virus genotypes: global distribution and clinical importance. World J Gastroenterol 2014;20(18):5427–34.

[26] Chu CJ, Keeffe EB, Han SH, et al. Hepatitis B virus genotypes in the United States: results of a nationwide study. Gastroenterology 2003;125(2):444–51.

[27] Organization WH. Global hepatitis report, 2017. 2017. Available at: http://www.who.int/hepatitis/publications/global-hepatitis-report2017/en/. Accessed April 8, 2018.

[28] Lok AS, McMahon BJ. Chronic hepatitis B: update 2009. Hepatology 2009;50(3):661–2.

[29] Terrault NA, Lok ASF, McMahon BJ, et al. Update on prevention, diagnosis, and treatment of chronic hepatitis B: AASLD 2018 hepatitis B guidance. Hepatology 2018;67(4):1560–99.

[30] Sorrell MF, Belongia EA, Costa J, et al. National Institutes of Health Consensus Development Conference Statement: management of hepatitis B. Ann Intern Med 2009;150(2):104–10.

[31] Valsamakis A. Molecular testing in the diagnosis and management of chronic hepatitis B. Clin Microbiol Rev 2007;20(3):426–39, Table of contents.

[32] Maasoumy B, Bremer B, Lehmann P, et al. Commutability and concordance of four hepatitis B virus DNA

assays in an international multicenter study. Therap Adv Gastroenterol 2017;10(8):609–18.

[33] Yeh ML, Huang CF, Hsieh MY, et al. Comparison of the Abbott RealTime HBV assay with the Roche Cobas AmpliPrep/Cobas TaqMan HBV assay for HBV DNA detection and quantification. J Clin Virol 2014;60(3):206–14.

[34] Chevaliez S, Dubernet F, Dauvillier C, et al. The new Aptima HCV Quant Dx real-time TMA assay accurately quantifies hepatitis C virus genotype 1-6 RNA. J Clin Virol 2017;91:5–11.

[35] Dolan A, Cunningham C, Hector RD, et al. Genetic content of wild-type human cytomegalovirus. J Gen Virol 2004;85(Pt 5):1301–12.

[36] Bate SL, Dollard SC, Cannon MJ. Cytomegalovirus seroprevalence in the United States: the national health and nutrition examination surveys, 1988-2004. Clin Infect Dis 2010;50(11):1439–47.

[37] Gandhi MK, Khanna R. Human cytomegalovirus: clinical aspects, immune regulation, and emerging treatments. Lancet Infect Dis 2004;4(12):725–38.

[38] Razonable RR, Humar A, AST Infectious Diseases Community of Practice. Cytomegalovirus in solid organ transplantation. Am J Transplant 2013;13(Suppl 4):93–106.

[39] Ljungman P, Boeckh M, Hirsch HH, et al. Definitions of cytomegalovirus infection and disease in transplant patients for use in clinical trials. Clin Infect Dis 2017;64(1):87–91.

[40] Confer DL, Abress LK, Navarro W, et al. Selection of adult unrelated hematopoietic stem cell donors: beyond HLA. Biol Blood Marrow Transplant 2010;16(1 Suppl):S8–11.

[41] Boeckh M, Ljungman P. How we treat cytomegalovirus in hematopoietic cell transplant recipients. Blood 2009;113(23):5711–9.

[42] Pergam SA, Xie H, Sandhu R, et al. Efficiency and risk factors for CMV transmission in seronegative hematopoietic stem cell recipients. Biol Blood Marrow Transplant 2012;18(9):1391–400.

[43] Milano F, Pergam SA, Xie H, et al. Intensive strategy to prevent CMV disease in seropositive umbilical cord blood transplant recipients. Blood 2011;118(20):5689–96.

[44] Pollack M, Heugel J, Xie H, et al. An international comparison of current strategies to prevent herpesvirus and fungal infections in hematopoietic cell transplant recipients. Biol Blood Marrow Transplant 2011;17(5):664–73.

[45] Boeckh M. Complications, diagnosis, management, and prevention of CMV infections: current and future. Hematology Am Soc Hematol Educ Program 2011;2011:305–9.

[46] Erard V, Guthrie KA, Seo S, et al. Reduced mortality of cytomegalovirus pneumonia after hematopoietic cell transplantation due to antiviral therapy and changes in transplantation practices. Clin Infect Dis 2015;61(1):31–9.

[47] Ljungman P, Hakki M, Boeckh M. Cytomegalovirus in hematopoietic stem cell transplant recipients. Hematol Oncol Clin North Am 2011;25(1):151–69.

[48] Beam E, Lesnick T, Kremers W, et al. Cytomegalovirus disease is associated with higher all-cause mortality after lung transplantation despite extended antiviral prophylaxis. Clin Transplant 2016;30(3):270–8.

[49] Kotton CN, Kumar D, Caliendo AM, et al. Updated international consensus guidelines on the management of cytomegalovirus in solid-organ transplantation. Transplantation 2013;96(4):333–60.

[50] Tomblyn M, Chiller T, Einsele H, et al. Guidelines for preventing infectious complications among hematopoietic cell transplantation recipients: a global perspective. Biol Blood Marrow Transplant 2009;15(10):1143–238.

[51] Boeckh M, Boivin G. Quantitation of cytomegalovirus: methodologic aspects and clinical applications. Clin Microbiol Rev 1998;11(3):533–54.

[52] Hayden RT, Yan X, Wick MT, et al. Factors contributing to variability of quantitative viral PCR results in proficiency testing samples: a multivariate analysis. J Clin Microbiol 2012;50(2):337–45.

[53] Babady NE, Cheng C, Cumberbatch E, et al. Monitoring of cytomegalovirus viral loads by two molecular assays in whole-blood and plasma samples from hematopoietic stem cell transplant recipients. J Clin Microbiol 2015;53(4):1252–7.

[54] Dioverti MV, Lahr BD, Germer JJ, et al. Comparison of standardized cytomegalovirus (CMV) viral load thresholds in whole blood and plasma of solid organ and hematopoietic stem cell transplant recipients with CMV infection and disease. Open Forum Infect Dis 2017;4(3):ofx143.

[55] Hayden RT, Preiksaitis J, Tong Y, et al. Commutability of the first World Health Organization international standard for human cytomegalovirus. J Clin Microbiol 2015;53(10):3325–33.

[56] Hayden RT, Sun Y, Tang L, et al. Progress in quantitative viral load testing: variability and impact of the WHO quantitative international standards. J Clin Microbiol 2017;55(2):423–30.

[57] Hirsch HH, Lautenschlager I, Pinsky BA, et al. An international multicenter performance analysis of cytomegalovirus load tests. Clin Infect Dis 2013;56(3):367–73.

[58] Hoteit R, Fermanian P, Abbas F, et al. Comparison of the Artus RotorGene and COBAS Ampliprep/COBAS TaqMan Platforms for the detection of cytomegalovirus: experience of a tertiary care center. Genet Test Mol Biomarkers 2016;20(4):167–9.

[59] Tsai HP, Tsai YY, Lin IT, et al. Comparison of two commercial automated nucleic acid extraction and integrated quantitation real-time PCR platforms for the detection of cytomegalovirus in plasma. PLoS One 2016;11(8):e0160493.

[60] Young LS, Rickinson AB. Epstein-Barr virus: 40 years on. Nat Rev Cancer 2004;4(10):757–68.

[61] Odumade OA, Hogquist KA, Balfour HH Jr. Progress and problems in understanding and managing primary Epstein-Barr virus infections. Clin Microbiol Rev 2011; 24(1):193–209.
[62] Loren AW, Porter DL, Stadtmauer EA, et al. Post-transplant lymphoproliferative disorder: a review. Bone Marrow Transplant 2003;31(3):145–55.
[63] Petrara MR, Giunco S, Serraino D, et al. Post-transplant lymphoproliferative disorders: from epidemiology to pathogenesis-driven treatment. Cancer Lett 2015; 369(1):37–44.
[64] Gulley ML, Tang W. Using Epstein-Barr viral load assays to diagnose, monitor, and prevent posttransplant lymphoproliferative disorder. Clin Microbiol Rev 2010; 23(2):350–66.
[65] Allen UD, Preiksaitis JK, AST Infectious Diseases Community of Practice. Epstein-Barr virus and posttransplant lymphoproliferative disorder in solid organ transplantation. Am J Transplant 2013;13(Suppl 4): 107–20.
[66] San-Juan R, Manuel O, Hirsch HH, et al. Current preventive strategies and management of Epstein-Barr virus-related post-transplant lymphoproliferative disease in solid organ transplantation in Europe. Results of the ESGICH Questionnaire-based Cross-sectional Survey. Clin Microbiol Infect 2015;21(6): 604.e1-9.
[67] Adams MJ, Carstens EB. Ratification vote on taxonomic proposals to the International Committee on Taxonomy of Viruses (2012). Arch Virol 2012;157(7): 1411–22.
[68] Zerr DM, Meier AS, Selke SS, et al. A population-based study of primary human herpesvirus 6 infection. N Engl J Med 2005;352(8):768–76.
[69] Pellett PE, Ablashi DV, Ambros PF, et al. Chromosomally integrated human herpesvirus 6: questions and answers. Rev Med Virol 2012;22(3):144–55.
[70] Razonable RR. Human herpesviruses 6, 7 and 8 in solid organ transplant recipients. Am J Transplant 2013; 13(Suppl 3):67–77 [quiz: 77–8].
[71] Hill JA, Myerson D, Sedlak RH, et al. Hepatitis due to human herpesvirus 6B after hematopoietic cell transplantation and a review of the literature. Transpl Infect Dis 2014;16(3):477–83.
[72] Yamane A, Mori T, Suzuki S, et al. Risk factors for developing human herpesvirus 6 (HHV-6) reactivation after allogeneic hematopoietic stem cell transplantation and its association with central nervous system disorders. Biol Blood Marrow Transplant 2007;13(1):100–6.
[73] Dulery R, Salleron J, Dewilde A, et al. Early human herpesvirus type 6 reactivation after allogeneic stem cell transplantation: a large-scale clinical study. Biol Blood Marrow Transplant 2012;18(7):1080–9.
[74] Zerr DM, Boeckh M, Delaney C, et al. HHV-6 reactivation and associated sequelae after hematopoietic cell transplantation. Biol Blood Marrow Transplant 2012; 18(11):1700–8.
[75] Olson AL, Dahi PB, Zheng J, et al. Frequent human herpesvirus-6 viremia but low incidence of encephalitis in double-unit cord blood recipients transplanted without antithymocyte globulin. Biol Blood Marrow Transplant 2014;20(6):787–93.
[76] Seeley WW, Marty FM, Holmes TM, et al. Post-transplant acute limbic encephalitis: clinical features and relationship to HHV6. Neurology 2007;69(2):156–65.
[77] Hill JA, Koo S, Guzman Suarez BB, et al. Cord-blood hematopoietic stem cell transplant confers an increased risk for human herpesvirus-6-associated acute limbic encephalitis: a cohort analysis. Biol Blood Marrow Transplant 2012;18(11):1638–48.
[78] Betts BC, Young JA, Ustun C, et al. Human herpesvirus 6 infection after hematopoietic cell transplantation: is routine surveillance necessary? Biol Blood Marrow Transplant 2011;17(10):1562–8.
[79] Ogata M, Satou T, Kawano R, et al. Plasma HHV-6 viral load-guided preemptive therapy against HHV-6 encephalopathy after allogeneic stem cell transplantation: a prospective evaluation. Bone Marrow Transplant 2008;41(3):279–85.
[80] Ishiyama K, Katagiri T, Hoshino T, et al. Preemptive therapy of human herpesvirus-6 encephalitis with foscarnet sodium for high-risk patients after hematopoietic SCT. Bone Marrow Transplant 2011;46(6):863–9.
[81] Hill JA, Zerr DM. Roseoloviruses in transplant recipients: clinical consequences and prospects for treatment and prevention trials. Curr Opin Virol 2014;9:53–60.
[82] Tomblyn M, Chiller T, Einsele H, et al. Guidelines for preventing infectious complications among hematopoietic cell transplant recipients: a global perspective. Preface. Bone Marrow Transplant 2009;44(8):453–5.
[83] Fernandez-Ruiz M, Kumar D, Husain S, et al. Utility of a monitoring strategy for human herpesviruses 6 and 7 viremia after liver transplantation: a randomized clinical trial. Transplantation 2015;99(1):106–13.
[84] Hill JA, Sedlak RH, Jerome KR. Past, present, and future perspectives on the diagnosis of Roseolovirus infections. Curr Opin Virol 2014;9:84–90.
[85] Sedlak RH, Cook L, Huang ML, et al. Identification of chromosomally integrated human herpesvirus 6 by droplet digital PCR. Clin Chem 2014;60(5):765–72.
[86] Lion T. Adenovirus infections in immunocompetent and immunocompromised patients. Clin Microbiol Rev 2014;27(3):441–62.
[87] Lynch JP 3rd, Kajon AE. Adenovirus: epidemiology, global spread of novel serotypes, and advances in treatment and prevention. Semin Respir Crit Care Med 2016;37(4):586–602.
[88] Florescu DF, Hoffman JA, AST Infectious Diseases Community of Practice. Adenovirus in solid organ transplantation. Am J Transplant 2013;13(Suppl 4):206–11.
[89] Lee YJ, Palomino-Guilen P, Babady NE, et al. Disseminated adenovirus infection in cancer patients presenting with focal pulmonary consolidation. J Clin Microbiol 2014;52(1):350–3.

[90] Rustia E, Violago L, Jin Z, et al. Risk factors and utility of a risk-based algorithm for monitoring cytomegalovirus, Epstein-Barr virus, and adenovirus infections in pediatric recipients after allogeneic hematopoietic cell transplantation. Biol Blood Marrow Transplant 2016;22(9):1646–53.

[91] Sive JI, Thomson KJ, Morris EC, et al. Adenoviremia has limited clinical impact in the majority of patients following alemtuzumab-based allogeneic stem cell transplantation in adults. Clin Infect Dis 2012;55(10):1362–70.

[92] Lee YJ, Huang YT, Kim SJ, et al. Adenovirus viremia in adult CD34(+) selected hematopoietic cell transplant recipients: low incidence and high clinical impact. Biol Blood Marrow Transplant 2016;22(1):174–8.

[93] Boeckh M, Gooley TA, Myerson D, et al. Cytomegalovirus pp65 antigenemia-guided early treatment with ganciclovir versus ganciclovir at engraftment after allogeneic marrow transplantation: a randomized double-blind study. Blood 1996;88(10):4063–71.

[94] Zaia JA. Prevention of cytomegalovirus disease in hematopoietic stem cell transplantation. Clin Infect Dis 2002;35(8):999–1004.

[95] Hill JA, Mayer BT, Xie H, et al. Kinetics of double-stranded DNA viremia after allogeneic hematopoietic cell transplantation. Clin Infect Dis 2018;66(3):368–75.

[96] Zaia J, Baden L, Boeckh MJ, et al. Viral disease prevention after hematopoietic cell transplantation. Bone Marrow Transplant 2009;44(8):471–82.

[97] Lion T, Kosulin K, Landlinger C, et al. Monitoring of adenovirus load in stool by real-time PCR permits early detection of impending invasive infection in patients after allogeneic stem cell transplantation. Leukemia 2010;24(4):706–14.

[98] Srinivasan A, Klepper C, Sunkara A, et al. Impact of adenoviral stool load on adenoviremia in pediatric hematopoietic stem cell transplant recipients. Pediatr Infect Dis J 2015;34(6):562–5.

[99] McMillen T, Lee YJ, Kamboj M, et al. Limited diagnostic value of a multiplexed gastrointestinal pathogen panel for the detection of adenovirus infection in an oncology patient population. J Clin Virol 2017;94:37–41.

[100] Moens U, Calvignac-Spencer S, Lauber C, et al. ICTV virus taxonomy profile: polyomaviridae. J Gen Virol 2017;98(6):1159–60.

[101] Helle F, Brochot E, Handala L, et al. Biology of the BKPyV: an update. Viruses 2017;9(11) [pii:E327].

[102] Hirsch HH, Steiger J. Polyomavirus BK. Lancet Infect Dis 2003;3(10):611–23.

[103] Hirsch HH, Randhawa P, AST Infectious Diseases Community of Practice. BK polyomavirus in solid organ transplantation. Am J Transplant 2013;13(Suppl 4):179–88.

[104] Scadden JR, Sharif A, Skordilis K, et al. Polyoma virus nephropathy in kidney transplantation. World J Transplant 2017;7(6):329–38.

[105] Lunde LE, Dasaraju S, Cao Q, et al. Hemorrhagic cystitis after allogeneic hematopoietic cell transplantation: risk factors, graft source and survival. Bone Marrow Transplant 2015;50(11):1432–7.

[106] Uhm J, Hamad N, Michelis FV, et al. The risk of polyomavirus BK-associated hemorrhagic cystitis after allogeneic hematopoietic SCT is associated with myeloablative conditioning, CMV viremia and severe acute GVHD. Bone Marrow Transplant 2014;49(12):1528–34.

[107] Lee YJ, Zheng J, Kolitsopoulos Y, et al. Relationship of BK polyoma virus (BKV) in the urine with hemorrhagic cystitis and renal function in recipients of T Cell-depleted peripheral blood and cord blood stem cell transplantations. Biol Blood Marrow Transplant 2014;20(8):1204–10.

[108] Hasan MR, Tan R, Al-Rawahi G, et al. Comparative evaluation of laboratory developed real-time PCR assays and RealStar((R)) BKV PCR Kit for quantitative detection of BK polyomavirus. J Virol Methods 2016;234:80–6.

[109] Greer AE, Forman MS, Valsamakis A. Comparison of BKV quantification using a single automated nucleic acid extraction platform and 3 real-time PCR assays. Diagn Microbiol Infect Dis 2015;82(4):297–302.

[110] Hassan S, Mittal C, Amer S, et al. Currently recommended BK virus (BKV) plasma viral load cutoff of >/=4 log10/mL underestimates the diagnosis of BKV-associated nephropathy: a single transplant center experience. Transpl Infect Dis 2014;16(1):55–60.

[111] WHO. First WHO international standard for BK virus DNA. Geneva (Switzerland): 2016.

[112] World Health Organization (WHO), Tan SK, Milligan S, Sahoo MK, et al. Calibration of BK virus nucleic acid amplification testing to the 1st WHO international standard for BK virus. J Clin Microbiol 2017;55(3):923–30.

Advances in Molecular Pathology 1 (2018) 81–89
ADVANCES IN MOLECULAR PATHOLOGY

The Current State of Metagenomics in Infectious Disease

Priyanka Uprety, MSPH, PhD[a,b,1], Stephanie L. Mitchell, PhD, D(ABMM)[c,d], Bryan L. Krock, PhD[a,b], Erin H. Graf, PhD, D(ABMM)[a,b,*]

[a]Department of Pathology and Laboratory Medicine, Children's Hospital of Philadelphia, 3401 Civic Center Boulevard, Philadelphia, PA 19104, USA; [b]Department of Pathology and Laboratory Medicine, Perelman School of Medicine at the University of Pennsylvania, Philadelphia, PA, USA; [c]Department of Pathology and Laboratory Medicine, Children's Hospital of Pittsburgh of UPMC, 4401 Penn Avenue, Main Hospital, Floor B, #269, Pittsburgh, PA 15224, USA; [d]Department of Pathology, University of Pittsburgh, School of Medicine, Pittsburgh, PA, USA

KEYWORDS

- Diagnostic metagenomics • Shotgun sequencing • Pathogen enrichment • Bioinformatics for metagenomics
- Contamination in metagenomics

KEY POINTS

- The low relative proportion of microbial nucleic acid, large number and incomplete catalog of reference genomes, and high rates of microbial nucleic acid contamination are challenges unique to diagnostic metagenomics.
- Enrichment of pathogen sequence over the background of human nucleic acid is an area of intense focus, but numerous published methods suffer from limitations and most show modest improvement.
- False-positive results are common in diagnostic metagenomics without careful control during the wet bench and analysis steps.
- There is a lack of standardization throughout all aspects of diagnostic metagenomics from sequence enrichment to data analysis.

INTRODUCTION

Culture remains the gold standard for the detection of many pathogens in diagnostic microbiology laboratories. Although culture is largely unbiased, it is insensitive and takes several days to weeks to provide a definitive result. Commercially available syndromic molecular panels (see Ryan F. Relich and April N. Abbott article, "Syndromic and Point of Care Molecular Testing", in this issue) provide rapid turnaround times and highly improved sensitivity compared with culture but, despite a large number of targets, are still biased to the most common or likely pathogens in a given source, limiting their clinical sensitivity. Moreover, only a limited number of sample types are approved by the US Food and Drug Administration for syndromic panels, restricting the clinical application of this approach. Given the current testing limitations, massively parallel sequencing-based assays have emerged as a single "test" that allows for simultaneous, and potentially highly sensitive, detection of all possible pathogens (bacteria, viruses, fungi, and parasites) in any sample type. In recognition of this promise, a large number of case reports and proof-of-concept studies have shown this technology's tremendous

Disclosure Statement: The authors listed have nothing to disclose.

[1] Present address: 3400 Spruce Street, Philadelphia, PA 19103.

*Corresponding author. 3401 Civic Center Boulevard, Philadelphia, PA 19104. *E-mail address:* grafe@email.chop.edu

https://doi.org/10.1016/j.yamp.2018.07.001
2589-4080/18/

clinical value by identifying etiologic agents that would have gone undetected by conventional testing [1–6]. The significance and impact of these clinical cases is expertly reviewed by Simner and colleagues [7]. In this review, we highlight select case reports and studies with focus on the impact of novel methods and analysis strategies on diagnostic microbiology.

SIGNIFICANCE

Metagenomics is the study of all genetic material (RNA and/or DNA) as it exists in a particular location or environment, such as a soil, seawater, or the human nasopharynx. Owing to the mixed nature of microbial communities, metagenomic studies historically were accomplished via amplification of conserved targets, cloning, and Sanger sequencing. Although meaningful clinical results could be derived from these approaches in humans [8], these methods were far too costly, laborious, and slow for clinical diagnostic application. The introduction of next-generation sequencing technologies over the last decade, associated simplified sample preparation methods, and subsequent dramatic decreases in sequencing costs per base have made diagnostic applications of metagenomics realistic. For the purposes of this review, we refer to this approach as metagenomic deep sequencing (MDS) because multiple technologies for massively parallel sequencing are now being applied to clinical diagnostics making the term next generation obsolete.

Deep sequencing has been used for the clinical diagnosis of genetic diseases for almost a decade. However, the application of this technology to infectious diseases suffers from distinctly different methods challenges. Unlike human genomics, human DNA is not of primary interest for diagnostic metagenomics, although it vastly predominates all clinical samples. Second, microbial contamination is inevitable and can arise from many sources, impacting results. Third, human genomics requires only 1 reference genome, whereas diagnostic metagenomics requires thousands of reference genomes, with a large number of pathogen genomes not yet sequenced or available for reference. This section reviews these topics; all of the methods described herein undoubtedly bias MDS and should be considered when reviewing clinical studies and case reports.

STRATEGIES TO OVERCOME THE ABUNDANCE OF HUMAN NUCLEIC ACIDS

Regardless of the sample type, human nucleic acids dominate the reads obtained by MDS for both DNAseq and RNAseq. This factor is most acute for highly human-cellular samples, such as tissues and sources with inflammatory responses in the setting of infection, but also presents a challenge for acellular sites such as plasma. In numerous clinical studies applying shotgun MDS to a variety of sample types, human reads typically constitute more than 99% of the data [1,2,4–6,9–12], limiting the recovery of rare pathogen sequence. Compensating through deeper sequencing can improve sensitivity, but comes at significant financial cost and potential time delay. Given that the majority of data in these shotgun datasets are ignored, there is tremendous focus on developing methods to enrich for pathogen nucleic acids before sequencing. These strategies are briefly described herein and compared in Table 1. Approaches range from user-friendly, commercially available kits to highly customized and complex laboratory developed methods.

Negative selection approaches include differential centrifugation to pellet human cells, most commonly applied to urine specimens [13], filtration of fluids to exclude larger human cells [14,15], and detergent-based selective lysis followed by enzymatic degradation of human nucleic acids [16,17]. The latter method has shown variable improvement from zero to several thousand-fold enrichment of pathogen sequence [3,16,17] and was recently used to discover a novel cause of chronic prosthetic joint infection. Thoendel and colleagues [3] applied differential lysis to fluid derived from sonication of the explanted prosthetic joint and obtained 1796 reads (0.0064% of total reads) aligning with *Mycoplasma salivarium*. However, this identification was confirmed without differential lysis, with 0.0084% of reads aligning with *M salivarium*, showing no benefit to enrichment. The variability of differential lysis efficiency may be due to differences in sample types, pathogens, and/or specific methods. Importantly, commercially available differential lysis kits also lyse virus particles, eliminating viral nucleic acid. All of these approaches require intact human cells and cannot remove nucleic acid from previously degraded cells. Consequently, these methods still result in greater than 90% of reads of human origin in the majority of clinical samples. Furthermore, these methods would not be appropriate for studies attempting to sequence intracellular pathogens [18].

Depletion of human nucleic acid via selective binding of methylated CpG DNA or probes targeting human ribosomal RNA have also shown variable performance, with almost no effect to 150-fold enrichment of bacterial or viral sequence [15,16,19–21]. A similar method takes advantage of the clustered regularly interspaced short palindromic repeats (CRISPR)/Cas9 system of

TABLE 1
Select Enrichment Approaches

	Pathogen Enrichment Method	Fold-Enrichment of Pathogen Sequence [References]	Limitations
Negative selection	Differential lysis of human cells	None to 9580× [3,16,17]	Requires intact cells, may remove viral nucleic acid
	Methylated CpG depletion	10× to 85× [16,20]	Eukaryotic pathogens can have high levels of methylated cytosines
	Human rRNA targeted probes	1.3× to150× [15,21]	Can result in depletion of eukaryotic pathogen rRNA
	CRISPR/Cas9	3.6× to10.3× [23]	Limited to RNAseq libraries
Positive selection	Amplification	1000× to >100,000× [25]	Must know sequence(s) of interest, reads will only contain what is amplified
	Bait capture	100× to 10,000× [15,30]	Expensive and time consuming (16-h incubation), may not be practical for all pathogens

Abbreviation: rRNA, ribosomal RNA.

targeted editing [22] to cleave specific short sequences from prepared libraries, resulting in noncleaved library amplification. Application to cerebrospinal fluid (CSF) samples, targeting subunits of human mitochondrial ribosomal RNA shown to be abundant in the same CSF samples, resulted in a 3- to 10-fold enrichment of pathogen sequence [23]. A kit-based human ribosomal RNA targeted CRISPR/Cas9 showed similar efficiency in plasma [24]. Doan and colleagues [4] applied this technique to ocular fluid, resulting in the detection of an unexpected pathogen in a case of chronic uveitis with numerous negative diagnostic tests. Sampling aqueous fluid from the right eye and vitreous fluid from the left eye, they detected 585 and 10 unique read pairs, respectively, of Rubella virus. Although this study shows the promise of the depletion method, the read counts of Rubella virus, and other known pathogens from samples included as positive controls, were still less than 1% of the total reads. Further, the CRISPR/Cas9 approach is only suited for RNAseq, because designing probes targeting the entire human genome is currently impractical for DNAseq.

Positive selection approaches include amplification of a few or many regions of microbial genomes and probe-hybridization capture. Amplicon sequencing, also referred to as targeted metagenomics, is one of the most efficient methods to reduce background human DNA (reviewed in Figure 2 of Simner and colleagues [7]) with reports of up to 100,000-fold enrichment [25]. This approach is the basis of microbiome studies targeting the 16S bacterial ribosome to estimate bacterial diversity. Amplification of the same target sequences has been used to detect bacterial pathogen sequence in synovial fluid from prosthetic joint infections [26] and blood from septic children [27], but with little to no improvement over culture. Larger primer sets targeting conserved regions of viruses have also been described to selectively amplify specific virus families present in a sample [25,28,29]. Although some of these methods may improve detection, they lead to significant bias, because the resulting sequence data will include only the region(s) amplified, which may not provide enough resolution to determine species-level identification and may not capture relevant antimicrobial resistance genes.

Solution-based bait–capture methods are well-described for human genomic diagnostics. Many small nucleic acid probes with designed complementarity tiled across a region of interest can pull out relevant DNA or RNA (complementary DNA) sequence, via streptavidin coupling, at extremely high specificity. For example, the human exome can be enriched several thousand-fold via bait–capture. Analogous probe sets have been designed targeting all vertebrate viruses with similar efficiency [15,30]. Importantly, these methods showed efficient enrichment even when virus sequences were approximately 40% different from the reference sequence used to generate the probe set, suggesting that highly divergent or perhaps novel viruses may be captured by these systems, a concern unique to diagnostic metagenomics. In another study, probe sets derived directly from extracted or amplified bacterial or viral (respectively) nucleic acid also showed efficient enrichment of pathogen RNA [31]. Unfortunately, despite being the most efficient enrichment approach to date aside from amplicon sequencing, bait–capture methods are expensive, time consuming, and require a large amount of high-quality starting material, requiring most diagnostic metagenomics studies to pool samples before hybridization, which is not yet practical for clinical diagnostic use owing to low sample throughput. Furthermore, capture of all possible pathogen sequences is impractical. Thus, studies targeting conserved regions common to groups of bacterial, fungal, and parasitic pathogens are needed to evaluate enrichment of these groups and potential bias.

Many of the approaches described herein can increase the overall contribution of microbial nucleic acid for analysis, but they all have limitations and associated biases (see Table 1); as a result, deeper sequencing may still be the preferred method. Additionally, many of these methods result in low amounts of DNA and/or RNA (complementary DNA) to carry in to library preparation or sequencing, often requiring secondary amplification that will add additional bias, selecting for libraries with smaller insert sizes. As stated in a recent review [32], more efficient and practical methods are needed. Finally, standardization of these approaches may become important as MDS evolves in diagnostic microbiology.

FACTORS THAT INFLUENCE THE ACCURACY OF DIAGNOSTIC METAGENOMICS

Contamination

Contamination with microbial nucleic acids is a well-described problem for MDS [33–36] (Table 2). Sources of contamination include introduction of environmental organisms and/or host flora at the time of specimen collection or later processing steps, a problem also shared by culture. Other preanalytical sources include nucleic acids present in containers or solutions used to collect patient samples. Contamination can also occur during the analytical phase within the laboratory, such as sample-to-sample contamination during nucleic acid extraction, library preparation, and/or cluster generation and microbial nucleic acids present in various laboratory reagents. With such a large window for contamination, appropriate negative controls are essential to pinpoint microbial signatures of contamination, which can be computationally and statistically managed at later stages of analysis. For example, a water-only control included at the step of nucleic acid extraction may capture reagent contamination but would miss contamination from sample collection processes and thus could lead to false-positive results. Several reports of possible or probable false-positive MDS results owing to contamination have been described. These include microbiome dysbiosis in the brain tissue of individuals with multiple sclerosis [37] as well as virus discovery in patients with hepatitis of unknown etiology [35,38].

TABLE 2
Sources of False-Positive Results and Recommended Controls for Analysis

Sources of False-Positive Reads [References]	Controls [References]
Sample contamination during collection, processing [45]	Uninfected samples collected and processed in the same manner
Reagent contamination [33–36]	No template control (eg, water)
Sample-to-sample contamination [9,12]	Contamination analysis software [56], orthogonal confirmation
Sequencer errors [39]	PhiX or other positive control
Bioinformatic pipeline error [33,39,45]	Manual analysis of positive hits, orthogonal confirmation

Even with controls that can detect known sources of contamination, the challenge remains to interpret results in this context. This concern is particularly important in samples with minimal starting nucleic acids, which are much more prone to domination by contaminating microbial nucleic acids (Fig. 1). To truly differentiate contamination from pathogen detection, computational methods are needed. Statistical approaches have been described to capture these contamination signatures and interpret test sample reads using specific cutoff criteria. One report validated a cutoff of a greater than 10-fold difference

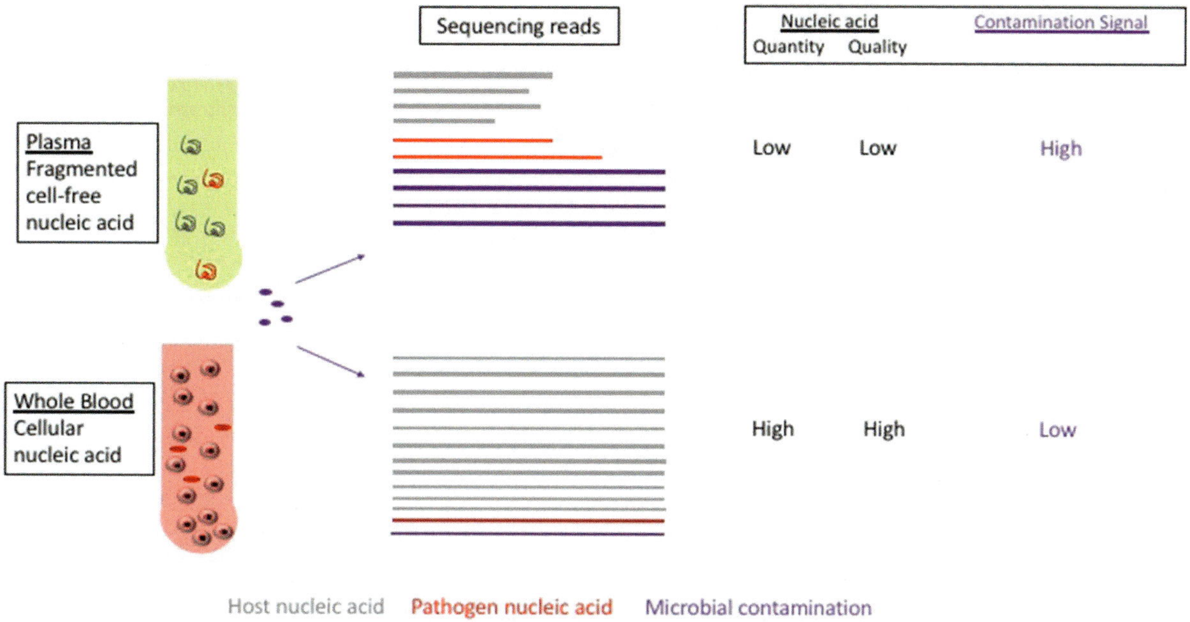

FIG. 1 Impact of contamination on samples with low nucleic acid input. Human nucleic acid is present at low levels in plasma and is highly degraded and fragmented (*top*). When libraries are prepared from this matrix, contaminating microbial nucleic acids may overwhelm the sequence data, masking the presence of pathogen reads. In contrast, whole blood contains high quantities of intact human chromosomes (*bottom*), producing better quality libraries and reducing the signal from contamination; however, pathogen sequence may be masked by the predominance of human reads.

when comparing reads of putative pathogen (per million total reads [RPM]) in the CSF to RPM of the same putative pathogen in a no-template control [39]. In another report, also applying diagnostic metagenomics to CSF, the authors compiled a large sampling of water controls and uninfected CSF samples, some from a subset of patients with noninfectious meningitis, to calculate an expected RPM for a given genus or species. They then applied these data to a Z-score based calculation to rank taxa detected in samples with suspected central nervous system infection. In a proof-of-concept case series, they were able to correctly rank top taxa compared with conventional diagnostic microbiology results. This included 1 case of *Histoplasma capsulatum* meningitis with just 33 read-pairs obtained via MDS. Although these proof-of-concept experiments have shown promise, the methods are highly individualized to the datasets within each study and may not be generalizable to all diagnostic metagenomics approaches. As with enrichment approaches, standardization of statistical approaches to interpret patient results in the setting of unavoidable contamination may become important.

Bioinformatics

A number of web-based and commercially available as well as published pipelines exist to process and analyze MDS data. A comprehensive review of each is not possible here, but readers should refer to the following citations for examples of commonly used pipelines [13,40–43]. Most are based on alignment to large databases of reference genomes, referred to as resequencing. An initial filter step removes human reads and then most analyze snapshots of length "k," called k-mers, from remaining reads to assign them to the lowest taxonomic level. In some pipelines analysis may be done at the protein coding level to provide more sensitive detection of divergent pathogens, particularly viruses. The sensitivity of a pipeline is depends on the reference sequences included in its database. As recently described by Greninger and colleagues [44], a particular pipeline would have missed identification of *Balamuthia mandrillaris* in a CSF sample owing to the fact that a whole genome reference sequence was not yet published for that organism. Specificity depends on a number of factors, including the length of the k-mer used for taxonomic classification as well as the efficiency of the initial human read filter. In the latter case, human reads that slip through often are misclassified to eukaryotic organisms that share some sequence homology. For example, in a few studies, human reads were misclassified as the parasite *Toxoplasma gondii*, which could have led to a false-positive diagnosis if not realized by manual analysis [33,45]; this concept is illustrated in Fig. 2. The error rate of the sequencer as well as the length of reads (number of cycles of sequencing) will also impact specificity. Although shorter reads reduce cost and turnaround time, they may contain fewer signature sequences to resolve species or even genus-level differences.

REGULATORY ASPECTS OF METAGENOMIC DEEP SEQUENCING

Despite the tremendous enthusiasm for MDS in the clinical microbiology laboratory, this approach has primarily been applied in research studies, with very few clinically validated diagnostic MDS tests. As MDS grows in clinical diagnostics, standards and guidelines for assay design, validation, and interpretation are acutely needed for the appropriate clinical implementation of this complex methodology, expertly reviewed by Schlaberg and colleagues [39] and Gargis and colleagues [46]. Human genomic diagnostics has primarily addressed deep sequencing validation by using a methods-based approach where a specific depth of coverage and quality metrics requirements must be reproducibly achieved for the genomic region of interest. Because diagnostic MDS relies on the detection of rare pathogen sequence, a primary feature will be to determine the number of sequencing reads required to achieve accurate results. In a recent review, a cutoff of just 3 reads, spanning 3 different genomic regions of a given virus, was validated for viral diagnosis in CSF [39]. Cutoffs will likely need to be sample-type and pathogen specific owing to overlap with the human genome or closely related nonpathogenic strains. These values can be derived empirically by spiking known microbes into various sample types, but endless combinations exist and not all can be practically tested. The risk of not testing all combinations is well illustrated in the same review by Schlaberg and colleagues [39] (see Figure 2 in that article). In this review, a simulated library was created containing dolphin morbillivirus "RNA" demonstrating alignment along many locations of the closely related measles virus genome, suggesting this hypothetical library could have been misclassified, potentially resulting in a very inaccurate diagnosis. Because validation of every possible pathogen and closely related genomes is not practical, alternative approaches may be needed. This process could include manual analysis with defined criteria and/or confirmation of positive results with a secondary method. Human genomics uses the latter approach to confirm pathogenic mutations via Sanger sequencing, although with more practice and comfort with these complex methodologies, this step is beginning to be used less often. The time frame of infections and endless possibilities for primer design make molecular confirmation approaches unrealistic for diagnostic microbiology.

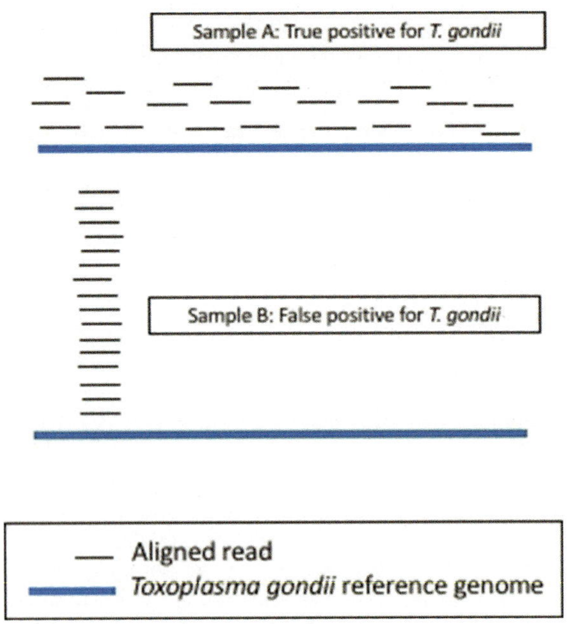

FIG. 2 Misclassification of human reads to a pathogen genome. A hypothetical example of manual alignment analysis of a sample with *Toxoplasma gondii* nucleic acid (*top*) and a sample with human reads misclassified as *T gondii* (*bottom*). In sample A, reads span different regions of the *T gondii* genome, whereas in sample B, reads stack in a single locus that shares identity with human nucleic acid. The latter would lead to a potential misdiagnosis if produced by a bioinformatic pipeline without manual review.

Owing to the complex readout of MDS data, significant efforts will be needed to define the normal microbial composition of each anatomic site and what constitutes dysbiosis. Defining normal variation is also a significant challenge in human genomics, which is being addressed by collecting genomic data from many thousands of individuals from many ancestries and making the dataset publicly available [47]. Similar data sharing efforts have been initiated by the Human Microbiome Project [48] and will be essential to broader implementation of MDS. In a strategy similar to conventional microbial culture, quantitative sequence information may play a role in interpretation. Several studies have published correlations between normalized reads of pathogens via MDS compared with pathogen loads determined by quantitative polymerase chain reaction [11,12,15]. Validation of quantitative MDS tests may prove most important for the interpretation of bacterial and/or fungal sequences found in nonsterile sources. Host response signatures may also aid in the interpretation of this complex data in nonsterile as well as sterile sites. Several studies have analyzed human gene expression in a variety of clinical conditions to attempt to identify pathogen-specific [49–51] or even genus-specific [52] markers. These approaches are a long way from widespread application. Further, as stated elsewhere in this article, RNAseq data obtained from diagnostic MDS may not contain relevant host messenger RNA reads for transcriptional profiling, thus, requiring additional methods optimization and validation.

Finally, the availability of microbial reference genome sequences is exponentially increasing, but remains incomplete. As described elsewhere in this article, many studies have pointed out reference genomes either missing or incorrectly defined (eg, wrong species) from public and private databases that could lead to false-negative or incorrect diagnoses. As databases evolve, there may be a role for reanalysis of MDS data to detect new pathogens previously missed or incorrectly identified. Although the time frame is not practical for most infectious conditions, it may help to identify novel pathogen associations.

PRESENT RELEVANCE AND FUTURE AVENUES TO CONSIDER OR TO INVESTIGATE

The common theme between the clinical studies, methods considerations, and regulatory aspects discussed in this review is the lack of standardization for diagnostic MDS. Furthermore, the accuracy of MDS as a standalone assay is limited by the presence and quantity of pathogen nucleic acid and reference databases used. Indeed, MDS may never be sensitive enough if the pathogen quantity is too low to be detected over background contamination or if the pathogen nucleic acid present is not informatically recognized. Furthermore, very few studies have applied MDS to large clinical cohorts to determine how often MDS provides a negative or uninterpretable result, particularly in a prospective setting. These data are needed to establish the clinical usefulness and limitations of this approach before widespread adoption of this methodology for clinical diagnostics is possible.

The primary additional barriers to widespread adoption of diagnostic MDS include cost and time. If diagnostic MDS is reserved only for cases in which all other diagnostic testing has proved to be negative, this would result in a small number of rare cases for most hospitals. Validation of an assay that would be used a handful of times per year may not be cost effective enough to justify internal adoption over send-out to a reference laboratory. A more practical short-term alternative would be to embed clinical MDS testing within genomic laboratories that already perform clinical deep sequencing, where MDS can benefit from higher sample flux in the sample preparation and sequencing steps, helping to reduce assay cost and turnaround time. However, this process may still require a costly validation for an infrequently used method and typical turnaround times for human genomic deep sequencing assays are currently days to weeks longer than infectious disease molecular testing. To justify adoption within clinical molecular microbiology operations, laboratories could start to examine whether other assays, such as syndromic polymerase chain reaction panels with double digit targets could be replaced with diagnostic MDS. For MDS to replace current polymerase chain reaction panels, the turnaround time may have to be on the scale of an hour, including library preparation. Deep sequencing platforms are emerging to meet these needs [53], but have not been clinically implemented to date. Despite these current impediments, the additional information gained via MDS could make this method more attractive to replace current polymerase chain reaction panels. For example, real-time tracking of viral or bacterial sequence could flag an outbreak earlier than current surveillance methods [54] and the detection of resistance markers could be performed at the time of pathogen detection [55].

SUMMARY

Given the tremendous clinical promise, MDS will no doubt find its place in the future of infectious disease diagnostics. The technical and interpretive challenges outlined in this review require careful consideration by laboratories adopting this methodology. The standardization of wet bench and informatics approaches between laboratories and/or in collaboration with professional organizations and regulatory agencies may also ensure the best outcomes for patient care.

REFERENCES

[1] Mongkolrattanothai K, Naccache SN, Bender JM, et al. Neurobrucellosis: unexpected answer from metagenomic next-generation sequencing. J Pediatric Infect Dis Soc 2017;6(4):393–8.

[2] Wilson MR, Naccache SN, Samayoa E, et al. Actionable diagnosis of neuroleptospirosis by next-generation sequencing. N Engl J Med 2014;370(25):2408–17.

[3] Thoendel M, Jeraldo P, Greenwood-Quaintance KE, et al. A novel prosthetic joint infection pathogen, Mycoplasma salivarium, identified by metagenomic shotgun sequencing. Clin Infect Dis 2017;65(2):332–5.

[4] Doan T, Wilson MR, Crawford ED, et al. Illuminating uveitis: metagenomic deep sequencing identifies common and rare pathogens. Genome Med 2016;8(1):90.

[5] Naccache SN, Peggs KS, Mattes FM, et al. Diagnosis of neuroinvasive astrovirus infection in an immunocompromised adult with encephalitis by unbiased next-generation sequencing. Clin Infect Dis 2015;60(6):919–23.

[6] Wilson MR, Suan D, Duggins A, et al. A novel cause of chronic viral meningoencephalitis: Cache Valley virus. Ann Neurol 2017;82(1):105–14.

[7] Simner PJ, Miller S, Carroll KC. Understanding the promises and hurdles of metagenomic next-generation sequencing as a diagnostic tool for infectious diseases. Clin Infect Dis 2018;66(5):778–88.

[8] Finkbeiner SR, Allred AF, Tarr PI, et al. Metagenomic analysis of human diarrhea: viral detection and discovery. PLoS Pathog 2008;4(2):e1000011.

[9] Doan T, Acharya NR, Pinsky BA, et al. Metagenomic DNA sequencing for the diagnosis of intraocular infections. Ophthalmology 2017;124(8):1247–8.

[10] Mai NTH, Phu NH, Nhu LNT, et al. Central nervous system infection diagnosis by next-generation sequencing: a glimpse into the future? Open Forum Infect Dis 2017; 4(2):ofx046.

[11] Zhou Y, Wylie KM, El Feghaly RE, et al. Metagenomic approach for identification of the pathogens associated with diarrhea in stool specimens. J Clin Microbiol 2016;54(2):368–75.

[12] Graf EH, Simmon KE, Tardif KD, et al. Unbiased detection of respiratory viruses by use of RNA sequencing-based metagenomics: a systematic comparison to a commercial PCR panel. J Clin Microbiol 2016;54(4):1000–7.

[13] Janes VAMS, Willemse N, Visser CE, et al. Metagenomic sequencing to replace semi-quantitative urine culture for detection of urinary tract infections: a proof of concept. bioRxivorg 2017. https://doi.org/10.1101/178178.

[14] Rosseel T, Ozhelvaci O, Freimanis G, et al. Evaluation of convenient pretreatment protocols for RNA virus metagenomics in serum and tissue samples. J Virol Methods 2015;222:72–80.

[15] Briese T, Kapoor A, Mishra N, et al. Virome capture sequencing enables sensitive viral diagnosis and comprehensive virome analysis. MBio 2015;6(5): e01491-15.

[16] Thoendel M, Jeraldo PR, Greenwood-Quaintance KE, et al. Comparison of microbial DNA enrichment tools for metagenomic whole genome sequencing. J Microbiol Methods 2016;127:141–5.

[17] Hasan MR, Rawat A, Tang P, et al. Depletion of human DNA in spiked clinical specimens for improvement of sensitivity of pathogen detection by next-generation sequencing. J Clin Microbiol 2016;54(4):919–27.

[18] Graham RMA, Donohue S, McMahon J, et al. Detection of spotted fever group rickettsia DNA by deep sequencing. Emerg Infect Dis 2017;23(11):1911–3.

[19] Street TL, Sanderson ND, Atkins BL, et al. Molecular diagnosis of orthopedic-device-related infection directly from sonication fluid by metagenomic sequencing. J Clin Microbiol 2017;55(8):2334–47.

[20] Feehery GR, Yigit E, Oyola SO, et al. A method for selectively enriching microbial DNA from contaminating vertebrate host DNA. PLoS One 2013;8(10):e76096.

[21] Manso CF, Bibby DF, Mbisa JL. Efficient and unbiased metagenomic recovery of RNA virus genomes from human plasma samples. Sci Rep 2017;7(1):4173.

[22] Cong L, Ran FA, Cox D, et al. Multiplex genome engineering using CRISPR/Cas systems. Science 2013; 339(6121):819–23.

[23] Gu W, Crawford ED, O'Donovan BD, et al. Depletion of abundant sequences by hybridization (DASH): using Cas9 to remove unwanted high-abundance species in sequencing libraries and molecular counting applications. Genome Biol 2016;17:41.

[24] Pan W, Ngo TTM, Camunas-Soler J, et al. Simultaneously monitoring immune response and microbial Infections during Pregnancy through Plasma cfRNA sequencing. Clin Chem 2017;63(11):1695–704.

[25] Brinkmann A, Ergunay K, Radonic A, et al. Development and preliminary evaluation of a multiplexed amplification and next generation sequencing method for viral hemorrhagic fever diagnostics. PLoS Negl Trop Dis 2017;11(11):e0006075.

[26] Tarabichi M, Shohat N, Goswami K, et al. Diagnosis of periprosthetic joint infection: the potential of next-generation sequencing. J Bone Joint Surg Am 2018; 100(2):147–54.

[27] Decuypere S, Meehan CJ, Van Puyvelde S, et al. Diagnosis of bacterial bloodstream infections: a 16S metagenomics approach. PLoS Negl Trop Dis 2016;10(2): e0004470.

[28] McGinnis J, Laplante J, Shudt M, et al. Next generation sequencing for whole genome analysis and surveillance of influenza A viruses. J Clin Virol 2016; 79:44–50.

[29] Tan le V, Tuyen NT, Thanh TT, et al. A generic assay for whole-genome amplification and deep sequencing of enterovirus A71. J Virol Methods 2015;215-216:30–6.

[30] Wylie TN, Wylie KM, Herter BN, et al. Enhanced virome sequencing using targeted sequence capture. Genome Res 2015;25(12):1910–20.

[31] Bent ZW, Tran-Gyamfi MB, Langevin SA, et al. Enriching pathogen transcripts from infected samples: a capture-based approach to enhanced host-pathogen RNA sequencing. Anal Biochem 2013;438(1):90–6.

[32] Schlaberg R. Toward noninvasive probing of maternal-fetal-microbial interactions during pregnancy. Clin Chem 2017;63(11):1669–70.

[33] Thoendel M, Jeraldo P, Greenwood-Quaintance KE, et al. Impact of contaminating DNA in whole-genome amplification kits used for metagenomic shotgun sequencing for infection diagnosis. J Clin Microbiol 2017;55(6): 1789–801.

[34] Moustafa A, Xie C, Kirkness E, et al. The blood DNA virome in 8,000 humans. PLoS Pathog 2017;13(3): e1006292.

[35] Naccache SN, Greninger AL, Lee D, et al. The perils of pathogen discovery: origin of a novel parvovirus-like hybrid genome traced to nucleic acid extraction spin columns. J Virol 2013;87(22):11966–77.

[36] Strong MJ, Xu G, Morici L, et al. Microbial contamination in next generation sequencing: implications for sequence-based analysis of clinical samples. PLoS Pathog 2014; 10(11):e1004437.

[37] Wilson MROD, BD, Gelfand JM, et al. Metagenomics for chronic meningitis: clarifying interpretation and diagnosis. bioRxivorg 2018. https://doi.org/10.1101/213561.

[38] Naccache SN, Hackett J Jr, Delwart EL, et al. Concerns over the origin of NIH-CQV, a novel virus discovered in Chinese patients with seronegative hepatitis. Proc Natl Acad Sci U S A 2014;111(11):E976.

[39] Schlaberg R, Chiu CY, Miller S, et al. Validation of metagenomic next-generation sequencing tests for universal pathogen detection. Arch Pathol Lab Med 2017;141(6): 776–86.

[40] Flygare S, Simmon K, Miller C, et al. Taxonomer: an interactive metagenomics analysis portal for universal pathogen detection and host mRNA expression profiling. Genome Biol 2016;17(1):111.

[41] Naccache SN, Federman S, Veeraraghavan N, et al. A cloud-compatible bioinformatics pipeline for ultrarapid pathogen identification from next-generation sequencing of clinical samples. Genome Res 2014; 24(7):1180–92.

[42] Wood DE, Salzberg SL. Kraken: ultrafast metagenomic sequence classification using exact alignments. Genome Biol 2014;15(3):R46.

[43] Minot SSKN, Greenfield NB. One codex: a sensitive and accurate data platform for genomic microbial identification. bioRxivorg 2015. https://doi.org/10.1101/027607.

[44] Greninger AL, Messacar K, Dunnebacke T, et al. Clinical metagenomic identification of Balamuthia mandrillaris encephalitis and assembly of the draft genome: the continuing case for reference genome sequencing. Genome Med 2015;7:113.

[45] Clarke EL, Lauder AP, Hofstaedter CE, et al. Microbial lineages in sarcoidosis. a metagenomic analysis tailored for low-microbial content samples. Am J Respir Crit Care Med 2018;197(2):225–34.

[46] Gargis AS, Kalman L, Lubin IM. Assuring the quality of next-generation sequencing in clinical microbiology and public health laboratories. J Clin Microbiol 2016; 54(12):2857–65.

[47] Lek M, Karczewski KJ, Minikel EV, et al. Analysis of protein-coding genetic variation in 60,706 humans. Nature 2016;536(7616):285–91.

[48] Human Microbiome Project C. A framework for human microbiome research. Nature 2012;486(7402): 215–21.

[49] Gliddon HD, Herberg JA, Levin M, et al. Genome-wide host RNA signatures of infectious diseases: discovery and clinical translation. Immunology 2018;153(2): 171–8.

[50] Herberg JA, Kaforou M, Wright VJ, et al. Diagnostic test accuracy of a 2-transcript host RNA signature for discriminating bacterial vs viral infection in febrile children. JAMA 2016;316(8):835–45.

[51] Hu X, Yu J, Crosby SD, et al. Gene expression profiles in febrile children with defined viral and bacterial infection. Proc Natl Acad Sci U S A 2013;110(31): 12792–7.

[52] Zaas AK, Chen M, Varkey J, et al. Gene expression signatures diagnose influenza and other symptomatic respiratory viral infections in humans. Cell Host Microbe 2009; 6(3):207–17.

[53] Judge K, Harris SR, Reuter S, et al. Early insights into the potential of the Oxford Nanopore MinION for the detection of antimicrobial resistance genes. J Antimicrob Chemother 2015;70(10):2775–8.

[54] Greninger AL, Waghmare A, Adler A, et al. Rule-out outbreak: 24-hour metagenomic next-generation sequencing for characterizing respiratory virus source for infection prevention. J Pediatric Infect Dis Soc 2017;6(2):168–72.

[55] Andersen H, Connolly N, Bangar H, et al. Use of shotgun metagenome sequencing to detect fecal colonization with multidrug-resistant bacteria in children. J Clin Microbiol 2016;54(7):1804–13.

[56] Jun G, Flickinger M, Hetrick KN, et al. Detecting and estimating contamination of human DNA samples in sequencing and array-based genotype data. Am J Hum Genet 2012;91(5):839–48.

Advances in Molecular Pathology 1 (2018) 91–96
ADVANCES IN MOLECULAR PATHOLOGY

Replacement of Culture with Molecular Testing for Diagnosis Infectious Diseases

Gerald A. Capraro, PhD
Clinical Microbiology Laboratory, Carolinas Pathology Group, Atrium Health, 5040 Airport Center Parkway, Building H, Suite A, Charlotte, NC 28208, USA

KEYWORDS
• Molecular diagnostics • PCR • Culture • Turnaround time • Improvement • Quality

KEY POINTS
- Molecular diagnostics are more sensitive and specific than traditional culture-based testing and there are many successful examples where nucleic acid amplification testing has replaced culture.
- Current, commercially available molecular testing has the capability to be performed in traditional microbiology laboratories, but laboratories would have to decide what makes sense for their facility.
- A thoughtful approach to the implementation of molecular testing is necessary when deciding to transition from culture to molecular testing.

INTRODUCTION

Despite significant advances in molecular testing platforms, in vitro cultivation of microbial pathogens on artificial media remains a hallmark of infectious disease diagnostics. Culture-based approaches allow for the recovery, identification, and antimicrobial susceptibility testing of a specific pathogen. However, there are many limitations to the use of culture. The growth of an organism can take days to weeks; definitive testing for identification can be performed only on pure culture or isolated colony, which may introduce additional delays; some organisms cannot be cultivated in vitro (eg, some viruses, parasites) or have specialized growth requirements that cannot be met by most routine clinical microbiology laboratories (eg, *Mycoplasma* species). Ultimately, culture is labor intensive and is associated with long turnaround times. Molecular testing has exquisite sensitivity and specificity and is associated with faster turnaround times. Limitations of molecular assays include high cost, the need for specific primer sequences based on an a priori knowledge of the pathogen target sequence, and laboratory personnel with specific expertise in molecular techniques. Nonetheless, there are many areas where laboratories have transitioned away from culture-based pathogen detection to molecular methods. This article discusses the considerations for adoption of molecular assays as a replacement (in whole or in part) for culture, and to highlight examples where this approach has been successfully implemented.

DISCUSSION

The movement away from culture-based testing to molecular testing for infectious diseases largely began in academic medical centers and specialized reference

Disclosure Statement: The author serves on Advisory Boards for DiaSorin Molecular, BioRad, BD, and Roche Diagnostics. He has received research funding from Quidel, DiaSorin Molecular, and DiaGenode and speaking honoraria from Quidel.

E-mail address: gerald.capraro@carolinashealthcare.org

https://doi.org/10.1016/j.yamp.2018.07.002
2589-4080/18/

laboratories, which implemented laboratory-developed molecular testing. Recently, there has been a shift in adoption of commercially available, sample-to-answer testing platforms for more routine pathogens. The nature of these tests allows use by smaller community hospitals and other laboratories located outside of large systems and academic centers. The decision to migrate culture-based diagnostic testing to molecular testing must include an assessment of several factors, including test volume, analytical performance, workflow and throughput, availability of trained personnel, and cost. Regulatory and accreditation factors must also be taken into consideration.

Early adoption of molecular testing as a replacement for culture occurred in the diagnostic virology laboratory. The ability to read cytopathic effect in cell culture and identify specific viruses based on the cytopathic effect observed in various cell lines is an expert skill that has waned in laboratories over time owing to staff attrition and a shortage of new medical laboratory scientists who are interested in microbiology. This situation has caused a shift in virology testing to shorter turnaround time and shell vial cultures, which require their own level of expertise to read immunofluorescent stains. The loss of skilled personnel and the inability to propagate some viruses in culture in vitro led to the replacement of culture-based virology testing with molecular testing. Viruses such as human immunodeficiency virus, hepatitis A, hepatitis B, and hepatitis C were among the first molecular tests used both for the diagnosis of infection and monitoring of viral load over time to determine the effectiveness of antiviral therapy. Testing for other clinically important viruses soon shifted to molecular testing. Respiratory virus testing, for example, has largely transitioned to multiplex molecular panels that allow for a diagnosis of influenza virus A, influenza virus B, and respiratory syncytial virus (as well as other respiratory viruses for which there are no specific antiviral therapies, such as human metapneumovirus) from a single specimen in a single test. The diagnosis of infectious diarrhea has also shifted from culture, specialized microscopy, and rapid antigen testing methods to multiplex molecular gastrointestinal panels. Etiologic causes of infectious gastroenteritis include bacteria, viruses, and parasites, and clinical presentation typically does not allow for a specific diagnosis because diarrhea is the predominant symptom. Therefore, a battery of tests must be ordered, yet often the causative agent remains unidentified. Gastrointestinal panels provide the laboratory with a single test for a single specimen and yield results for a breadth of infectious agents. Performance of these culture-independent diagnostic tests is reported to be excellent [1,2], with a sensitivity of greater than 95% and a specificity of greater than 97%. Despite the improved turnaround time and improvement in the use of infection control practices [3], culture-independent diagnostic tests have created a quandary with regard to the public health [4]. The replacement of culture with culture-independent diagnostic tests has resulted in laboratories no longer routinely recovering isolates of *Salmonella* and other pathogens of public health importance, which must be submitted to public health laboratories for outbreak tracking and other epidemiologic purposes. Some states continue to require submission of an isolate to the public health laboratory, whereas others have allowed submission of the primary specimen that tested positive by a culture-independent diagnostic test. As laboratories work through this diagnostic transitional period, it is critical that the lines of communication between diagnostic laboratories and public health laboratories remain open.

One of the earliest transitions to molecular diagnostics for bacteria was for the sexually transmitted pathogens *Neisseria gonorrhoeae* and *Chlamydia trachomatis*. Molecular probe assays and polymerase chain reaction provide exquisite sensitivity and specificity and provide faster time to result compared with culture. Most laboratories now use molecular methods for the screening of patients with suspected *C trachomatis-N gonorrhoeae* infection. Several molecular assays cleared by the US Food and Drug Administration (FDA) are commercially available and demonstrate excellent performance for urogenital specimens from both males and females (Table 1). Infections in men who have sex with men and other high-risk patients can be diagnosed by testing oropharyngeal, ocular, and/or rectal specimens [5,6]. These alternative specimen types have not received FDA clearance; therefore, testing would require validation by individual laboratories. The drawback to molecular testing for these pathogens is that there is no isolate available for antimicrobial susceptibility testing. However, current standard therapeutic regimens recommended by the Centers for Disease Control and Prevention include ceftriaxone, 250 mg administered intramuscularly, and azithromycin, 1 g orally, for uncomplicated infection [7]. The gonococcal isolate surveillance project tracks resistance patterns in the United States by partnering with sexually transmitted disease clinics and publishing resistance patterns for various regions. Clinicians in these locales may rely on gonococcal isolate surveillance project data to provide appropriate empiric therapy of suspected gonorrhea infections.

TABLE 1
Commercially Available Nucleic Acid Amplification Tests for the Detection of *Neisseria gonorrhoeae* and *Chlamydia trachomatis*

Test Name	Manufacturer	Method	Specimen Types	Sensitivity (%)	Specificity (%)	References
BD ProbeTec	BD	SDA	U, ECS, US, V	>96	>99	[27]
Aptima Combo 2	Hologic	TMA	U, ECS, US, V	>94	>97	[28]
Abbott RealTime CT/NG	Abbott Molecular	PCR	U, ECS, US, V	>92	>99	[29]
Cobas 4800 CT/NG	Roche Molecular	PCR	U, ECS, V	>98	>99	[30]
Cepheid CT/NG Xpert	Cepheid	PCR	U, ECS, V	>95	>99	[31]

Abbreviations: ECS, endocervical swab; PCR, polymerase chain reaction; SDA, strand displacement amplification; TMA, transcription-mediated amplification; U, urine; US, urethral swab; V, vaginal swab.

In cases of suspected failure of empiric treatment, the Centers for Disease Control and Prevention recommend culture of appropriate specimens, with antimicrobial susceptibility testing of recovered gonococcal isolates [7]; however, with the transition to molecular testing, many laboratories no longer have the expertise or reagents to perform this testing on site and would have to send specimens to a reference laboratory.

The evolution of diagnostic tests for *Clostridioides difficile* [8] continues today. Anaerobic toxigenic culture methods were time consuming, and results were often reported too late during a patient's hospital course to make clinically actionable decisions. To shorten the turnaround time, culture was removed from the testing strategy, and toxin neutralization testing performed directly on filtered liquid stool became standard of care. However, this approach was labor intensive and was fraught with false-negative results. A liquid-based, enzyme-linked immunosorbent assay to determine the presence of *C difficile* toxin in a filtered stool specimen was fast and easy to perform and soon replaced toxin neutralization as the diagnostic modality of choice. This test was associated with an unacceptable rate of both false-positive and false-negative results, so to achieve an acceptable level of analytical sensitivity, 3 patient specimens were required. The lack of confidence in this test by clinicians led to a culture of repeat testing for *C difficile*, and the order for "Cdiff × 3" is something that laboratories still contend with. Currently, many laboratories have implemented a 2-step diagnostic algorithm for laboratory detection of *C difficile* [9] using an immunochromatographic cartridge to determine the presence of both the glutamate dehydrogenase enzyme and toxins A and B as a primary screen for *C difficile* infection, and molecular testing as the confirmatory assay for indeterminate results (ie, GDH-positive, toxin A/B-negative). The American Society for Microbiology and the Infectious Diseases Society of America have issued guidance documents to assist laboratories in this testing strategy [10,11]. The use of molecular testing as a standalone assay for *C difficile* detection has shown to be of benefit and can shorten the turnaround time compared with the multistep diagnostic algorithm; however, as with all *C difficile* testing, it is incumbent on the laboratory to restrict these tests to diarrheal stools only and to reject nonliquid stool specimens.

The use of molecular testing for *Mycobacterium tuberculosis* (MTB) complex organisms, which cause pulmonary disease, would not replace conventional culture methods, per se. It would, however, provide a rapid result to the clinician and infection preventionist and allow for the appropriate isolation of only those patients who test positive for MTB by molecular testing. Culture of the specimen would continue to be required to obtain an isolate for antimicrobial susceptibility testing. Molecular testing for MTB has performed well compared with culture, with a reported sensitivity and specificity of 98.6% and 100%, respectively [12]. Use of the Xpert MTB/RIF Ultra assay (Cepheid, Sunnyvale, CA), a second-generation molecular test with a shorter turnaround time was shown to have a sensitivity of 87.5% and a specificity of 98.7% compared with culture when used at the point of care [13]. This assay has decreased sensitivity against smear-negative pulmonary specimens; however, in cases of culture-confirmed tuberculosis where the acid fast bacillus smear was reported as negative, the Xpert MTB/RIF assay had a sensitivity of 73.1%, an improvement of 36.5%, and may be used to accurately diagnose pulmonary tuberculosis in low prevalence areas [14]. One limitation of the commercially available molecular tests for MTB is that only respiratory specimens have received FDA clearance. Individual laboratories would be required to self-validate other clinically relevant specimen types (eg, cerebrospinal fluid, kidney biopsy material) to report results obtained from these specimens, because this use of the test would be considered off label.

There are several commercially available nucleic acid amplification tests (NAATs) for the detection of *Streptococcus agalactiae* (group B *Streptococcus* [GBS]). Except for one, each of these requires a specimen to be inoculated to an enrichment broth, such as Todd Hewitt, Todd Hewitt with Colistin, and Nalidixic Acid (LIM Broth), or Carrot Broth, for an overnight incubation before being tested by the molecular assay, to allow for maximum analytical sensitivity and specificity. The lone commercial assay for the direct detection of GBS in clinical specimens is the Xpert GBS assay (Cepheid) and has a reported sensitivity of between 78% and 86% in published studies [15,16], which is inferior to polymerase chain reaction assays performed on enriched specimens. Other commercially available molecular assays for detection of GBS are shown in Table 2. The benefit to molecular detection of GBS is improved turnaround time and laboratory workflow, particularly if a colorimetric enrichment broth or other enhanced culture method is used [17–19]. Laboratories would need to continue to provide culture and susceptibility testing results for isolates from patients with penicillin allergy, so the complete replacement of GBS culture with molecular techniques may not be possible.

In a similar fashion, molecular tests for *Streptococcus pyogenes* (group A *Streptococcus*) are commercially available and present a significant improvement in turnaround time. Studies have shown these assays to have superior analytical performance as compared with rapid antigen detection assays [20,21] and they can be placed in the laboratory or located at the point of care (Table 3). With improved sensitivity, the need for culture confirmation of negative results may no longer be necessary [22].

From an infection prevention perspective, the use of molecular testing over culture for surveillance of specific pathogens presents the opportunity to act quickly to prevent the spread of communicable diseases and/or antimicrobial resistance mechanisms. Methicillin-resistant *Staphylococcus aureus*, vancomycin-resistant *Enterococcus* species, *C difficile*, carbapenem-resistant *Enterobacteriaceae*, and other multidrug-resistant organisms present significant threats to the health care environment. Hand hygiene plays a role in mitigating the spread of these organisms; however, organism-specific surveillance strategies can augment infection prevention strategies [23,24]. Some hospitals have chosen to screen patients upon admission and at certain regular frequencies to isolate or cohort colonized patients. Support from the microbiology laboratory is essential to the success of infection prevention strategies. Culture-based surveillance has been the presumed gold standard owing to its excellent specificity and relatively low cost to perform. Molecular assays for these organisms are now available and present improvements over culture in analytical performance, turnaround time, and laboratory workflow. Many results can be available in approximately 1 hour from receipt of the specimen, which allows for the rapid isolation of colonized patients and deisolation of patients found to be negative for colonization with multidrug-resistant organisms. In a similar fashion, patients scheduled for orthopedic or cardiac surgery may be screened for methicillin-resistant *S aureus* colonization. If found to be colonized, a treatment regimen including chlorhexidine and mupirocin leads to decolonization before the surgical

TABLE 2
Commercially Available Nucleic Acid Amplification Tests for the Detection of *Streptococcus agalactiae* (Group B *Streptococcus*)

Test Name	Manufacturer	Method	Sensitivity (%)	Specificity (%)	References
ARIES GBS Assay	Luminex	PCR	96	91	[32]
BD Max GBS Assay	BD	PCR	100	95.8	[33]
Xpert GBS Assay LB	Cepheid	PCR	99	92.4	[15]
Solana GBS Assay	Quidel	HDA	100	95.9	PI
Illumigene GBS Assay	Meridian Bioscience	LAMP	90.9	97.9	[33]

Abbreviations: HDA, helicase-dependent amplification; LAMP, loop-mediated isothermal amplification; PCR, polymerase chain reaction; PI, package insert (assay recently cleared by the US Food and Drug Administration).

TABLE 3
Commercially Available Nucleic Acid Amplification Tests for the Detection of *Streptococcus pyogenes* (Group A *Streptococcus*)

Test Name	Manufacturer	Method	Sensitivity (%)	Specificity (%)	References
Simplexa GAS Direct	DiaSorin Molecular	PCR	100	100	[34]
Cobas LIAT Strep A	Roche Molecular	PCR	97.7	93.3	[10]
Xpert Xpress Strep A	Cepheid	PCR	100	94.1	PI
Solana GAS Assay	Quidel	HDA	98.2	97.2	[35]
Illumigene GAS Assay	Meridian Bioscience	LAMP	100	99.2	[36]

Abbreviations: HDA, helicase-dependent amplification; LAMP, loop-mediated isothermal amplification; PCR, polymerase chain reaction; PI, package insert (assay recently cleared by the US Food and Drug Administration).

procedure and has been shown to mitigate surgical site infections with methicillin-resistant *S aureus* [25,26].

Molecular diagnostic assays are replacing conventional, culture-based methods for the diagnosis of infectious diseases. NAATs are associated with higher sensitivity and specificity, shorter turnaround times, and the use of NAATs for diagnosis of infectious diseases is associated with improved patient outcomes. However, the implementation of NAATs as a replacement for culture must be done in a thoughtful way by laboratories that have considered the costs associated with these improved tests, the level of technical expertise that must be perpetually available in the laboratory, the amount of clinician education that is necessary for appropriate use of these tests, and the regulatory and accreditation requirements necessary for performance of molecular testing.

REFERENCES

[1] Buss SN, Leber A, Chapin K, et al. Multicenter evaluation of the BioFire FilmArray Gastrointestinal Panel for etiologic diagnosis of infectious gastroenteritis. J Clin Microbiol 2015;53:915–25.

[2] Binnicker MJ. Multiplex molecular panels for diagnosis of gastrointestinal infection: performance, result interpretation, and cost-effectiveness. J Clin Microbiol 2015;53:3723–8.

[3] Rand KH, Tremblay EE, Hoidal M, et al. Multiplex gastrointestinal pathogen panels: implications for infection control. Diagn Microbiol Infect Dis 2015;82:154–7.

[4] Prakash VP, LeBlanc L, Alexander-Scott NE, et al. Use of a culture-independent gastrointestinal multiplex PCR panel during a shigellosis outbreak: considerations for clinical laboratories and public health. J Clin Microbiol 2015;53:1048–9.

[5] Cosentino LA, Danby CS, Rabe LK, et al. Use of nucleic acid amplification testing for diagnosis of extragenital sexually transmitted infections. J Clin Microbiol 2017;55:2801–7.

[6] Dize L, West SK, Mkocha H, et al. Evaluation of pooled ocular and vaginal swabs by the Cepheid GeneXper CT/NG assay for the detection of Chlamydia trachomatis and Neisseria gonorrhoeae compared to the GenProbe Aptima Combo 2 assay. Diagn Microbiol Infect Dis 2015;81:102–4.

[7] CDC. Sexually transmitted diseases treatment guidelines. MMWR Recomm Rep 2015;64(No. 3).

[8] Lawson PA, Citron DM, Tyrrell KL, et al. Reclassification of Clostridium difficile as Clostridioides difficile (Hall and O'Toole 1935) Prevot 1938. Anaerobe 2016;40:95–9.

[9] Culbreath K, Ager E, Nemeyer RJ, et al. Evolution of testing algorithms at a university hospital for detection of Clostridium difficile infections. J Clin Microbiol 2012;50:3073–6.

[10] ASM. A practical guidance document for the laboratory detection of toxigenic Clostridium difficile. 2010.

[11] McDonald LC, Gerding DN, Johnson S, et al. Clinical practice guidelines for Clostridium difficile infection in adults and children: 2017 update by the Infectious Diseases Society of America (IDSA) and Society for Healthcare Epidemiology of America (SHEA). Clin Infect Dis 2018;66:987–94.

[12] Pandey P, Pant ND, Rijal KR, et al. Diagnostic accuracy of GeneXpert MTB/RIF assay in comparison to conventional drug susceptibility testing method for the diagnosis of multidrug-resistant tuberculosis. PLoS One 2017;12:e0169798.

[13] Chakravorty S, Simmons AM, Rowneki M, et al. The new Xpert MTB/RIF Ultra: improving detection of Mycobacterium tuberculosis and resistance to rifampin in an assay suitable for point-of-care testing. Mbio 2017;29:812–7.

[14] Lombardi G, DiGregori V, Girometti N, et al. Diagnosis of smear-negative tuberculosis is greatly improved by Xpert MTB/RIF. PLoS One 2017;12:e0176186.

[15] Buchan BW, Faron ML, Fuller D, et al. Multicenter clinical evaluation of the Xpert GBS LB assay for detection

of group B Streptococcus in prenatal screening specimens. J Clin Microbiol 2015;53:443–8.

[16] Plainvert C, Al Alaoui F, Tazi A, et al. Intrapartum group B Streptococcus screening in the labor ward by Xpert GBS real-time PCR. Eur J Clin Microbiol Infect Dis 2018;37:265–70.

[17] Church DL, Baxter H, Lloyd T, et al. Evaluation of StrepB carrot broth versus Lim broth for detection of group B Streptococcus colonization status of near-term pregnant women. J Clin Microbiol 2008;46:2780–2.

[18] da Gloria Carvalho M, Facklam R, Jackson D, et al. Evaluation of three commercial broth media for pigment detection and identification of a group B Streptococcus (Streptococcus agalactiae). J Clin Microbiol 2009;47:4161–3.

[19] Berg BR, Houseman JL, Garrasi MA, et al. Culture-based method with performance comparable to that of PCR-based methods for detection of Group B Streptococcus in screening samples from pregnant women. J Clin Microbiol 2013;51:1253–5.

[20] Cohen DM, Russo ME, Jaggi P, et al. Multicenter clinical evaluation of the novel Alere i Strep A isothermal nucleic acid amplification test. J Clin Microbiol 2015;53:2258–61.

[21] Wang F, Tian Y, Chen L, et al. Accurate detection of Streptococcus pyogenes at the point of care using the Cobas Liat Strep A nucleic acid test. Clin Pediatr (Phila) 2017;56:1128–34.

[22] Webb KH, Needham CA, Kurtz SR. Use of a high-sensitivity rapid strep test without culture confirmation of negative results: 2 years' experience. J Fam Pract 2000;49:34–8.

[23] McLaws ML. The relationship between hand hygiene and health care-associated infection: it's complicated. Infect Drug Resist 2015;8:7–18.

[24] Backman C, Zoutman DE, Marck PB. An integrative review of the current evidence on the relationship between hand hygiene interventions and the incidence of health care-associated infections. Am J Infect Control 2008;36:333–48.

[25] Thompson P, Houston S. Decreasing methicillin-resistant Staphylococcus aureus surgical site infections with chlorhexidine and mupirocin. Am J Infect Control 2013;41:629–33.

[26] George S, Leasure AR, Horstmanshof D. Effectiveness of decolonization with chlorhexidine and mupirocin in reducing surgical site infections: a systematic review. Dimens Crit Care Nurs 2016;35:204–22.

[27] Van Der Pol B, Taylor SN, Lebar W, et al. Clinical evaluation of the BD ProbeTec Neisseria gonorrhoeae Qx amplified DNA assay on the BD Viper system with XTR technology. Sex Transm Dis 2012;39:147–53.

[28] Gaydos CA, Quinn TC, Willis D, et al. Performance of the APTIMA Combo 2 assay for detection of Chlamydia trachomatis and Neisseria gonorrhoeae in female urine and endocervical swab specimens. J Clin Microbiol 2003;41:304–9.

[29] Gaydos CA, Cartwright CP, Colaninno P, et al. Performance of the Abbott Real Time CT/NG for detection of Chlamydia trachomatis and Neisseria gonorrhoeae. J Clin Microbiol 2010;48:3236–43.

[30] Bromhead C, Miller A, Jones M, et al. Comparison of the Cobas 4800 CT/NG test with culture for detecting Neisseria gonorrhoeae in genital and nongenital specimens in a low-prevalence population in New Zealand. J Clin Microbiol 2013;51:1505–9.

[31] Gaydos CA, Van Der Pol B, Jett-Goheen M, et al. Performance of the Cepheid CT/NG Xpert Rapid PCR Test for detection of Chlamydia trachomatis and Neisseria gonorrhoeae. J Clin Microbiol 2013;51:1666–72.

[32] Hernandez DR, Wolk DM, Walker KL, et al. Multicenter diagnostic accuracy evaluation of the Luminex ARIES Real-Time PCR Assay for Group B Streptococcus detection in Lim-enriched samples. J Clin Microbiol 2018. https://doi.org/10.1128/JCM.01768-17.

[33] Miller SA, Deak E, Humphries R. Comparison of the AmpliVue, BD Max System, and illumigene molecular assays for detection of group B Streptococcus in antenatal screening specimens. J Clin Microbiol 2015;53:1938–41.

[34] Church DL, Lloyd T, Larios O, et al. Evaluation of Simplexa Group A Strep Direct kit compared to Hologic Group A Streptococcal Direct Assay for detection of Group A Streptococcus in throat swabs. J Clin Microbiol 2018;56 [pii:e01666-17].

[35] Uphoff TS, Buchan BW, Ledeboer NA, et al. Multicenter evaluation of the Solana Group A Streptococcus assay: comparison with culture. J Clin Microbiol 2016;54:2388–90.

[36] Henson AM, Carter D, Todd K, et al. Detection of Streptococcus pyogenes by use of illumigene Group A Streptococcus assay. J Clin Microbiol 2013;51:4207–9.

Advances in Molecular Pathology 1 (2018) 97–113
ADVANCES IN MOLECULAR PATHOLOGY

Syndromic and Point-of-Care Molecular Testing

Ryan F. Relich, PhD, D(ABMM), MLS(ASCP)SM[a,*], April N. Abbott, PhD, D(ABMM)[b]
[a]Division of Clinical Microbiology, Indiana University Health Pathology Laboratory, Indiana University Health and Indiana University School of Medicine, Suite 6027E, 350 West 11th Street, Indianapolis, IN 46202, USA; [b]Department of Laboratory Medicine, Deaconess Hospital, 600 Mary Street, Evansville, IN 47747, USA

KEYWORDS
• Syndromic panels • Point-of-care molecular diagnostics • Multiplex PCR • Group A *Streptococcus*
• Influenza-like illness • Meningitis • Gastroenteritis • Blood stream infections

KEY POINTS

- Syndromic and point-of-care molecular diagnostic testing methods have revolutionized infectious disease testing by permitting the simultaneous detection of multiple pathogens and drug resistance mechanisms directly from clinical specimens and positive blood cultures.
- Syndromic testing panels currently include those designed for the detection of pathogens responsible for bloodstream, central nervous system, gastrointestinal tract, and respiratory tract infections as well as some biothreat agents.
- Point-of-care molecular diagnostic systems afford providers the ability to generate laboratory-quality results without the need for confirmatory testing of negative specimens.
- Implementation of syndromic and point-of-care molecular infectious disease testing methods has curbed the unnecessary use of antibiotics, strengthening antimicrobial stewardship practices.
- Development of methods for the detection of infectious diseases beyond those that are detectable by current technologies is an area of investigation.

INTRODUCTION

For decades, the clinical laboratory diagnosis of many infectious diseases relied solely on time-consuming and often labor-intensive manual cultivation-based, microscopic, and immunoserologic methods that required experienced technical personnel to perform and interpret. The introduction of semiautomated and fully automated microbial phenotyping systems in the later part of the 20th century vastly improved the processes of bacterial and yeast isolate workup by decreasing identification and antimicrobial susceptibility testing turnaround times (TATs); however, the detection of many viruses and parasites still required traditional techniques. Subsequent improvements to automated platforms, including the refinement of the automated expert systems used by these devices to generate and interpret data, led to further decreases in TATs and a concomitant increase in culture throughput.

In the 1990s, the era of molecular diagnostics was ushered in with the introduction of nucleic acid analysis methods, including the hybridization protection assay (eg, AccuProbe, Salem, MA) for the identification of isolates and polymerase chain reaction (PCR) for the detection of pathogens directly from patient specimens [1–7]. Later, the implementation of real-time nucleic acid amplification chemistries permitted both faster pathogen detection and the enablement of nucleic acid quantitation [8]. These methods quickly migrated from research

*Corresponding author, *E-mail address:* rrelich@iupui.edu

https://doi.org/10.1016/j.yamp.2018.07.007

laboratories into clinical laboratories, first as laboratory-developed tests or so-called home brew tests. This revolution enabled laboratorians to more precisely identify the causes of infectious diseases by detecting pathogen-specific nucleotide sequences in cultured isolates and clinical specimens. Many of these methods proved to be far superior in terms of accuracy and result TAT compared with cultivation-dependent approaches, especially for the identification of viruses. Over time, these methods also underwent refinements that included the adaptation of several assays to automated platforms, allowing users to minimize the manual handling of specimens and reaction components.

One recent advancement in pathogen detection is the syndromic approach in which groups of pathogens are tested for simultaneously in a single reaction vessel. These assays incorporate components of older methods, including real-time PCR; however, rather than ordering separate tests for various pathogens, the syndromic tests allow simultaneous detection of a variety of agents that are associated with a specific disease syndrome [9].

The newest systems are those that allow users to perform laboratory-quality molecular testing at the point of patient care, a major advancement that has moved molecular pathology to the forefront of modern diagnostics. Many Clinical Laboratory Improvement Amendments (CLIA)-waived point-of-care (POC) systems are now available and permit rapid result reporting, enabling prescription of targeted treatment at the time of clinic visit. The current assays on these platforms largely target infections diagnosed in the ambulatory setting such as influenza and streptococcal pharyngitis.

SIGNIFICANCE

Syndromic and POC molecular testing methods have revolutionized the diagnosis of infectious diseases by increasing the accuracy of microbial detection, substantially decreasing the time needed to generate clinically useful laboratory test results, and enabling the performance of laboratory-quality testing at or near the point of care by nonlaboratorians [9]. In return, patients are able to receive appropriate treatment sooner, avoiding prolonged exposure to unnecessary antimicrobial drugs, thereby avoiding the selection of drug-resistant pathogens and strengthening antimicrobial stewardship practices [9–11]. In addition, many of these methods permit the rapid detection of pathogens that pose significant infection control and public health hazards, including high-consequence and travel-related pathogens (eg, *Bacillus anthracis*, Ebola virus, and *Plasmodium* spp.) that can be associated with either naturally acquired infections or infections resulting from the deliberate release of these agents. As a consequence of the rapid TATs of these tests, containment and epidemiologic interventions can be instituted very soon after specimen acquisition.

In addition to the syndromic and POC molecular testing solutions available for aiding in the identification of pathogens, many test panels are also capable of detecting antimicrobial resistance mechanisms [9,12,13], the rapid detection of which affords clinicians and infection control practitioners the ability to quickly implement appropriate therapies and infection control precautions. The diagnostic power of these technologies coupled with their user friendliness have made them highly attractive alternatives to traditional methods that rely on the procurement of isolates. As a consequence, methods such as viral culture and direct immunofluorescence have largely disappeared from modern clinical microbiology laboratories. With these methods removed, many laboratories have streamlined the workup of clinical specimens by using one syndromic testing platform for the analysis of a variety of specimen types for a large array of pathogens.

PRESENT RELEVANCE AND FUTURE AVENUES TO CONSIDER/INVESTIGATE

Currently, numerous diagnostic product manufacturers market infectious disease syndromic panels and POC molecular tests that are available in a variety of formats, including customizable panels, single-analyte tests, and CLIA-waived and moderate complexity systems. These tests were designed to provide all of the advantages that traditional molecular diagnostic tests offer plus the benefits of rapid result delivery, portability, and ease of use. The ability of many of these test platforms to be successfully used by nonlaboratorians have made them amenable to deployment in patient care facilities such as clinics and hospital emergency departments, which are traditionally not staffed by medical laboratory scientists.

Several syndromic and POC testing systems that provide qualitative results are described herein. Please note that not all available systems are mentioned, but those with a visible market presence in the United States are discussed.

Currently Available Syndromic Panel Platforms

BD MAX system

The BD MAX System (BD Diagnostics, Quebec, Canada; Fig. 1) is an automated real-time PCR platform using TaqMan hydrolysis probes for detection. In addition

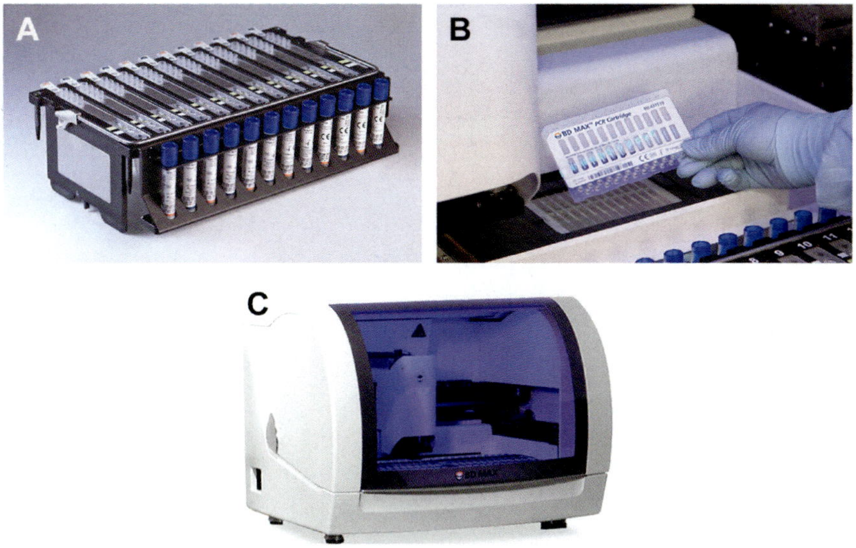

FIG. 1 The BD MAX System, which is comprised of (**A**) a rack for holding specimens (blue-capped tubes in front) and reagent strip, (**B**) the PCR cartridge, and (**C**) the BD MAX instrument. (*Courtesy of* BD, Sparks, MD; with permission.)

to syndromic panels (see Table 1 and Table 3), the system is designed to run singleplex and user-defined assays. To perform testing, specimens in sample buffer, reagents, extraction wells, pipette tips, and a real-time PCR microfluidic cartridge is placed on board the BD MAX instrument, which automates all sample handling and real-time PCR steps (see Fig. 1). Up to 24 assays can be run simultaneously and results are available within 3 hours. Panel performance characteristics are reviewed in refs. [14–17].

ePlex, ePlex NP, and eSensor XT-8 systems

The ePlex, ePlex NP, and XT-8 systems (GenMark Diagnostics, Inc., Carlsbad, CA; Fig. 2) use patented eSensor technology to detect a variety of pathogens directly from patient specimens (ePlex and ePlex NP systems) and amplified nucleic acid mixtures (eSensor XT-8 system).

For the ePlex system, the specimen in a buffer solution is added to the ePlex panel in which all liquid handling steps are performed by digital microfluidics technology (electrowetting) [14]. Electrochemical detection of ferrocene-labeled PCR amplicons occurs via capture probes that have been immobilized on gold-plated electrodes [15]. Results are generally available within 90 minutes, and anywhere from 3 to 24 assays can be ran simultaneously, depending on the instrument configuration (the ePlex NP performs a maximum of 3 tests at once). In contrast, the eSensor XT-8 system, the predecessor of the ePlex system, is designed to simultaneously interrogate up to 24 samples that have undergone offline nucleic acid amplification; results are available within 30 minutes [15]. Analytes detectable by the current panels are listed in Table 2 and performance characteristics and impacts of these systems are discussed in refs. [18–21].

FilmArray system

The FilmArray system (BioFire Diagnostics and BioFire Defense, LLC, Salt Lake City, UT; Fig. 3) family of syndromic panels includes several assays that are cleared by the US Food and Drug Administration (FDA) and several research use only assays (Box 1, see Table 2; Tables 3 and 4). Of note, BioFire Defense offers research-use-only reagents panels that are designed for detection of high-consequence and emerging pathogens whose detection could signal possible bioterrorism events, and for pathogens associated with travel to areas of the world where certain infectious diseases that are rare in the United States are endemic (Table 5).

The FilmArray System incorporates lyophilized reagents and assay reaction vessels on a small plastic

TABLE 1
Overview of Analytes Detected by the BD MAX Women's Health Panels, CT/GC/TV, and Vaginal Panel

Analyte	FDA Cleared?	*Atopobium vaginae*	Bacterial Vaginosis-Associated Bacteria-2	*Candida* spp.[a]	*Chlamydia trachomatis*	*Gardnerella vaginalis*	*Lactobacillus* spp.[b]	*Megasphaera*-1	*Neisseria gonorrhoeae*	*Trichomonas vaginalis*
BD MAX CT/GC/TV	+	–	–	–	+	–	–	–	+	+
BD MAX Vaginal Panel[c]	+	+	+	+	–	+	+	+	–	+

Abbreviations: CT/GC/VT, *Chlamydia trachomatis*/gonococcus (*Neisseria gonorrhoeae*)/*Trichomonas vaginalis*; FDA, US Food and Drug Administration.

Symbols: +, yes or present on panel; -, no or absent from panel.

[a] The BD MAX vaginal panel detects *Candida albicans*, *C dubliniensis*, *C glabrata*, *C krusei*, *C parapsilosis*, and *C tropicalis* but reports them as "*Candida* group" for all except *C glabrata* and *C krusei*, which it reports individually.

[b] The BD MAX Vaginal Panel detects *Lactobacillus crispatus* and *L jensenii*, which are grouped as *Lactobacillus* species.

[c] Detection of 1 or more bacterial analytes are reported as positive or negative for bacterial vaginosis.

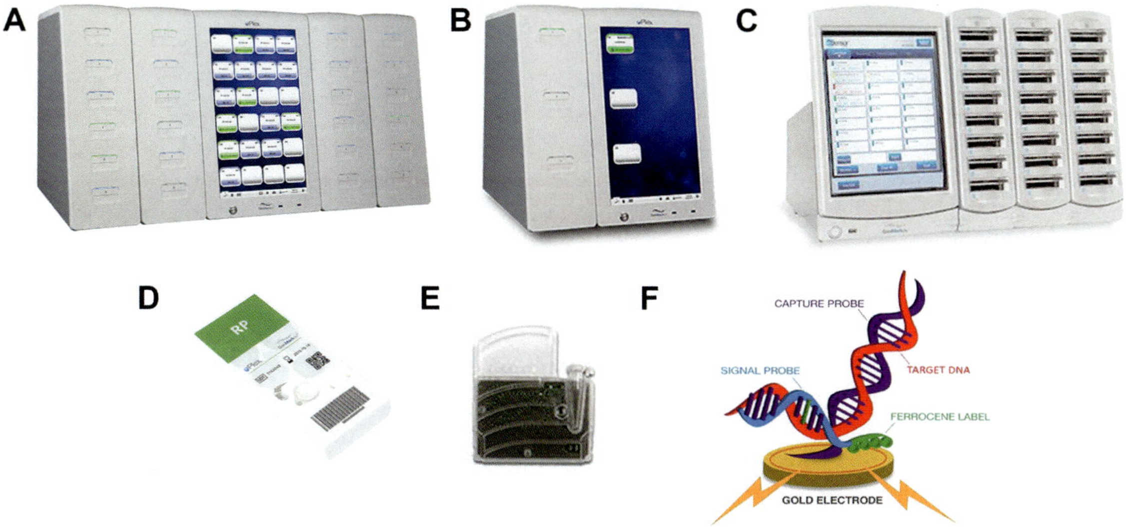

FIG. 2 The ePlex (**A**), ePlex NP (**B**), and eSensor XT-8 (**C**) systems available from GenMark Diagnostics. Also shown are examples of ePlex (**D**) and XT-8 (**E**) panels. The nucleic acid hybridization complex described in the text is shown in (**F**). (*Courtesy of* GenMark Diagnostics, Carlsbad, CA; with permission.)

film pouch topped by a solid plastic reagent housing (Fig. 3A). After reagent rehydration, the sample in buffer is added to a pouch that is then loaded into a FilmArray instrument for automated nucleic acid extraction, real-time PCR, detection, and high-resolution melt steps. The hands-on time of this system is minimal (approximately 2 minutes) and results are generally available in approximately 60 minutes [18]. Like the ePlex system, the FilmArray 2.0 and Torch instruments are scalable. With the exception of the FilmArray BCID Panel, which is meant for testing blood culture broths, all other panels are amenable to the direct testing of clinical specimens. The FilmArray BioThreat Panel, BioThreat-E Test, and Global Fever Panel are designed to test a variety of sample types, which are listed in the notes in Box 1. Numerous studies describing the performance characteristics and benefits of the FilmArray System have been published; examples can be found in refs. [13,22–31].

Unyvero system

The Unyvero Lower Respiratory Tract Panel (Curetis USA Inc., San Diego, CA; Fig. 4), known as the Pneumonia Panel in Europe, is the first multiplex lower respiratory tract infection testing system to receive FDA clearance as of April 2018. This system uses PCR to detect an array of bacterial pathogens and antimicrobial resistance genes (Table 6) directly from tracheal aspirates in 4 to 5 hours. The Unyvero system is composed of 3 hardware components: a sample lysis device (Unyvero L4 Lysator), a panel analyzer (Unyvero A50 Analyzer), and a touchscreen computer interface and barcode scanner (Unyvero C8 Cockpit). Performance characteristics are described in refs. [32,33].

VERIGENE system

The VERIGENE system (Luminex Corporation. Austin, TX; Fig. 5) consists of VERIGENE Processor *SP* modules and the VERIGENE Reader, designed around a family of FDA-cleared syndromic panels. Multiple Processor *SP* units can be combined with a single Reader to accommodate the simultaneous testing of multiple samples. The extraction tray containing the sample, test cartridge (see Tables 2 and 3 for cartridges and analytes), tip holder assembly, and utility tray are loaded into the Processor *SP* for automated nucleic acid extraction, purification, target amplification (if required by the specific assay), and hybridization of the target molecules to a glass detection array in the test cartridge. NanoGrid Technology is used to capture, detect, and identify target molecules. After the processing step, the test cartridge array is placed into the VERIGENE Reader to obtain results, which may be selectively reported. Total hands-on, automated processing, and test interpretation time is less than 3 hours. Performance characteristics are described in refs. [34,35].

TABLE 2
Syndromic Panels that Are Currently Available in the United States for the Detection of Upper Respiratory Tract Pathogens

Analyte	**FDA Cleared?**	**Adenovirus**	**Adenovirus Subtyping**	***Bordetella bronchiseptica***	***Bordetella holmesii***	***Bordetella pertussis/B. parapertussis***	***Chlamydophila pneumoniae***	**Coronavirus HKU1**	**Coronavirus NL63**	**Coronavirus 229E**	**Coronavirus OC43**	**Enterovirus/Rhinovirus**	**Human Bocavirus**	**Human Metapneumovirus**	**Human Metapneumovirus Subtyping**	**Human Parainfluenza Virus 1**	**Human Parainfluenza Virus 2**	**Human Parainfluenza Virus 3**	**Human Parainfluenza Virus 4**	**Influenza A**	**Influenza A Subtyping**	**Influenza B**	***Legionella pneumophila***	***Mycoplasma pneumoniae***	**Respiratory Syncytial Virus**	**Respiratory Syncytial Virus Subtyping**
ePlex RP	+	+	−	−	−	−/−	+	+	+	+	+	+	−	+	−	+	+	+	+	+	+	+	−	+	+	+
eSensor RVP	+	+	+	−	−	−	−	−	−	−	−	+[c]	−	+	−	+	+	+	−	+	+	+	−	−	+	+
FilmArray RP Panel	+	+	−	−	−	+/−	+	+	+	+	+	+	−	+	−	+	+	+	+	+	+	+	−	+	+	−
FilmArray RP2 Panel	+	+	−	−	−	+/+	+	+	+	+	+	+	−	+	−	+	+	+	+	+	+	+	−	+	+	−
FilmArray RP EZ[a]	+	+	−	−	−	+/−	+	+	+	+	+	+/+	−	+	−	+	+	+	+	+	+	+	−	+	+	−
NxTAG RPP[b]	+	+	−	−	−	−/−	+	+	+	+	+	+	+	+	−	+	+	+	+	+	+	+	−	−	+	+
VERIGENE RP *Flex*[b]	+	+	−	+	+	+/+	−	−	−	−	−	+[c]	−	+	−	+	+	+	+	+	+	+	−	−	+	+

Abbreviations: FDA, US Food and Drug Administration; RPP, respiratory pathogen panel.

Symbols: +, yes or present on panel; -, no or absent from panel.

[a] The FilmArray RP EZ assay tests for human coronaviruses HKU1, NL63, 229E, and OC43 and human parainfluenza viruses 1, 2, 3, and 4, but it reports those analytes as coronavirus and parainfluenza virus, respectively.

[b] The NxTAG and VERIGENE RP *flex* assays allow users to selectively report targets.

[c] Rhinovirus alone is reported by the eSensor RVP, VERIGENE RP *flex*, US versions of the NxTAG RVP assays.

BOX 1
Central Nervous System Pathogens Detected by the FilmArray ME Panel

Bacteria

Escherichia coli K1

Haemophilus influenzae

Listeria monocytogenes

Neisseria meningitidis

Streptococcus agalactiae

Streptococcus pneumoniae

Fungi[a]

Cryptococcus neoformans/C gattii

Viruses

Cytomegalovirus

Enterovirus

Herpes simplex virus 1

Herpes simplex virus 2

Human herpes virus 6

Human parechovirus

Varicella-zoster virus

[a] The FilmArray ME Panel detects *C neoformans* and *C gattii* but reports them together as *C neoformans/C gattii*.

xTAG technology

In addition to the VERIGENE system, Luminex offers FDA-cleared bead hybridization-based (xTAG) assays that require offline nucleic acid extraction followed by multiplex PCR and bead hybridization in 96-well plates. Analysis of beads is carried out by the MAGPIX instrument (Fig. 6). The MAGPIX instrument interrogates beads in each well of the reaction plate to detect fluorescent reporters that are linked to bead-hybridized target molecules. The total time required to perform a run is approximately 5 hours, so batch testing of samples is required. The NxTAG next-generation Respiratory Pathogen Panel allows users to selectively report analytes (see Table 2) whereas the xTAG Gastrointestinal Pathogen Panel (see Table 3) does not. See refs. [36–38] for performance characteristics.

Brief Description of Currently Available Syndromic Panels

Blood culture

Accurate diagnosis and early, appropriate treatment of sepsis is a life-saving event. Syndromic panels are designed to use the exponential growth of organisms in broth-based blood culture systems to detect the most common causes of bacteremia and key resistance mechanisms that would alter therapeutic management (eg, methicillin resistance). The performance of these systems has been thoroughly reviewed elsewhere [39]. Of note, FilmArray and VERIGENE correctly detect more than 95% of identifiable organisms in monomicrobial cultures when compared with conventional methods. The Achilles heel of blood culture syndromic panels is miscalls, which are associated with polymicrobial cultures and, more specifically, those errors associated with antimicrobial resistance.

Central nervous system

Infectious meningitis and encephalitis are often medical emergencies requiring prompt and accurate diagnosis and intervention for favorable outcomes. Culture is suboptimal for detecting many etiologies; however, most laboratories lack the infrastructure to perform laboratory-developed molecular tests and, therefore, rely on reference laboratories for viral detection in the cerebrospinal fluid or when the patient is on antimicrobials. Widespread early adoption has been plagued by concerns around performance in a setting where misdiagnosis could be catastrophic. As with the respiratory panel, the correlation of results without a sensitive and specific gold standard is challenging. A multicenter evaluation established a high percent agreement (>99%) with comparator testing; however, the percent agreement for positive results was only 84.4% [40]. Furthermore, reports of false-negative (eg, potential suboptimal detection of herpesviruses and *Cryptococcus*) and false-positive results (eg, *Streptococcus pneumoniae* and herpes simplex virus-1) have resulted in delayed or missed meningitis diagnoses [41].

Gastrointestinal

Acute gastroenteritis presents a clinical and public health dilemma because the symptoms of infectious and noninfectious causes of diarrhea overlap. Traditional diagnostics (eg, culture, microscopy, antigen detection) are time consuming and may require multiple specimens for optimal sensitivity. Studies have reproducibly shown that 2 to 3 times more pathogens are detected when a molecular assay is used, compared with traditional methods [39]. This is due in part to an enhanced range of the targets, an increase in sensitivity of the assays over traditional methods, and the recognition of co-infections that were previously unrecognized. Sensitivity and specificity of these assays, overall, is high, with few exceptions. Notably, detection of rotavirus, *Campylobacter* spp., and *Salmonella* spp. may be problematic with VERIGENE; one publication noted

TABLE 3
Syndromic Panels that Are Currently Available in the United States for the Detection of Gastrointestinal Tract Pathogens

Analyte	FDA Cleared?	Adenovirus F 40/41	Astrovirus	*Campylobacter* spp.	*Clostridium difficile* (Toxin A/B)	*Cryptosporidium* spp.	*Cyclospora cayetanensis*	*Entamoeba histolytica*	*Escherichia coli* O157	*E coli* (EAEC)	*E coli* (EPEC)	*E coli* (EIEC)	*E coli* (ETEC)	*E coli* (STEC) or *stx1* and *stx2*	*Giardia intestinalis* (*G lamblia*)	Norovirus	*Plesiomonas shigelloides*	Rotavirus	*Salmonella* spp.	Sapovirus	*Shigella* spp.	*Vibrio cholerae*	*Vibrio parahaemolyticus*	*Vibrio vulnificus*	*Yersinia enterocolitica*
BD MAX Enteric Bacterial Panel	+	−	−	+	−	−	−	−	+	−	−	+	−	+	−	−	−	−	+	−	+	−	−	−	−
BD MAX Extended Enteric Bacterial Panel	+	−	−	+	−	−	−	−	+	−	−	−	+	+	−	−	+	−	+	−	+	+	+	+	+
BD MAX Enteric Parasite Panel	+	−	−	−	−	+	−	+	−	−	−	−	−	−	+	−	−	−	−	−	−	−	−	−	−
FilmArray GI Panel[a]	+	+	+	+	+	+	+	+	+	+	+	+	+	+	+	+	+	+	+	+	+	+	+	+	+
VERIGENE EP Test[b]	+	−	−	+	−	−	−	−	−	−	−	−	−	+	−	+	−	+	+	−	+	+	+	−	+
xTAG GPP[c]	+	+	−	+	+	+	−	+	+	−	−	−	+	+	+	+	−	+	+	−	+	+	−	−	−

Abbreviations: EIEC, *Shigella*/enteroinvasive *E coli*; EAEC, Enteroaggregative *E coli*; EPEC, Enteropathogenic *E coli;* ETEC, Enterotoxigenic *E coli*; STEC, Shiga Toxin-producing *E coli*; FDA, US Food and Drug Administration; GI, gastrointestinal; GPP, gastrointestinal pathogen panel.

Symbols: +, yes or present on panel; -, no or absent from panel.

[a] The FilmArray GI panel detects *Campylobacter jejuni*, *C coli*, and *C upsaliensis* and reports them as "*Campylobacter* (*jejuni*, *coli* and *upsaliensis*)." *Shigella* spp. are reported along with *E coli* (EIEC) as "*Shigella*/enteroinvasive *E coli* (EIEC)." *V cholerae*, *V parahaemolyticus*, and *V vulnificus* are detected and are reported as "*Vibrio* (*parahaemolyticus*, *vulnificus* and *cholerae*); however, *V cholerae* is also reported independently if it alone is detected. Norovirus genogroups I and II are detected, and astrovirus genotypes I, II, IV, and V are detected.

[b] The *VERIGENE* EP test detects *C jejuni*, *C coli*, and *C lari* and reports them as *Campylobacter* group. *Shigella boydii*, *S dysenteriae*, *S flexneri*, and *S sonnei* are detected and reported as *Shigella* spp. *V cholerae* and *V parahaemolyticus* are detected and reported as *Vibrio* group. Norovirus genogroups I and II are detected.

[c] The xTAG GPP detects *C jejuni*, *C coli*, and *C lari* and reports them as *Campylobacter*; *Cryptosporidium parvum* and *C hominis*, and reports them as *Cryptosporidium*; and *S boydii*, *S dysenteriae*, *S flexneri*, and *S sonnei*, and reports them as *Shigella*.

TABLE 4
Syndromic Panels that Are Currently Available in the United States for the Detection of Bloodstream Infection Pathogens

Analyte	FilmArray BCID Panel	VERIGENE GN BC Test	VERIGENE GP BC Test
FDA Cleared?	+	+	+
Acinetobacter baumannii or *Acinetobacter* spp.	+	+	×
Candida spp.	+	×	×
Citrobacter spp.	-	+	×
Enterobacteriaceae	+	-	×
Enterobacter spp.	+	-	×
Enterococcus spp.	+	×	+
Escherichia coli	+	+	×
Haemophilus influenzae	+	-	×
Klebsiella oxytoca	+	-	×
Klebsiella pneumoniae	+	+	×
Listeria spp.	+	×	×
Micrococcus spp.	-	×	+
Neisseria meningitidis	+	-	×
Proteus spp.	+	+	×
Pseudomonas aeruginosa	+	+	×
Serratia spp.	+	+	×
Staphylococcus spp.	+	×	+
Staphylococcus aureus	+	×	+
Streptococcus spp.	+	×	+
Streptococcus agalactiae	+	×	+
Streptococcus pneumoniae	+	×	+
Streptococcus pyogenes	+	×	+
Carbapenemase Genes	+	+	×
Extended-Spectrum β-Lactamase Genes	-	+	×
mecA	+	×	+
vanA/vanB	+	×	+

Abbreviation: FDA, US Food and Drug Administration.
Symbols: +, yes or present on panel; -, no or absent from panel.

TABLE 5
Multiplex Nucleic Acid Amplification Panels Available for the Detection of High-Consequence and Travel-Associated Pathogens

Analyte	FDA Cleared?	*Bacillus anthracis*	*Brucella melitensis*	*Burkholderia mallei /B pseudomallei*	Chikungunya Virus	*Clostridium botulinum*	*Coxiella burnettii*	Crimean-Congo Hemorrhagic Fever Virus	Dengue Virus	Ebola Virus (*Zaire ebolavirus*)	EEE Virus	*Francisella tularensis*	Lassa Virus	*Leptospira* spp.	*Leishmania* spp.	Marburg Virus	Orthopox Virus	*Plasmodium* spp.	*Ricinus communis*	*Rickettsia prowazekii*	*Salmonella enterica* Serovar. Paratyphi A	*S enterica* Serovar. Typhi	Variola Virus	VEE Virus	WEE Virus	Yellow Fever Virus	*Yersinia pestis*	West Nile Virus	Zika Virus
FilmArray BioThreat Panel[a]	–	+	+	+	–	+	+	–	–	+	+	+	–	–	–	+	+	–	+	+	–	–	+	+	+	–	+	–	–
FilmArray BioThreat–E Test[b]	–[c]	–	–	–	–	–	–	–	–	+	–	–	–	–	–	–	–	–	–	–	–	–	–	–	–	–	–	–	–
FilmArray Global Fever Panel[d]	–	+	–	–	+	–	–	+	+	+	–	+	+	+	+	+	–	+[e]	–	–	+	+	–	–	–	+	–	+	+

Abbreviations: EEE virus, eastern equine encephalitis virus; FDA, US Food and Drug Administration; VEE virus, Venezuelan equine encephalitis virus; WEE, western equine encephalitis virus.

Symbols: +, yes or present on panel/test; -, no or absent from panel/test.

[a] The FilmArray BioThreat Panel is designed to detect analytes from swab, liquid, culture, and powder samples.

[b] The FilmArray BioThreat-E Test is designed to detect Ebola virus (*Zaire ebolavirus*) in blood and urine samples.

[c] The FilmArray BioThreat-E Test was granted FDA EUA status in 2014 and it is only authorized for use by CLIA moderate and high complexity laboratories throughout the duration of the EUA. This test is intended to detect Ebola virus (*Zaire ebolavirus*) from blood and urine specimens.

[d] The FilmArray Global Fever Panel is designed to detect analytes in whole blood.

[e] The FilmArray Global Fever Panel detects and reports *Plasmodium* spp. and it also distinguishes *Plasmodium falciparum* from *Plasmodium ovale/Plasmodium vivax* and reports them as such.

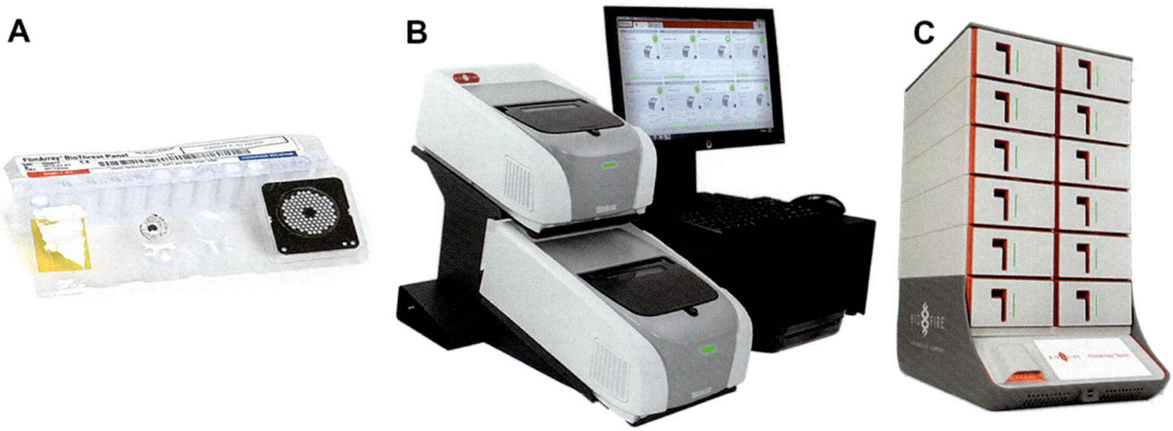

FIG. 3 The FilmArray system. The FilmArray pouch (**A**) and (**B**) the FilmArray 2.0 and (**C**) Torch instruments. (*Courtesy of* BioFire Diagnostics, Salt Lake City, UT; with permission.)

false positivity with norovirus using BioFire. Overall, these platforms allow timely, accurate diagnosis of diarrhea and can assist with pathogen-directed therapy [42].

Respiratory

Owing to a relative paucity of accurate and rapid diagnostics, pathogen determination in acute respiratory illness had traditionally fallen to clinical presentation, despite its poor prognostic value. Rapid, accurate diagnosis is critical for antibiotic stewardship, informing the clinician if antivirals are warranted, and infection control initiatives (eg, isolation, cohorting). Unsurprisingly, respiratory illness has been a key target for syndromic testing (see Table 2). Performance characteristics have been reviewed in depth elsewhere [39], with key attributes highlighted herein. All commercially available respiratory panels significantly outperform traditional methods of detection and have expanded our recognition of coinfections (approximately 5% of samples tested). At present, no gold standard method for comparison of these assays has hampered exact determination of performance; however, the generally accepted overall agreement between molecular methods is between 85% and 99% for each target, with some exceptions. Accurate detection of adenovirus is problematic in many first-generation assays; however, a multicenter analysis of the FilmArray RP2 [43] indicates increased sensitivity with this assay.

Sexually transmitted infections/women's health

Sexually transmitted infections, bacterial vaginosis, and vaginal yeast infections are associated with significant morbidity and can have long-term consequences, including infertility. The diagnosis of these highly prevalent infectious diseases once required the use of

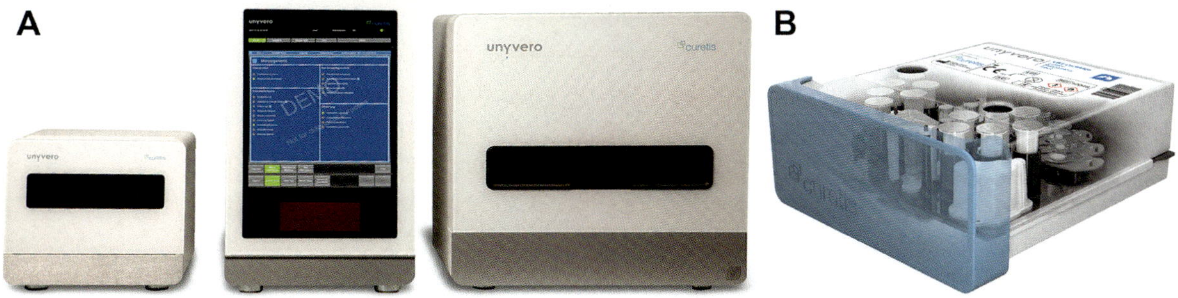

FIG. 4 The Curetis Unyvero system, composed of the Unyvero L4 Lysator (**A**, *left*), the Unyvero C8 Cockpit (**A**, *middle*), and the Unyvero A50 Analyzer (**A**, *right*), and the Unyvero LRT panel (**B**). (*Courtesy of* Curetis, San Diego, CA; with permission.)

TABLE 6
Curetis Unyvero Lower Respiratory Tract Panel for the Diagnosis of Community-Acquired and Health Care-Associated Pneumonia

Microbial Targets	Antimicrobial Resistance Genes
Acinetobacter spp.	bla_{TEM}
Chlamydophila pneumoniae	bla_{SHV}
Citrobacter freundii	bla_{VIM}
Enterobacter cloacae complex	bla_{NDM}
Escherichia coli	bla_{KPC}
Haemophilus influenzae	$bla_{CTX\text{-}M}$
Klebsiella oxytoca	$bla_{OXA\text{-}23}$
Klebsiella pneumoniae	$bla_{OXA\text{-}24}$
Klebsiella variicola	$bla_{OXA\text{-}48}$
Legionella pneumophila	$bla_{OXA\text{-}58}$
Moraxella catarrhalis	*gyrA*83 mutation (of *Escherichia coli*)
Morganella morganii	*gyrA*87 mutation (of *E coli*)
Mycoplasma pneumoniae	*gyrA*83 mutation (of *Pseudomonas aeruginosa*)
Proteus spp.	*gyrA*87 mutation (of *P aeruginosa*)
Pseudomonas aeruginosa	*mecA*
Serratia marcescens	
Staphylococcus aureus	
Stenotrophomonas maltophilia	
Streptococcus pneumoniae	

multiple testing methods such as microscopy, culture, and nucleic acid amplification testing; however, the advent of syndromic testing systems for these pathogens (eg, BD MAX CT/GC/TV and BD MAX Vaginal Panel; see Table 1) has streamlined their detection. Overall, both of the assays listed in Table 1 outperform traditional methods, including *Chlamydia trachomatis* culture and microscopic screening for bacterial vaginosis, candidiasis, and trichomoniasis. In one study that evaluated the performance of the BD MAX CT/GC/TV assay, the sensitivities for detection of all three analytes were 91.5% or greater and the specificities were 98.6% or greater [14]. According to clinical trial data of the BD MAX Vaginal Panel, the sensitivities for analytes ranged from 75.9% (analyte [collection method]: *Candida glabrata* [clinician-collected specimens]) to 100% (*C glabrata* [simulated specimens] and *Candida krusei* [simulated specimens]) and specificities ranged from 84.5% (bacterial vaginosis [self-collected specimens]) to 100% (*C glabrata* [simulated specimens] and *C krusei* [self-collected and simulated specimens]) [44]. Overall, sexually transmitted infection/women's health syndromic panels outperform traditional methods in terms of sensitivity, specificity, and TATs.

Currently Available Point-of-Care Molecular Methods

The push to get faster diagnostic answers to guide admission or discharge strategies and therapeutics is likely to propel multiplex testing into the realm of

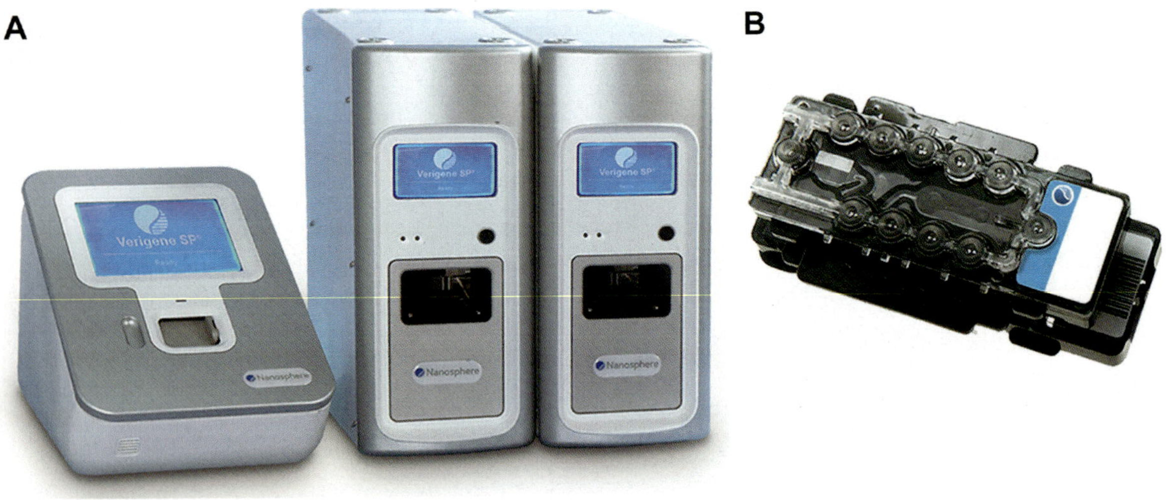

FIG. 5 The Luminex VERIGENE system, composed of (**A**, *left*) the VERIGENE Reader, (**A**, *right*) VERIGENE Processor *SP* (**A**, *right*), and (**B**) a VERIGENE Test Cartridge. (*Courtesy of* Luminex, Austin, TX; with permission.)

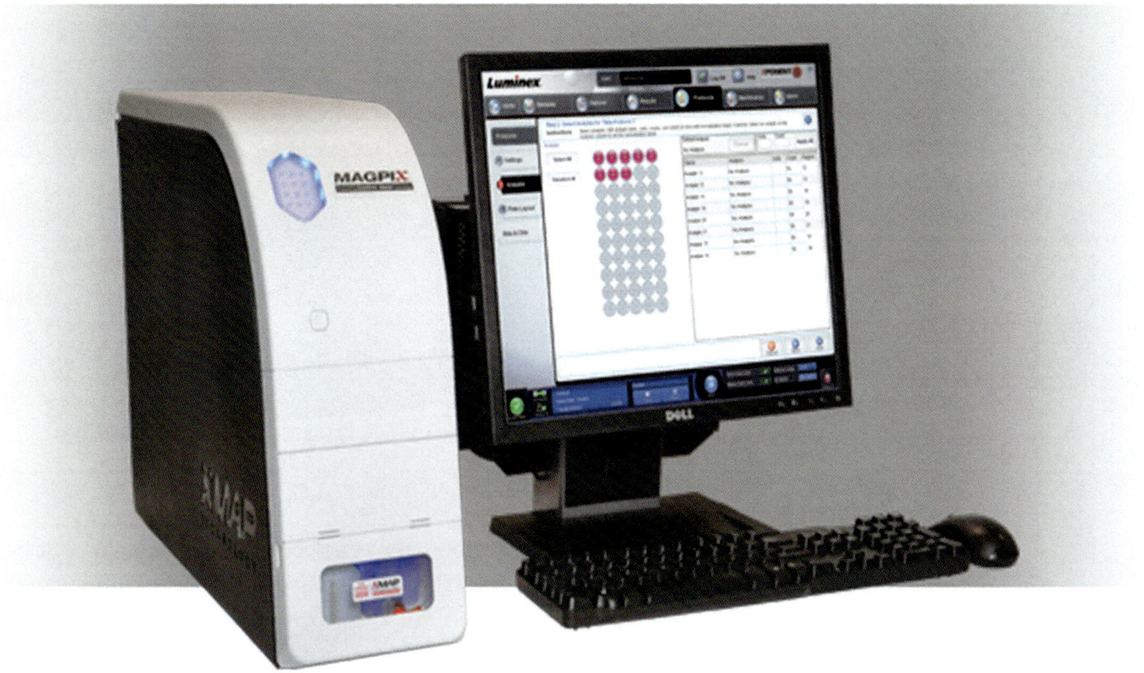

FIG. 6 The Luminex MAGPIX instrument and computer for NxTAG and xTAG assays. (*Courtesy of* Luminex, Austin, TX; with permission.)

POC testing. At present, issues with contamination, quality control performance and monitoring, interpretation of results, and overall good laboratory practices as technologies migrate into a less controlled setting is an obvious concern. Current CLIA-waived platforms are discussed briefly, because these systems may be readily adaptable to multiplex syndromic testing in the POC setting.

Alere i

The Alere i (Alere Scarborough, Inc., Scarborough, ME; Fig. 7) system uses nicking enzyme amplification reaction technology, an isothermal amplification method, to detect nucleic acids of target pathogens, including influenza A and B viruses, respiratory syncytial virus, and group A *Streptococcus*, either directly from swabs or from swab eluates in transport media. The consumable is a 3-component system that consists of a reagent

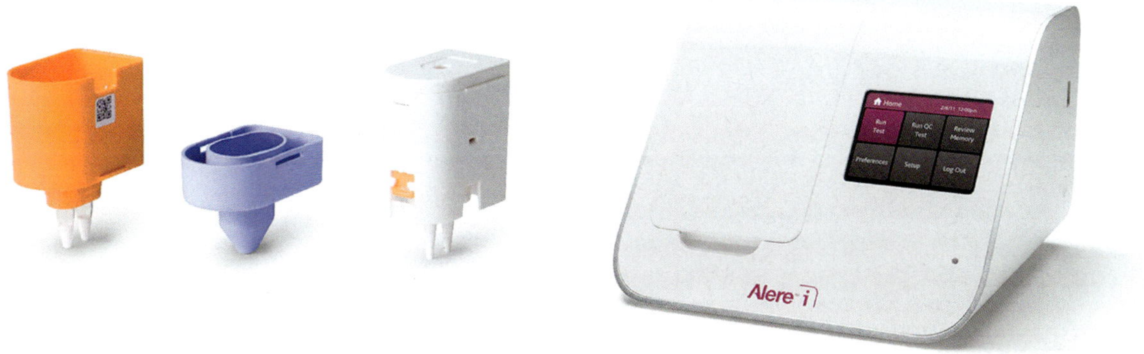

FIG. 7 The Alere i system, including the 3-part test cartridge (*left*) and the Alere i instrument (*right*). (*Courtesy of* Alere, Waltham, MA; with permission.)

base, elution buffer container, and transfer cartridge that is assembled on the Alere i instrument. Positive results are available within 8 to 15 minutes (depending on the assay type). Performance characteristics and additional details are described in refs. [45–50].

cobas Liat system

The cobas Liat System (Roche Diagnostics, Indianapolis, IN; Fig. 8) integrates all reagents necessary for nucleic acid purification and amplification (by real-time PCR) into a segmented soft plastic tube housed within a rigid plastic frame. After specimen collection (eg, nasopharyngeal swab) and elution into a suitable specimen transport medium (eg, viral transport medium), a small aliquot of the specimen is pipetted into the tube, the tube is capped, and the entire tube-frame assembly is loaded into the cobas Liat instrument, which automates all reaction and amplicon detection steps. Results for influenza detection are available within 20 minutes, and those for group A *Streptococcus* are available within 15 minutes of assay initiation. Currently, three FDA-cleared, CLIA-waived assays are available for the detection of influenza A/B viruses alone, influenza A/B viruses and respiratory syncytial virus, and group A *Streptococcus*. Performance characteristics are discussed in refs. [45,51–53].

Solana

The Solana system (Quidel Corporation, San Diego, CA; Fig. 9) uses isothermal, helicase-dependent amplification and fluorescent-probe detection of target nucleic acids. Currently, FDA-approved assays are available for the detection of *Clostridium difficile*, groups A and B streptococci, herpes simplex viruses, varicella-zoster virus, influenza viruses, respiratory syncytial virus, human metapneumovirus, and *Trichomonas vaginalis*.

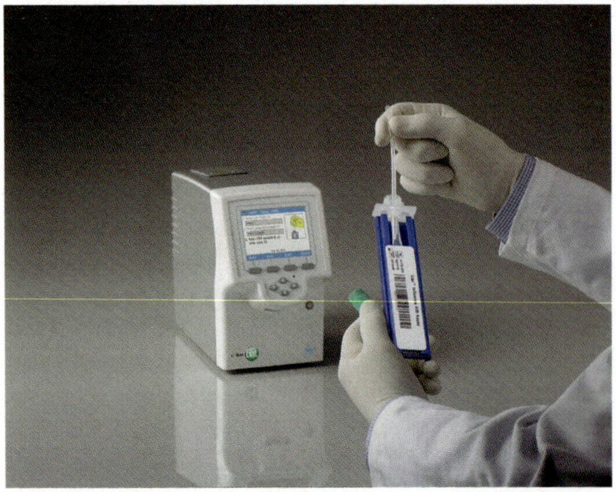

FIG. 8 The cobas Liat system from Roche Diagnostics includes the test cartridge (*foreground*) and the Liat instrument (*background*). (*Courtesy of* Roche Diagnostics, Indianapolis, IN; with permission.)

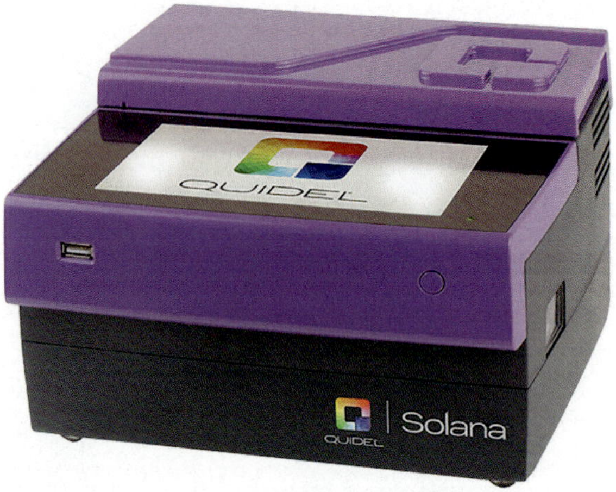

FIG. 9 The Quidel Solana instrument. (*Courtesy of* Quidel, San Diego, CA; with permission.)

To perform testing, a patient specimen (eg, nasal swab in viral transport medium) in Process Buffer is heated before transfer to a reaction tube. The reaction tube contains all reagents needed for amplification and detection in a lyophilized form. The reaction tube is next inserted into the Solana instrument where amplification and detection are performed. Results are available in 30 minutes or less. Up to 12 Solana diagnostic assays can be analyzed simultaneously. Relevant performance characteristics are described in ref. [54] and in assay package inserts available on the Quidel website (https://www.quidel.com).

The Future of Syndromic Testing and Point-of-Care Molecular Diagnostics

Each of these systems, plus those that have not been described herein, are constantly undergoing refinement to ensure their continued relevance in the molecular diagnostics marketplace. Test systems are continuously challenged with new strains of pathogens and antimicrobial resistance mechanisms to evaluate their inclusivity and/or exclusivity, and panels are frequently updated to include additional analytes. Also, new assays that enable detection and quantitation of pathogens associated with disease processes besides those mentioned previously are in development. The goal of most manufacturers is to offer infectious disease diagnostic testing solutions that allow identification of the greatest breadth of pathogens associated with a specific disease process or syndrome. To that end, future applications of these technologies include the enhancement of currently available systems, the development of additional panels that are amenable to the diagnosis other infectious processes, and the development of tests that enable users to comprehensively profile the antimicrobial susceptibility of pathogens.

SUMMARY

The use of multiplex panels for pathogen detection provides several advantages over traditional laboratory diagnostic approach. Providers tout multiplex assays as a means to simplify the ordering process, decrease the number of required specimens, detect pathogens that may not be part of the initial diagnostic differential owing to rarity of the agent or inaccessibility of an alternative in-house test method, and provide results in a clinically actionable timeframe. The incorporation of molecular multiplex panels is of financial and logistical benefit to the laboratory. Specifically, one can decrease the number of methods needed to detect the same diversity of infectious agents and decrease technologist hands-on time, which results in a simplified workflow for the purposes of training, competency, use, and often cost. For the patient, these assays provide superior accuracy over traditional approaches and a greater breadth of targeted pathogens, which may decrease the number of medical visits, interventions, and durations of diagnosis. Certain multiplex assays provide benefits beyond direct patient care, such as early recognition of drug-resistant pathogens for swift implementation of infection control measures or improved detection of gastrointestinal pathogens that may impact outbreak investigations. Finally, rapid pathogen detection and the potential for improved, early intervention has been shown to positively impact associated costs by aiding in selective test use and reduced length of stay [39].

Taken together, the benefits of molecular syndromic panels and POC tests vastly outweigh any disadvantages, which is centered around cost to the health care system, namely, to the hospital or patient. The claim that this so-called shotgun approach adds unnecessary cost to the patient is an oversimplification. Although molecular multiplex assays are often more costly in terms of reagents and patient billing compared with a single culture- or serology-based assay, when multiple diagnostic tests are ordered, the multiplex assay is often less expensive than the full battery of traditional tests. Anecdotally, physicians desire to provide the patient with a definitive diagnosis and treatment plan, which may inadvertently lead to the overuse of medical resources such as injudicious antibiotic use and additional diagnostic tests (eg, imaging) to help establish a diagnosis when the causative pathogen is not easily identified. Therefore, the ability to rapidly and accurately provide a cause for the patient's illness may improve both physician and patient satisfaction.

At present, FDA-cleared syndromic and POC molecular assays center around a few syndromes; however, this menu is likely to expand in the coming years as laboratories rapidly adopt this approach to testing. When combined with consultation (eg, antimicrobial stewardship intervention), the implementation of these assays has been shown to decrease the time to appropriate therapy, improve patient survival, and decrease overall health care-associated costs [9]. Care must be taken in the selection and appropriate use of multiplex panels. Specifically, one must balance the potential for increased laboratory reagent and equipment costs against the potential for reduced labor costs and increased revenue. To provide the highest quality of care while limiting unnecessary expense, laboratories must develop algorithms that assist providers in test ordering and use.

REFERENCES

[1] Daly JA, Clifton NL, Seskin KC, et al. Use of rapid, nonradioactive DNA probes in culture confirmation tests to detect *Streptococcus agalactiae*, *Haemophilus influenza*, and *Enterococcus* spp. from pediatric patients with significant infections. J Clin Microbiol 1991;29: 80–2.

[2] Davis TE, Fuller DD. Direct identification of bacterial isolates in blood cultures by using a DNA probe. J Clin Microbiol 1991;29:2193–6.

[3] Lumb R, Lanser JA, Lim IS. Rapid identification of mycobacteria by the Gen-Probe Accuprobe system. Pathology 1993;25:313–5.

[4] Padhye AA, Smith G, Standard PG, et al. Comparative evaluation of chemilluminescent DNA probe assays and exoantigen tests for rapid identification of *Blastomyces dermatitidis* and *Coccidioides immitis*. J Clin Microbiol 1994;32:867–70.

[5] Sninsky JJ. The polymerase chain reaction (PCR): a valuable method for retroviral detection. Lymphology 1990; 23:92–7.

[6] Persing DH, Mathiesen D, Marshall WF, et al. Detection of *Babesia microti* by polymerase chain reaction. J Clin Microbiol 1992;30:2097–103.

[7] Karron RA, Froehlich JL, Bobo L, et al. Rapid detection of parainfluenza virus type 3 RNA in respiratory specimens: use of reverse-transcription-PCR-enzyme immunoassay. J Clin Microbiol 1994;32:484–8.

[8] Orlando C, Pinzani P, Pazzagli M. Developments in quantitative PCR. Clin Chem Lab Med 1998;36:255–69.

[9] Abbott AN, Fang FC. Clinical impact of multiplex syndromic panels in the diagnosis of bloodstream, gastrointestinal, respiratory, and central nervous system infections. Clin Microbiol Newsl 2017;39:133–42.

[10] Messacar K, Hurst AL, Child J, et al. Clinical impact and provider acceptability of real-time antimicrobial stewardship decision support for rapid diagnostics in children with positive blood culture results. J Pediatric Infect Dis Soc 2016;6:267–74.

[11] Rappo U, Schuetz AN, Jenkins SG, et al. Impact of early detection of respiratory viruses by multiplex PCR assay on clinical outcomes in adult patients. J Clin Microbiol 2016;54:2096–103.

[12] Ward C, Stocker K, Begum J, et al. Performance evaluation of the Verigene® (Nanosphere) and FilmArray® (BioFire®) molecular assays for identification of causative organisms in bacterial bloodstream infections. Eur J Clin Microbiol Infect Dis 2015;34:487–96.

[13] Salimnia H, Fairfax MR, Lephart PR, et al. Evaluation of the FilmArray blood culture identification panel: results of a multicenter controlled trial. J Clin Microbiol 2016; 54:687–98.

[14] Van Der Pol B. Profile of the triplex assay for detection of chlamydia, gonorrhea, and trichomonas using the BD MAX system. Expert Rev Mol Diagn 2017;17:539–47.

[15] Madison-Antenucci S, Relich RF, Doyle L, et al. Multicenter evaluation of the BD MAX enteric parasite real-time PCR assay for detection of *Giardia duodenalis, Cryptosporidium hominis, Cryptosporidium parvum,* and *Entamoeba histolytica*. J Clin Microbiol 2016;54:2681–8.

[16] Knabl L, Grutsch I, Orth-Höller D. Comparison of the BD MAX enteric pathogen panel with conventional diagnostic procedures in diarrheal stool samples. Eur J Clin Microbiol Infect Dis 2016;35:131–6.

[17] Simner PJ, Oethinger M, Stellrecht KA, et al. Multisite evaluation of the BD MAX extended enteric bacterial panel for detection of *Yersinia enterocolitica*, enterotoxigenic *Escherichia coli, Vibrio*, and *Plesiomonas shigelloides* from stool specimens. J Clin Microbiol 2017;55: 3258–66.

[18] Nijhuis RHT, Guerendiain D, Claas ECJ. Comparison of the ePlex respiratory pathogen panel with laboratory-developed real-time PCR assays for detection of respiratory pathogens. J Clin Microbiol 2017;55:1938–45.

[19] Pierce VM, Hodinka RL. Comparison of the GenMark diagnostics eSensor respiratory viral panel to real-time PCR for detection of respiratory viruses in children. J Clin Microbiol 2012;50:3458–65.

[20] Babady NE, England MR, Jurcic Smith KL, et al. Multicenter evaluation of the ePlex respiratory pathogen panel for the detection of viral and bacterial respiratory tract pathogens in nasopharyngeal swabs. J Clin Microbiol 2018;56 [pii:e01658-17].

[21] Van Rijn AL, Nijhuis RHT, Bekker V, et al. Clinical implications of rapid ePlex respiratory pathogen panel testing compared to laboratory-developed real-time PCR. Eur J Clin Microbiol Infect Dis 2018;37:571–7.

[22] McCoy MH, Relich RF, Davis TE, et al. Performance of the FilmArray blood culture identification panel utilized by non-expert staff compared to conventional microbial identification and antimicrobial resistance gene detection from positive blood cultures. J Med Microbiol 2016;65:619–25.

[23] Rogers BB, Shankar P, Jerris RC, et al. Impact of a rapid respiratory panel test on patient outcomes. Arch Pathol Lab Med 2015;139:636–41.

[24] Kanack KJ. Rapid respiratory panel testing influences patient management and clinical outcomes. MLO Med Lab Obs 2014;46:16.

[25] MacVane SH, Nolte FS. Benefits of adding a rapid PCR-based blood culture identification panel to an established antimicrobial stewardship program. J Clin Microbiol 2016;54:2455–63.

[26] Southern TR, Van Schooneveld TC, Bannister DL, et al. Implementation and performance of the BioFire FilmArray blood culture identification panel with antimicrobial treatment recommendations for bloodstream infections at a midwestern academic tertiary hospital. Diagn Microbiol Infect Dis 2015;81:96–101.

[27] Buss SN, Leber A, Chapin K, et al. Multicenter evaluation of the BioFire FilmArray gastrointestinal panel for etiologic diagnosis of infectious gastroenteritis. J Clin Microbiol 2015;53:915–25.

[28] Prakash VP, LeBlanc L, Alexander-Scott NE, et al. Use of a culture-independent gastrointestinal multiplex PCR panel during a shigellosis outbreak: considerations for clinical laboratories and public health. J Clin Microbiol 2015;53:1048–9.

[29] Hanson KE, Slechta ES, Killpack JA, et al. Preclinical assessment of a fully automated multiplex PCR panel for detection of central nervous system pathogens. J Clin Microbiol 2016;54:785–7.

[30] Duff S, Hasbun R, Ginocchio CC, et al. Economic analysis of rapid multiplex polymerase chain reaction testing for meningitis/encephalitis in pediatric patients. Future Microbiol 2018;13:617–29.

[31] Gay-Andrieu F, Magassouba N, Picto V, et al. Clinical evaluation of the BioFire FilmArray BioThreat-E test for the diagnosis of Ebola virus disease in Guinea. J Clin Virol 2017;92:20–4.

[32] Papan C, Meyer-Buehn M, Laniado G, et al. Assessment of the multiplex PCR-based assay Unyvero pneumonia application for detection of bacterial pathogens and antibiotic resistance genes in children and neonates. Infection 2018;46:189–96.

[33] Personne Y, Ozongwu C, Platt G, et al. 'Sample-in, answer-out'? Evaluation and comprehensive analysis of the Unyvero P50 pneumonia assay. Diagn Microbiol Infect Dis 2016;86:5–10.

[34] Ledeboer NA, Lopansri BK, Dhiman N, et al. Identification of Gram-negative bacteria and genetic resistance determinants from positive blood culture broths by use of the Verigene Gram-negative blood culture multiplex microarray-based molecular assay. J Clin Microbiol 2015;53:2460–72.

[35] Buchan BW, Ginocchio CC, Manii R, et al. Multiplex identification of Gram-positive bacteria and resistance determinants directly from positive blood culture broths: evaluation of an automated microarray-based nucleic acid test. PLoS Med 2013;10:e1001478.

[36] Esposito S, Principi N. The role of the NxTAG respiratory pathogen panel assay and other multiplex platforms in clinical practice. Expert Rev Mol Diagn 2017;17:9–17.

[37] Tang YW, Gonsalves S, Sun JY, et al. Clinical evaluation of the Luminex NxTAG respiratory pathogen panel. J Clin Microbiol 2016;54:1912–4.

[38] Huang RS, Johnson CL, Pritchard L, et al. Performance of the Verigene enteric pathogens test, BioFire FilmArray gastrointestinal panel and Luminex xTAG gastrointestinal pathogen panel for detection of common enteric pathogens. Diagn Microbiol Infect Dis 2016;86:336–9.

[39] Ramanan P, Bryson AL, Binnicker MJ, et al. Syndromic panel-based testing in clinical microbiology. Clin Microbiol Rev 2017;31 [pii:e00024-17].

[40] Leber AL, Everhart K, Balada-Llasat JM, et al. Multicenter evaluation of BioFire FilmArray Meningitis/Encephalitis Panel for detection of bacteria, viruses, and yeast in cerebrospinal fluid specimens. J Clin Microbiol 2016;54(9): 2251–61.

[41] Dien Bard J, Alby K. Point-counterpoint: meningitis/encephalitis syndromic testing in the clinical laboratory. J Clin Microbiol 2018;56(4) [pii:e00018-18].

[42] Cybulski RJ Jr, Bateman AC, Bourassa L, et al. Clinical impact of a multiplex gastrointestinal PCR panel in patients with acute gastroenteritis. Clin Infect Dis 2018. https://doi.org/10.1093/cid/ciy357.

[43] Leber AL, Everhart K, Daly JA, et al. Multicenter evaluation of BioFire FilmArray Respiratory Panel 2 for detection of viruses and bacteria in nasopharyngeal swab samples. J Clin Microbiol 2018;25(6):56 [pii:e01945-17].

[44] Kawa D, Paradis S, Yu JH, et al. Evaluating the standard of care for women's health: the BD MAX Vaginal Panel and management of vaginal infections (white paper). 2017. Available at: http://moleculardiagnostics.bd.com/wp-content/uploads/2017/08/MAX-Vaginal-Panel-White paper.pdf. Accessed June 25, 2018.

[45] Young S, Illescas P, Nicasio J, et al. Diagnostic accuracy of the real-time PCR cobas Liat influenza A/B assay and the Alere i influenza A&B NEAR isothermal nucleic acid amplification assay for the detection of influenza using adult nasopharyngeal specimens. J Clin Virol 2017;94: 86–90.

[46] Davis S, Allen AJ, O'Leary R, et al. Diagnostic accuracy and cost analysis of the Alere i influenza A&B near-patient test using throat swabs. J Hosp Infect 2017;97: 301–9.

[47] Hassan F, Hays LM, Bonner A, et al. Multicenter clinical evaluation of the Alere i respiratory syncytial virus isothermal nucleic acid amplification assay. J Clin Microbiol 2018;56 [pii:e01777-17].

[48] Schnee SV, Pfeil J, Ihling CM, et al. Performance of the Alere i RSV assay for point-of-care detection of respiratory syncytial virus in children. BMC Infect Dis 2017; 17:767.

[49] Cohen DM, Russo ME, Jaggi P, et al. Multicenter clinical evaluation of the novel Alere i Strep A isothermal nucleic acid amplification test. J Clin Microbiol 2015;53: 2258–61.

[50] Berry GJ, Miller CR, Prats MM, et al. Comparison of the Alere i Strep A test and the BD Veritor system in the detection of group A *Streptococcus* and the hypothetical impact of results on antibiotic utilization. J Clin Microbiol 2018;56 [pii:e01310-17].

[51] Melchers WJG, Kuijpers J, Sickler JJ, et al. Lab-in-a-tube: real-time molecular point-of-care diagnostics for influenza A and B using the cobas Liat system. J Med Virol 2017;89:1382–6.

[52] Gibson J, Schechter-Perkins EM, Mitchell P, et al. Multicenter evaluation of the cobas Liat Influenza A/B & RSV assay for rapid point of care diagnosis. J Clin Virol 2017;95:5–9.

[53] Ling L, Kaplan SE, Lopez JC, et al. Parallel validation of three molecular devices for simultaneous detection and identification of influenza A and B and respiratory syncytial viruses. J Clin Microbiol 2018;56 [pii: e01691-17].

[54] Gaydos CA, Schwebke J, Dombrowski J, et al. Clinical performance of the Solana point-of-care trichomonas assay from clinician-collected vaginal swabs and urine specimens from symptomatic and asymptomatic women. Expert Rev Mol Diagn 2017;17:303–6.

Pharmacogenomics

Advances in Molecular Pathology 1 (2018) 115–124
ADVANCES IN MOLECULAR PATHOLOGY

Applications of Pharmacogenomics in Oncology

Yuan Ji, PhD
Department of Pathology, ARUP Laboratories, University of Utah School of Medicine, Mail Code 115, 500 Chipeta Way, Salt Lake City, UT 84108, USA

KEYWORDS
• Pharmacogenetics • Pharmacogenomics • Germline variants • Single-nucleotide polymorphism • SNP • Somatic mutation • Companion diagnostics • Targeted therapy

KEY POINTS

- Testing germline PGx variants allows tailoring chemotherapy for patients with cancer to avoid toxicity, whereas detecting somatic changes aids in the selection of patients who will likely respond to targeted therapies.
- Pharmacogenetics or pharmacogenomics research applied to oncology has helped drive the development of PGx as a discipline.
- Two sets of genomes in a patient with cancer, tumor and germline, should both be taken into consideration when applying PGx to oncology.
- Professional guidelines are helpful in terms of providing dosing recommendations based on PGx genotypes; additional guidelines to facilitate standardization of clinical PGx testing and reporting are warranted.

INTRODUCTION

The concept of "one-size fits all" does not apply to pharmacologic therapy in oncology. Instead, individual responses to therapy, including the potential for toxicity, depend on the size of the therapeutic window of a medication, along with internal factors, such as comorbidities and concomitant medications, and with environmental factors. In addition, it is now generally accepted that an individual's genetic makeup may predispose some patients to a higher risk for adverse drug events (ADEs) or lack of efficacy, clinical presentations of which manifest only on drug administration. Pharmacogenetics (PGx), often interchangeably called pharmacogenomics, refers to the study of the role of inherited or acquired genomic changes in the drug response phenotype [1]. Although the concept of PGx has become embedded in many domains of medicine including oncology and is widely considered as a "critical component of personalized medicine," the field of PGx is still young and rapidly growing.

The clinical applications of PGx is summarized into two major categories: to avoid or minimize drug-induced toxicities or ADEs; and to maximize efficacy. Together, the ultimate clinical goal of PGx is to give the right medication to the right patient, at the right dose. In the recent Food and Drug Administration Table of Pharmacogenomic Biomarkers in Drug Labeling (https://www.fda.gov/Drugs/ScienceResearch/ucm572698.htm; accessed on April 25, 2018) (Fig. 1), there are greater than 200 drug entries with meaningful PGx associations. Not surprisingly, oncology is the major (32%) area of medicine represented with the

Disclosure Statement: The author has no commercial or financial conflicts of interest to disclose. Funding: University of Utah School of Medicine Department of Pathology Faculty Development Funds; ARUP Laboratories Medical Director Development Funds.
E-mail address: yuan.ji@aruplab.com

https://doi.org/10.1016/j.yamp.2018.06.007
2589-4080/18/

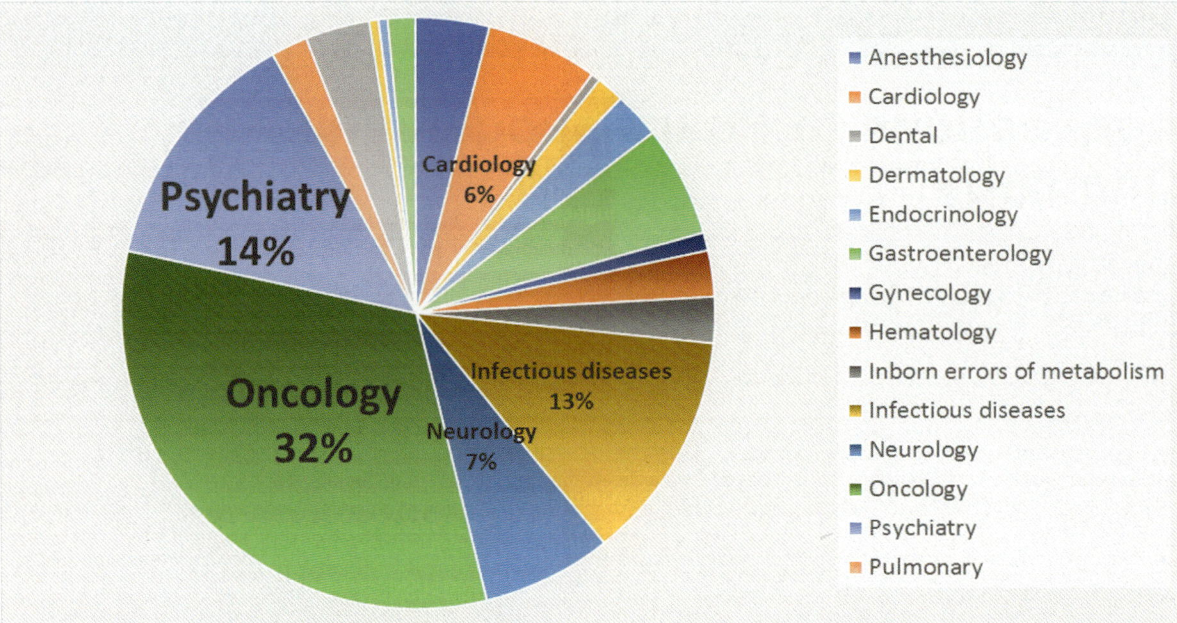

FIG. 1 A summary of applications of clinical PGx testing by specialty. (*Data from* US Food & Drug Administration. Table of pharmacogenomic biomarkers in drug labeling. Available at: https://www.fda.gov/Drugs/ScienceResearch/ucm572698.htm. Accessed April 25, 2018.)

most PGx applications, followed by psychiatry (14%). These PGx biomarkers related to anticancer drugs are further divided into two major categories based on whether the genetic variation is present in the germline or is a tumor-specific somatic alteration.

The use of molecular diagnostics to identify somatic variants in solid tumors and in hematologic malignancies to select targeted therapies has been rapidly expanding in recent years, largely driven by rapid developments in high throughput sequencing and increasing understanding of underlying biologic pathways leading to increasing numbers of targeted therapies. This field has rapidly adopted next-generation sequencing (NGS) as a mainstream testing platform, used for purposes ranging from multigene cancer hotspot panels to whole-exome sequencing (WES) to whole-genome sequencing (WGS). Professional societies from several disciplines, including pathology/laboratory medicine and oncology, have come together to develop guidelines for the use of this information and to promote standardization [2–7].

In this article, classic examples and recent developments of the integration of PGx into oncology are summarized from research and clinical implementation standpoints. Although somatic alterations are of great interest and importance in modern PGx for predicting response to therapeutic agents commonly used in oncology, the focus is on germline PGx variants. Although PGx is important in oncology, research in oncology has also shaped PGx; therefore, this article begins by highlighting PGx-oncology history, then discusses current applications and testing strategies, and ends by projecting future directions for this discipline.

SIGNIFICANCE

Pharmacogenetics at the Bench

PGx research, by nature, has been translational since the beginning of the field more than half century ago. Clinical observations of large individual variation in drug treatment outcomes and plasma drug concentrations provided the initial hint that there might be underlying genetic factors.

The influence of thiopurine S-methyltransferase (TPMT) genetic polymorphisms on risk for cytotoxicity during treatment with thiopurine drugs serves as one of the most striking examples of the critical role of inheritance in contributing to individualized drug therapy. This classic example highlights the evolution of PGx research strategies (Fig. 2) that began with a "phenotype-to-genotype" approach, transitioned to a

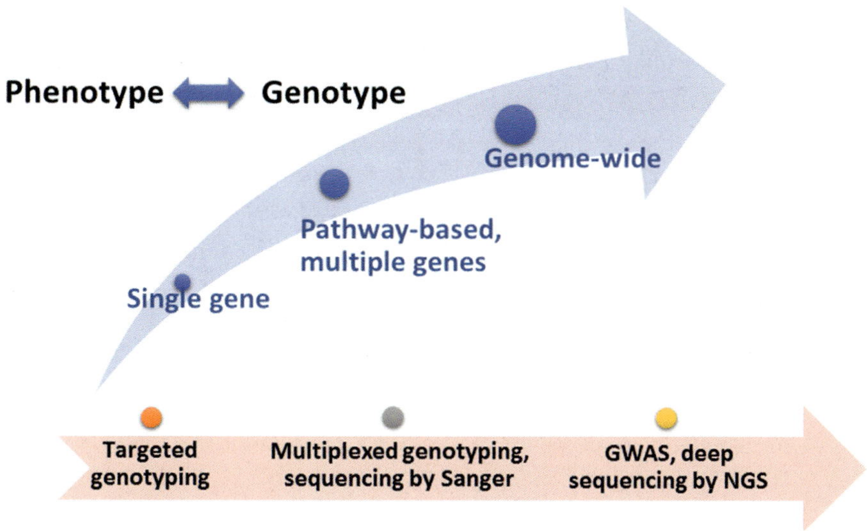

FIG. 2 Evolution of PGx research. Research strategies "phenotype-to-genotype" and "genotype-to-phenotype" are complementary to each other. Research has increased in scales from a few variants in a single gene, to pathway-based, finally to the whole genome. Genotyping techniques have also evolved from targeting a few variants, to multiplex testing of many targeted variants or sequencing of a whole gene, to genome-wide association studies (GWAS), and ultimately to large-scale deep sequencing by NGS.

"genotype-to-phenotype" approach, and ultimately evolved to the current approach involving both strategies concurrently.

PGx of aromatase inhibitors represents a more recent example and highlights how rapid developments in molecular techniques have driven the evolution of PGx research from studies of a single gene to multiple genes and pathway-based approaches, and finally to the whole-genome scale.

Example 1: thiopurines and thiopurine S-methyltransferase

TPMT plays a major role in metabolizing thiopurine drugs including 6-mercaptopurine and azathioprine. These cytotoxic purine analogues are widely used in the treatment of acute lymphoblastic leukemia of childhood and several other nononcologic indications, but have a narrow therapeutic index and can lead to life-threatening myelotoxicity in some individuals. A trimodal distribution of TPMT enzyme activity in red blood cells from 298 randomly selected white blood donors identified by Pazmino and coworkers [8] was the initial hint that genetic variation in a single gene may be related to the toxicities observed in some patients. Further work confirmed that inheritance of defective *TPMT* alleles in an autosomal codominant pattern was associated with the distribution of TPMT activity in red blood cells [9,10]; furthermore, TPMT activity in red blood cells correlates well with the clinical phenotype of myelosuppression and is the basis of TPMT enzyme activity assays in use clinically today [11–13].

The most common functional *TPMT* alleles (**3A, *3B, *3C,* and **2*) have been extensively characterized and account for more than 95% of inherited TPMT deficiencies in the white population [14,15]. In the nearly four decades since the initial in-depth studies by Weinshilboum and others, not only have additional common *TPMT* polymorphisms been identified by resequencing the entire *TPMT* gene in different ethnic populations, but also a further understanding of the mechanisms underlying the low-activity and null alleles has been attained [9,10,16]. Through TPMT functional studies and several other examples it has been demonstrated that a major mechanism by which nonsynonymous coding single-nucleotide polymorphisms (SNPs) affect enzyme activity is by decreasing the quantity of protein, most often because of protein misfolding followed by rapid degradation [16–19]. The successful clinical implementation of *TPMT* PGx was driven primarily by the clinical significance, the extensive research work including functional characterization, the ability to develop robust clinical-grade laboratory tests, and by continuous dialogue between the PGx research community and clinicians.

Finally, the TPMT story also highlights the transition from single-gene studies to whole-genome-based studies. A recent genome-wide association study (GWAS) reaffirmed erythrocyte TPMT activity as a monogenetic trait [20]. In addition, *NUDT15* was recently identified through a genome-wide analysis as an additional polymorphic gene that alters thiopurine metabolism, particularly among Asian and Hispanic populations [21,22]. *NUDT15* genetic testing is already on a fast track to becoming standard practice along with *TPMT* testing before prescription of thiopurine medications.

Example 2: aromatase inhibitors pharmacogenetics

For nearly a decade before the era of NGS, GWAS has been a powerful tool accelerating PGx discoveries by moving beyond a single-gene or a pathway-based approach to SNPs across the whole genome. Through GWAS associations involving many variants in genes/pathways previously known or thought to be important in the pharmacokinetic or pharmacodynamic pathways of specific drug were confirmed, but also GWAS had the tremendous advantage of allowing for discoveries of novel genomic loci underlying individual variation in drug response and ADEs through an unbiased analysis approach (ie, variants in genes/pathways not known to be related to the drug studied were also included in the analysis) [23].

PGx of aromatase inhibitors is an excellent example of GWAS applied to oncology. Ingle and colleagues [24] performed GWAS using DNA samples from MA.27, which was one of the largest clinical trials for aromatase inhibitors in women with breast cancer, to identify genetic variation associated with the severe musculoskeletal pain developed by some women that often leads to discontinuation of therapy. The strongest associations identified were markers in the gene cluster encoding T-cell leukemia-lymphoma proteins (eg, *TCL1A* gene). By extensive functional characterization, the authors of the study were able to link the ADE of severe musculoskeletal pain to *TCL1A* regulation by estrogen exposure *in vitro*, and to expression of inteleukin-17 receptor A and nuclear factor-κB transcriptional activity [25]. Although not routinely tested as PGx markers for aromatase inhibitors yet, these intriguing functional studies around *TCL1A* have illustrated a successful research strategy where associations identified by GWAS can be moved beyond simply reporting "*P*-values" to functional studies that provide further insight into the underlying mechanism.

The aromatase study used a model system of Epstein-Barr-virus-transformed lymphoblastoid cell lines from white Americans, African Americans, and Han Chinese Americans that have been well-characterized with rich data including genome-wide SNPs, gene resequencing of select pharmacogenes, whole-transcriptome expression data, and cytotoxicity profiles of several commonly used chemotherapeutic agents. This model system has served as an extremely valuable tool for the functional studies performed in the aromatase inhibitors PGx study [24,25] and many other discovery studies related to PGx in oncology [26–31].

Pharmacogenetics at the Bedside

Clinical applications of PGx in oncology include testing for somatic changes in tumors and germline variants to either select targeted therapy to optimize efficacy or to tailor therapy to avoid ADEs. In reality, when the term "pharmacogenomics" is used in oncology, it typically refers to testing for germline variants, whereas other terms, including theranostics (combining molecular diagnostics and therapeutic strategy), are usually used to describe genetic testing of somatic variants. The following sections focus on the current status of clinical applications of germline PGx in oncology, testing platforms, existing professional guidelines, and special considerations for this patient population.

Pharmacogenetics testing options

PGx tests are offered by a variety of Clinical Laboratory Improvement Amendments–approved clinical laboratories including large reference laboratories to small boutique laboratories that may only offer PGx tests. Direct-to-consumer PGx testing has also recently emerged on the market. A search of the Genetic Testing Registry (https://www.ncbi.nlm.nih.gov/gtr; last accessed April 25, 2018) using "pharmacogenomics" or "pharmacogenetics" as keywords revealed 160 PGx tests including single-gene tests targeting a specific drug (eg, *TPMT* testing for thiopurines) and panel-based PGx testing for many medications. Even for a single gene, tests were highly variable. Taking *TPMT* testing as an example, tests ranged from SNP-based genotyping of a few variants to full gene sequencing by Sanger or NGS with or without deletion/duplication analysis. At present, although the costs of NGS are rapidly decreasing, most clinically available PGx tests use a targeted genotyping approach, often in the form of a multiplex assay with a few to hundreds of PGx variants.

Professional guidelines

Variation among clinical laboratories in terms of the testing platform used, gene/allele selection, and interpretation and reporting can lead to frustration and confusion by ordering providers. Recently, an international group has outlined some of these challenges and begun to propose solutions to work toward standardization [32]. Building on this work, the Association for Molecular Pathology Clinical Practice Committee established a PGx working group consisting of clinical PGx testing experts to develop recommendations specific to laboratory testing. In the first document published by this group, the authors focused on clinical cytochrome P-450 2C19 (*CYP2C19*) PGx testing, and as a first step to standardize PGx tests, they recommend a panel of specific variant alleles that should be included at a minimum in clinical *CYP2C19* PGx tests [33]. This is the first time that a list of "must test" alleles has been proposed for a PGx gene; it is hoped that more genes will be included and these recommendations will be adopted by clinical laboratories.

In addition to recent work to standardize the testing itself, several organizations have developed clinical guidelines for the use of germline pharmacogenomic test results, including use in oncology [14,15,34–39]. Not including those medications related to other non-neoplastic complications in patients with cancer, currently there are 19 PGx dosing guidelines available for 11 cancer drugs (Table 1). The available practice guidelines, such as those published by the Clinical Pharmacogenetics Implementation Consortium (CPIC, https://cpicpgx.org/guidelines; last accessed April 25, 2018), the Royal Dutch Association for the Advancement of Pharmacy - Pharmacogenetics Working Group, and the Canadian Pharmacogenomics Network for Drug Safety are readily accessed through the Pharmacogenomics Knowledgebase (PharmGKB, https://www.pharmgkb.org/guidelines; last accessed April 25, 2018). Generally, these dosing guidelines are developed with a goal of helping clinicians understand how to use PGx test results to optimize drug therapy, and they are not designed to address whether the tests should be ordered or how the PGx tests should be designed and performed.

These guidelines are based on expert consensus and are reviewed and updated as needed. For example, the updated CPIC dihydropyrimidine dehydrogenase (*DYPD*)-fluoropyrimidine dosing guideline was recently updated [34]. This guideline focuses on the known functional consequences of a few variants (c.1905+1G>A, c.1679T>G, c.2846A>T, c.1129–5923C>G), providing genetic-based recommendations to use standard dosing, a decreased dose potentially with therapeutic drug monitoring (TDM), or to avoid fluoropyrimidines. Although these recommendations are helpful, they do not explicitly state whether testing should be performed before prescription, and they may be difficult to apply when variants are detected that are not yet well-characterized.

TABLE 1
Dosing Guidelines for Cancer Chemotherapeutic Drugs

Drug	CPIC[a]	DPWG[b]	CPNDS[c]	Others
Azathioprine	*TPMT*	*TPMT*		
Capecitabine	*DPYD*	*DPYD*		
Cisplatin			*TPMT*	
Daunorubicin			*RARG*, *SLC28A3*, *UGT1A6*	
Doxorubicin			*RARG*, *SLC28A3*, *UGT1A6*	
Fluorouracil	*DPYD*	*DPYD*		
Irinotecan		*UGT1A1*		*UGT1A1*
Mercaptopurine	*TPMT*	*TPMT*		
Tamoxifen	*CYP2D6*	*CYP2D6*		
Tegafur (prodrug of 5-fluorouracil)		*DPYD*		
Thioguanine	*TPMT*	*TPMT*		

[a] Clinical Pharmacogenetics Implementation Consortium.
[b] Royal Dutch Association for the Advancement of Pharmacy - Pharmacogenetics Working Group.
[c] Canadian Pharmacogenomics Network for Drug Safety.
From PharmGKB. Dosing guidelines. Available at: https://www.pharmgkb.org/guidelines; with permission from PharmGKB and Stanford University.

Another example of a PGx guideline relevant in oncology is the recently published CYP2D6-tamoxifen guideline [35]. Although genetic variation in *CYP2D6* has been known to be important in drug metabolism for many years, there is still a lack of consensus in the field regarding the assignment of predicted phenotype based on genotype; however, work to establish an enzyme activity scoring system and to harmonize *CYP2D6* genetic test interpretation among laboratories is underway [40]. Of note, in the CYP2D6-tamoxifen guideline, the phenotype assignment based on CYP2D6 activity scores differs from the scheme used in prior CYP2D6-related guidelines, suggesting that CYP2D6 substrate specificity may add further to the complexity of PGx. Although CYP2D6 is known to convert tamoxifen into metabolites with greater antiestrogen properties, because of many confounding factors, such as genotyping accuracy, study design, and interaction with other medications, results from tamoxifen outcome association studies have not been consistent [41]. Goetz and colleagues [42] reported a retrospective study of a prospective, randomized phase III trial and reported that CYP2D6 metabolizer status is a predictor of tamoxifen clinical outcome and treatment-related hot flashes in postmenopausal women. Later, a meta-analysis of 4973 patients treated with tamoxifen in the International Tamoxifen Pharmacogenomics Consortium provided additional evidence supporting the link between *CYP2D6* with tamoxifen treatment [43]. The recently published CPIC dosing guideline on *CYP2D6*-tamoxifen summarizes additional literature and provides therapeutic recommendations based on *CYP2D6* genotype [35]. This guideline also extends beyond the genetic recommendation by including a comment regarding avoidance of CYP2D6 inhibitors to avoid potential alteration in metabolizer status caused by drug-drug interaction, which is called "phenoconversion."

Special pharmacogenetics considerations for patients with malignancy

Patients with cancer have at least two genomes to consider: germline genome and tumor genome. Genetic alterations in both genomes may contribute to treatment outcomes and ADE; however, these two genomes are typically examined independently when evaluating PGx biomarkers in patients with cancer. This is in part because the specimen type optimal for evaluation differs with blood and/or buccal specimens often used for germline variant testing and the necessity to use tumor tissue for detection of somatic variants. McWhinney and McLeod [44] reviewed publications that examined the concordance of PGx genotyping results between germline DNA and somatic DNA, and concluded that there is high (>93%) concordance between germline and somatic DNA. Although this suggests that it may be possible to obtain reasonably accurate germline PGx results by testing tumor, given that the differences may be clinically significant and germline DNA is easy to obtain, it may be ideal to continue to test separate specimens when possible.

Although patients with cancer are often exposed to polypharmacy, this population is much less discussed than the elderly, which is a population reported to have greatly increased risk for ADEs because of polypharmacy [45]. Multiple medications including but not limited to antineoplastics, pain medications, antiemetics, and antidepressants are often prescribed to patients with cancer to control tumor growth and to manage symptoms. Because of potential drug-drug interactions, patients taking several medications are more likely to have ADEs and/or reduced efficacy. A systematic review and meta-analysis have showed that approximately 58% of patients taking four or more medications are prone to ADEs and that approximately 90% of ADEs are preventable [46]. Currently, when clinical PGx testing for patients with cancer is performed, testing usually focuses on one or one group of medications and consideration of complications caused by polypharmacy is unlikely to be included in the PGx report. Furthermore, because patients with cancer are often on many supportive therapies for which well-established PGx testing is available, this patient population is particularly likely to benefit from PGx testing to reduce trial and error prescribing and to improve quality of life [47].

Enzyme activity assays and therapeutic drug monitoring as complementary strategies

PGx testing is most appropriate before prescription to predict the most appropriate dose and/or to suggest that an alternate medication should be considered. In addition to genetic tests that predict enzyme activity, tests that measure the enzyme activity itself are also available for some enzymes, such as TPMT. In the case of TPMT, the two tests (phenotyping and genotyping) are complementary each with advantages and limitations; however, physicians generally prefer one over the other rather than using them together [48,49].

After initial dose prediction, patients may still require further dose adjustment to obtain optimal efficacy. TDM is useful in this setting because it allows for the measurement of drug concentrations *in vivo*, monitoring compliance, and determining ratios among metabolites. In addition, TDM is useful in a research setting for pharmacokinetic-pharmacodynamic modeling. In a 2016 study by Hertz and coworkers [50], an increased dose of tamoxifen was given to patients with breast cancer who were *CYP2D6* intermediate metabolizers or poor metabolizers and the concentration of the active metabolite endoxifen was measured. This study demonstrated that an increased dose was able to eliminate the differences in endoxifen concentration, without any obvious increases in treatment-related toxicity.

Despite the potential utility of combining TDM with PGx, both are available for only a subset of medications, including thiopurines-*TPMT* and potentially 5-fluoroucacil-*DPYD* [51,52].

PROPOSED FUTURE PHARMACOGENETICS TESTING MODEL FOR ONCOLOGY: A REFERENCE LABORATORY PERSPECTIVE

Although most patients are expected to have potentially actionable PGx variants [53,54], PGx is generally underused with only a small subset of patients who could benefit actually undergoing testing. In oncology, somatic PGx testing for selection of targeted therapy is more broadly applied, whereas germline PGx testing is less frequently used; these tests are currently ordered and performed independently, despite both having an impact on response to oncologic therapy. A novel model for future PGx testing in oncology that accounts for both genomes of these patients and integrates results into a final recommendation should be considered.

Increasing clinical use of WES/WGS in either blood or tumor specimens represents a potential opportunity to identify additional variants, both somatic and germline, that may impact therapy. For example, Apelániz-Ruiz and colleagues [55] reported that using an unbiased WES approach allowed for discovery of germline variants in *CYP3A4* that are related to paclitaxel dose-limiting neuropathy. A study by Li and colleagues [56] also used WES to interrogate tumor and blood samples from patients with non–small cell lung cancer and resistance to epidermal growth factor receptor (EGFR) tyrosine kinase inhibitors, but who were negative for the *EGFR* T790M mutation and *cMET*-unamplified. Using the powerful tool of WES, they identified several candidate genes (*BRAF, FGFR1, PAK1, PCNT, PEBP4*, and *SOX3*) with variants that may lead to EGFR tyrosine kinase inhibitor resistance [56]. A comprehensive study of 121 patients who went through both germline and tumor DNA WES was published by Parsons and colleagues from Baylor College of Medicine [57]. In this study, somatic mutations of established clinical utility (categories I and II) were detected in 27% of 121 patients, whereas at least one PGx variant was observed in 89% of the patients. Of

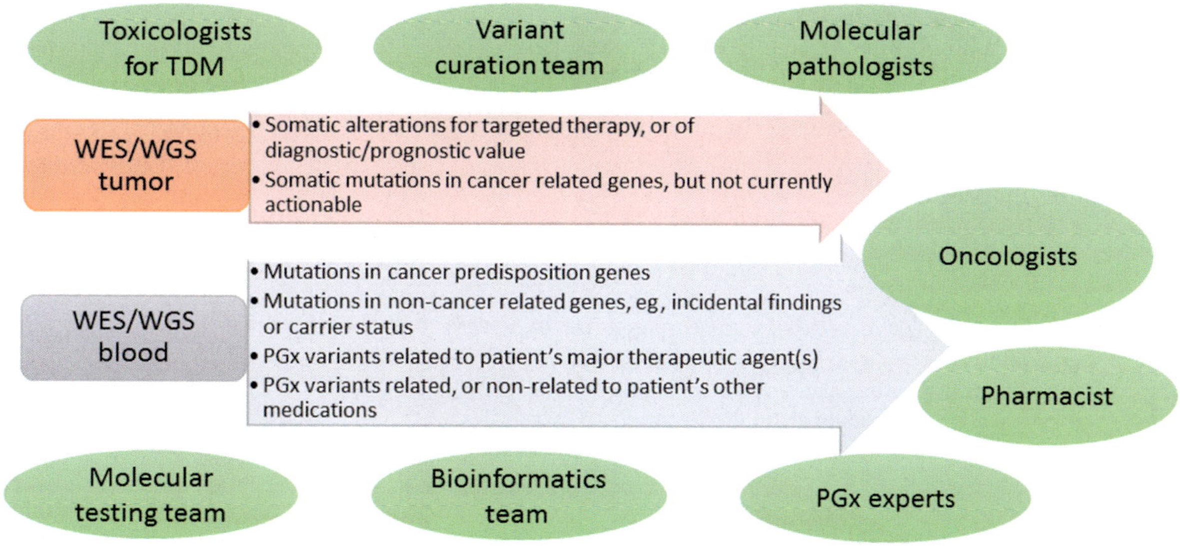

FIG. 3 An integrated model for future oncology PGx testing through WES/WGS. Looking to the future, tumor and germline genomes will likely be sequenced through WES or WGS. Germline and somatic variants will be analyzed and an integrated report describing features of the disease and relevant PGx recommendations will be developed by multidisciplinary teams for optimal cancer care. TDM, Therapeutic drug monitoring.

note, the PGx analysis was limited to *CYP2C19*, *CYP2C9*, and *VKORC1*; however, even though these variants were not specific for oncology, with such a high percentage of patients harboring variants, this study suggests the potential value of an integrated approach. A recent review by Nath and colleagues [58] further argues for an integrated approach by describing the influence of germline and somatic variants on response to targeted therapy in chronic myelogenous leukemia.

Future studies using modern technology to identify additional relevant variants (somatic and germline) and to develop and test integrated models to further individualize therapy for patients with cancer are warranted. A team-based approach at the testing laboratory that consists of key personnel with expertise in the molecular and morphologic characteristics of tumors, pharmacogenomics, TDM assays, and bioinformatics is essential to optimize care of patients with cancer through an integrated model of oncology testing (Fig. 3). Effective, real-time communication with ordering providers is also necessary as part of this model. Informative and productive dialogues already exist in other diagnostic settings, such as rapid WES/WGS for neonatal critical care settings [59,60], and should be applied in oncology.

SUMMARY

Several early examples of PGx were identified through translational research efforts and involve medications used in oncology, such as thiopurines, fluoropyrimidines, and irinotecan. Translational PGx research continues to drive the field of PGx. New discoveries of important biomarkers allow for the introduction of new clinical tests to benefit patients. Other translational studies generate the critical evidence to demonstrate the usefulness of this information, allowing for patient access to testing through ensuring provider awareness and increased willingness to cover testing by payers. Guidelines have been developed to aid health care providers in the use of PGx test results, and to standardize the interpretation and increase consistency among clinical laboratory tests. Finally, an integrated approach of sequencing tumor and germline genomes of patients with cancer is proposed for a more personalized cancer care in the near future.

REFERENCES

[1] Wang L, McLeod HL, Weinshilboum RM. Genomics and drug response. N Engl J Med 2011;364(12):1144–53.

[2] Li MM, Datto M, Duncavage EJ, et al. Standards and guidelines for the interpretation and reporting of sequence variants in cancer: a joint consensus recommendation of the association for molecular pathology, American Society of Clinical Oncology, and College of American Pathologists. J Mol Diagn 2017;19(1):4–23.

[3] Jennings LJ, Arcila ME, Corless C, et al. Guidelines for validation of next-generation sequencing-based oncology panels: a joint consensus recommendation of the association for molecular pathology and College of American Pathologists. J Mol Diagn 2017;19(3):341–65.

[4] Kalemkerian GP, Narula N, Kennedy EB, et al. Molecular testing guideline for the selection of patients with lung cancer for treatment with targeted tyrosine kinase inhibitors: American Society of Clinical Oncology Endorsement of the College of American Pathologists/International Association for the Study of Lung Cancer/Association for Molecular Pathology Clinical Practice Guideline Update. J Clin Oncol 2018;36(9):911–9.

[5] Sepulveda AR, Hamilton SR, Allegra CJ, et al. Molecular biomarkers for the evaluation of colorectal cancer: guideline from the American Society for Clinical Pathology, College of American Pathologists, Association for Molecular Pathology, and American Society of Clinical Oncology. Arch Pathol Lab Med 2017;141(5):625–57.

[6] Arber DA, Borowitz MJ, Cessna M, et al. Initial diagnostic workup of acute leukemia: guideline from the College of American Pathologists and the American Society of Hematology. Arch Pathol Lab Med 2017;141(10):1342–93.

[7] Bartley AN, Washington MK, Ventura CB, et al. HER2 testing and clinical decision making in gastroesophageal adenocarcinoma: guideline from the College of American Pathologists, American Society for Clinical Pathology, and American Society of Clinical Oncology. Am J Clin Pathol 2016;146(6):647–69.

[8] Pazmino PA, Sladek SL, Weinshilboum RM. Thiol S-methylation in uremia: erythrocyte enzyme activities and plasma inhibitors. Clin Pharmacol Ther 1980; 28(3):356–67.

[9] Loennechen T, Yates CR, Fessing MY, et al. Isolation of a human thiopurine S-methyltransferase (TPMT) complementary DNA with a single nucleotide transition A719G (TPMT*3C) and its association with loss of TPMT protein and catalytic activity in humans. Clin Pharmacol Ther 1998;64(1):46–51.

[10] Krynetski EY, Schuetz JD, Galpin AJ, et al. A single point mutation leading to loss of catalytic activity in human thiopurine S-methyltransferase. Proc Natl Acad Sci U S A 1995;92(4):949–53.

[11] Krynetski E, Evans WE. Drug methylation in cancer therapy: lessons from the TPMT polymorphism. Oncogene 2003;22(47):7403–13.

[12] McLeod HL, Relling MV, Liu Q, et al. Polymorphic thiopurine methyltransferase in erythrocytes is indicative of activity in leukemic blasts from children with acute lymphoblastic leukemia. Blood 1995;85(7):1897–902.

[13] Lennard L. Implementation of TPMT testing. Br J Clin Pharmacol 2014;77(4):704–14.

[14] Relling MV, Gardner EE, Sandborn WJ, et al. Clinical pharmacogenetics implementation consortium guidelines for thiopurine methyltransferase genotype and thiopurine dosing: 2013 update. Clin Pharmacol Ther 2013;93(4):324–5.
[15] Relling MV, Gardner EE, Sandborn WJ, et al. Clinical pharmacogenetics implementation consortium guidelines for thiopurine methyltransferase genotype and thiopurine dosing. Clin Pharmacol Ther 2011;89(3): 387–91.
[16] Salavaggione OE, Wang L, Wiepert M, et al. Thiopurine S-methyltransferase pharmacogenetics: variant allele functional and comparative genomics. Pharmacogenet Genomics 2005;15(11):801–15.
[17] Wang L, Sullivan W, Toft D, et al. Thiopurine S-methyltransferase pharmacogenetics: chaperone protein association and allozyme degradation. Pharmacogenetics 2003; 13(9):555–64.
[18] Wang L, Nguyen TV, McLaughlin RW, et al. Human thiopurine S-methyltransferase pharmacogenetics: variant allozyme misfolding and aggresome formation. Proc Natl Acad Sci U S A 2005;102(26):9394–9.
[19] Ji Y, Salavaggione OE, Wang L, et al. Human phenylethanolamine N-methyltransferase pharmacogenomics: gene re-sequencing and functional genomics. J Neurochem 2005;95(6):1766–76.
[20] Liu C, Yang W, Pei D, et al. Genomewide approach validates thiopurine methyltransferase activity is a monogenic pharmacogenomic trait. Clin Pharmacol Ther 2017;101(3):373–81.
[21] Moriyama T, Nishii R, Perez-Andreu V, et al. NUDT15 polymorphisms alter thiopurine metabolism and hematopoietic toxicity. Nat Genet 2016;48(4):367–73.
[22] Yang JJ, Landier W, Yang W, et al. Inherited NUDT15 variant is a genetic determinant of mercaptopurine intolerance in children with acute lymphoblastic leukemia. J Clin Oncol 2015;33(11):1235–42.
[23] Motsinger-Reif AA, Jorgenson E, Relling MV, et al. Genome-wide association studies in pharmacogenomics: successes and lessons. Pharmacogenet Genomics 2013; 23(8):383–94.
[24] Ingle JN, Schaid DJ, Goss PE, et al. Genome-wide associations and functional genomic studies of musculoskeletal adverse events in women receiving aromatase inhibitors. J Clin Oncol 2010;28(31):4674–82.
[25] Liu M, Wang L, Bongartz T, et al. Aromatase inhibitors, estrogens and musculoskeletal pain: estrogen-dependent T-cell leukemia 1A (TCL1A) gene-mediated regulation of cytokine expression. Breast Cancer Res 2012;14(2):R41.
[26] Fasching PA, Haberle L, Rack B, et al. Clinical validation of genetic variants associated with in vitro chemotherapy-related lymphoblastoid cell toxicity. Oncotarget 2017;8(44):78133–43.
[27] Niu N, Schaid DJ, Abo RP, et al. Genetic association with overall survival of taxane-treated lung cancer patients: a genome-wide association study in human lymphoblastoid cell lines followed by a clinical association study. BMC Cancer 2012;12:422.
[28] Li L, Fridley B, Kalari K, et al. Gemcitabine and cytosine arabinoside cytotoxicity: association with lymphoblastoid cell expression. Cancer Res 2008;68(17): 7050–8.
[29] Gamazon ER, Lamba JK, Pounds S, et al. Comprehensive genetic analysis of cytarabine sensitivity in a cell-based model identifies polymorphisms associated with outcome in AML patients. Blood 2013;121(21): 4366–76.
[30] Wheeler HE, Dolan ME. Lymphoblastoid cell lines in pharmacogenomic discovery and clinical translation. Pharmacogenomics 2012;13(1):55–70.
[31] Wheeler HE, Gorsic LK, Welsh M, et al. Genome-wide local ancestry approach identifies genes and variants associated with chemotherapeutic susceptibility in African Americans. PLoS One 2011;6(7):e21920.
[32] Kalman LV, Agundez J, Appell ML, et al. Pharmacogenetic allele nomenclature: international workgroup recommendations for test result reporting. Clin Pharmacol Ther 2016;99(2):172–85.
[33] Pratt VM, Del Tredici AL, Hachad H, et al. Recommendations for clinical CYP2C19 genotyping allele selection: a report of the association for molecular pathology. J Mol Diagn 2018;20(3):269–76.
[34] Amstutz U, Henricks LM, Offer SM, et al. Clinical pharmacogenetics implementation consortium (CPIC) guideline for dihydropyrimidine dehydrogenase genotype and fluoropyrimidine dosing: 2017 update. Clin Pharmacol Ther 2018;103(2):210–6.
[35] Goetz MP, Sangkuhl K, Guchelaar HJ, et al. Clinical pharmacogenetics implementation consortium (CPIC) guideline for CYP2D6 and tamoxifen therapy. Clin Pharmacol Ther 2018;103(5):770–7.
[36] Swen JJ, Nijenhuis M, de Boer A, et al. Pharmacogenetics: from bench to byte–an update of guidelines. Clin Pharmacol Ther 2011;89(5):662–73.
[37] Lee JW, Pussegoda K, Rassekh SR, et al. Clinical practice recommendations for the management and prevention of cisplatin-induced hearing loss using pharmacogenetic markers. Ther Drug Monit 2016;38(4):423–31.
[38] Aminkeng F, Ross CJ, Rassekh SR, et al. Recommendations for genetic testing to reduce the incidence of anthracycline-induced cardiotoxicity. Br J Clin Pharmacol 2016;82(3):683–95.
[39] Etienne-Grimaldi MC, Boyer JC, Thomas F, et al. UGT1A1 genotype and irinotecan therapy: general review and implementation in routine practice. Fundam Clin Pharmacol 2015;29(3):219–37.
[40] Hicks JK, Swen JJ, Gaedigk A. Challenges in CYP2D6 phenotype assignment from genotype data: a critical assessment and call for standardization. Curr Drug Metab 2014;15(2):218–32.
[41] Goetz MP, Ingle JN. CYP2D6 genotype and tamoxifen: considerations for proper nonprospective studies. Clin Pharmacol Ther 2014;96(2):141–4.

[42] Goetz MP, Rae JM, Suman VJ, et al. Pharmacogenetics of tamoxifen biotransformation is associated with clinical outcomes of efficacy and hot flashes. J Clin Oncol 2005;23(36):9312–8.

[43] Province MA, Goetz MP, Brauch H, et al. CYP2D6 genotype and adjuvant tamoxifen: meta-analysis of heterogeneous study populations. Clin Pharmacol Ther 2014; 95(2):216–27.

[44] McWhinney SR, McLeod HL. Using germline genotype in cancer pharmacogenetic studies. Pharmacogenomics 2009;10(3):489–93.

[45] Budnitz DS, Lovegrove MC, Shehab N, et al. Emergency hospitalizations for adverse drug events in older Americans. N Engl J Med 2011;365(21):2002–12.

[46] Johansson T, Abuzahra ME, Keller S, et al. Impact of strategies to reduce polypharmacy on clinically relevant endpoints: a systematic review and meta-analysis. Br J Clin Pharmacol 2016;82(2):532–48.

[47] Patel JN, Wiebe LA, Dunnenberger HM, et al. Value of supportive care pharmacogenomics in oncology practice. Oncologist 2018;23(8):956–64.

[48] Weitzel KW, Smith DM, Elsey AR, et al. Implementation of standardized clinical processes for TPMT testing in a diverse multidisciplinary population: challenges and lessons learned. Clin Transl Sci 2018;11(2):175–81.

[49] Zur RM, Roy LM, Ito S, et al. Thiopurine S-methyltransferase testing for averting drug toxicity: a meta-analysis of diagnostic test accuracy. Pharmacogenomics J 2016; 16(4):305–11.

[50] Hertz DL, Deal A, Ibrahim JG, et al. Tamoxifen dose escalation in patients with diminished CYP2D6 activity normalizes endoxifen concentrations without increasing toxicity. Oncologist 2016;21(7):795–803.

[51] Boisdron-Celle M, Capitain O, Faroux R, et al. Prevention of 5-fluorouracil-induced early severe toxicity by pre-therapeutic dihydropyrimidine dehydrogenase deficiency screening: assessment of a multiparametric approach. Semin Oncol 2017;44(1):13–23.

[52] Lee JJ, Beumer JH, Chu E. Therapeutic drug monitoring of 5-fluorouracil. Cancer Chemother Pharmacol 2016; 78(3):447–64.

[53] Van Driest SL, Shi Y, Bowton EA, et al. Clinically actionable genotypes among 10,000 patients with preemptive pharmacogenomic testing. Clin Pharmacol Ther 2014; 95(4):423–31.

[54] Ji Y, Skierka JM, Blommel JH, et al. Preemptive pharmacogenomic testing for precision medicine: a comprehensive analysis of five actionable pharmacogenomic genes using next-generation DNA sequencing and a customized CYP2D6 genotyping cascade. J Mol Diagn 2016; 18(3):438–45.

[55] Apellániz-Ruiz M, Lee MY, Sanchez-Barroso L, et al. Whole-exome sequencing reveals defective CYP3A4 variants predictive of paclitaxel dose-limiting neuropathy. Clin Cancer Res 2015;21(2):322–8.

[56] Li C, Liu H, Zhang B, et al. Whole-exome sequencing identifies key mutated genes in T790M wildtype/ cMET-unamplified lung adenocarcinoma with acquired resistance to first-generation EGFR tyrosine kinase inhibitors. J Cancer Res Clin Oncol 2018;144(6): 1079–86.

[57] Parsons DW, Roy A, Yang Y, et al. Diagnostic yield of clinical tumor and germline whole-exome sequencing for children with solid tumors. JAMA Oncol 2016;2(5): 616–24.

[58] Nath A, Wang J, Stephanie Huang R. Pharmacogenetics and pharmacogenomics of targeted therapeutics in chronic myeloid leukemia. Mol Diagn Ther 2017; 21(6):621–31.

[59] Farnaes L, Hildreth A, Sweeney NM, et al. Rapid whole-genome sequencing decreases infant morbidity and cost of hospitalization. NPJ Genom Med 2018; 3:10.

[60] Meng L, Pammi M, Saronwala A, et al. Use of exome sequencing for infants in intensive care units: ascertainment of severe single-gene disorders and effect on medical management. JAMA Pediatr 2017;171(12):e173438.

Advances in Molecular Pathology 1 (2018) 125–134
ADVANCES IN MOLECULAR PATHOLOGY

Building Evidence for Clinical Use of Pharmacogenomics and Reimbursement for Testing

Larisa H. Cavallari, PharmD[a,*], Victoria M. Pratt, PhD[b]
[a]Department of Pharmacotherapy and Translational Research, Center for Pharmacogenomics, University of Florida, PO Box 100486, Gainesville, FL 32610-0486, USA; [b]Pharmacogenomics and Molecular Genetics Laboratories, Department of Medical and Molecular Genetics, Indiana University School of Medicine, 975 W. Walnut Street, IB-344B, Indianapolis, IN 46202, USA

KEYWORDS
• Pharmacogenomics • Genotype • Evidence • Outcomes • Reimbursement

KEY POINTS

- The evidence gap in outcomes with pharmacogenomic testing and testing reimbursement are major challenges to pharmacogenomic implementation.
- Although randomized controlled trials (RCTs) are considered the gold standard for establishing clinical utility and informing treatment guidelines, few have been done in pharmacogenomics.
- Conducting an RCT for each gene-drug pair is impractical from a time and cost perspective, and more efficient approaches are needed for evidence generation.
- Outcomes data with pharmacogenomic testing are emerging from pragmatic and observational studies, and further data are expected from ongoing pragmatic clinical trials.
- It is expected that reimbursement will follow evidence for benefit with pharmacogenomic testing.

INTRODUCTION

In his 2015 State of the Union Address, former President Obama announced the Precision Medicine Initiative signaling continued US government support toward individualized disease detection, prevention, and management strategies [1]. Pharmacogenomics is one component of precision medicine and promises to optimize drug therapy through the incorporation of an individual's genetic information in drug prescribing decisions. Genotype specifically influences pharmacokinetics and pharmacodynamics and allows for prediction of risk for adverse drug effects and likelihood of drug effectiveness.

Following decades of research into genetic determinants of drug response, pharmacogenomics is entering clinical practice at institutions across the United States and Europe [2–11]. Guidelines by the Clinical Pharmacogenetics Implementation Consortium (CPIC) and Dutch Pharmacogenetics Working Group (DPWG) have facilitated the adoption of genotype-guided

Disclosure: The authors have nothing to disclose.
Funding: This work is supported by NIH/NHGRI grant U01 HG007269 and NIH/NCATS grant UL1 TR001427 to L.H. Cavallari. V. M. Pratt is supported by NIH/NHGRI grant U01HG007762 and the Indiana University Health – Indiana University School of Medicine Strategic Research Initiative. The Indiana University School of Medicine Pharmacogenomics Laboratory is a fee-for-service clinical laboratory that offers clinical pharmacogenetic testing.

*Corresponding author, *E-mail address:* lcavallari@cop.ufl.edu

https://doi.org/10.1016/j.yamp.2018.06.008
2589-4080/18/

therapy by informing implementation priorities and strategies [12,13]. These guidelines specifically provide recommendations for how to translate genotype results to prescribing decisions for gene-drug pairs with evidence supporting their incorporation in clinical practice.

Clinical validity is well established for gene-drug pairs addressed by the CPIC and DPGW. However, evidence supporting the clinical utility of testing is much more limited. Although randomized controlled trials (RCTs) are considered the gold standard for establishing clinical utility and informing treatment guidelines, few have been done in pharmacogenomics. Some in fact argue that RCTs should not be the level of evidentiary support required for pharmacogenomic implementation [14–16]. Rather, genotype may be viewed as one of the several patient-specific factors that influence drug response, as shown in Fig. 1. Laboratory tests such as serum creatinine, hemoglobin, and serum potassium are routinely ordered before initiating drug therapy to guide drug and dose selection in the absence of RCT evidence to support this approach. Genotype is essentially another laboratory test that can be considered in the context of other patient-specific factors to enable individualized drug therapy. Nonetheless, demonstrating value with genotype-guided therapy is needed to influence policy makers and key stakeholders in genomic medicine, including providers and third party payers. In this article, the authors discuss existing data and ongoing efforts to generate evidence in support of genotype-guided therapy approaches and reimbursement for pharmacogenomic testing.

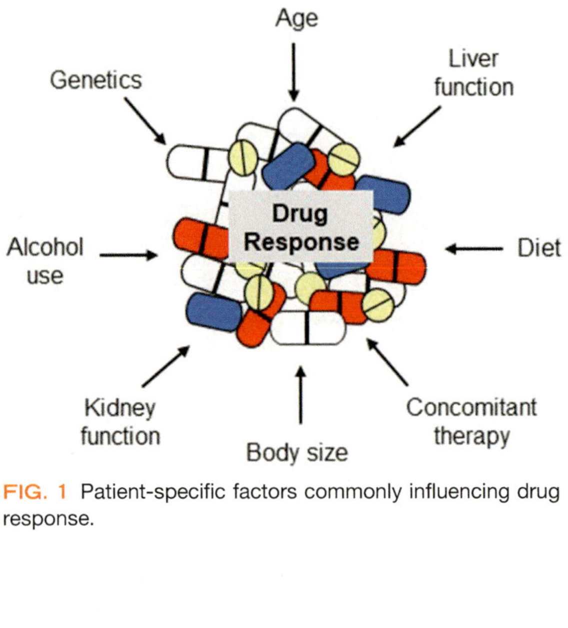

FIG. 1 Patient-specific factors commonly influencing drug response.

BUILDING EVIDENCE TO SUPPORT PHARMACOGENOMIC IMPLEMENTATION

Randomized Controlled Trial Evidence

Table 1 summarizes gene-drug pairs investigated in RCTs, which include *HLA-B*57:01*-abacavir, *TPMT*-thiopurines, and *CYP2C9/VKORC1*-warfarin. In the case of abacavir, the PREDICT-1 trial of nearly 2000 patients showed that prospective screening for the *HLA-B*57:01* allele, with avoidance of abacavir in patients testing positive for the allele, resulted in a significant reduction in the risk for immunologically confirmed hypersensitivity reactions, with a 100% negative predictive value [17]. Based on these data, the Food and Drug Administration (FDA), European Medicines Agency, CPIC, DPWG, and Human Immunodeficiency Virus treatment guidelines recommend *HLA-B*57:01* screening before initiation of abacavir-containing regimens [18]. Similarly, *TPMT*-guided thiopurine dosing was shown to reduce the risk for adverse hematologic reactions in variant allele carriers, with CPIC and DPWG guidelines available and *TPMT* genotyping routinely incorporated into thiopurine dosing decisions at many institutions [3,7,8,19–21].

Genotype-guided warfarin dosing is probably the most extensively studied pharmacogenomic intervention, with 3 large RCTs investigating the efficacy of genotype-guided warfarin dosing [22–24]. Only the most recent trial, Genetics InFormatics Trial (GIFT), had sufficient power to examine clinical outcomes with warfarin pharmacogenomics, whereas previous trials focused on the endpoint of time in therapeutic range. Among patients who underwent elective hip or knee arthroplasty, GIFT demonstrated a 27% relative risk reduction in the composite outcome of death, venous thromboembolism, major bleeding, or an international normalized ratio (INR) greater than or equal to 4 with a genotype-guided dosing approach versus dosing based on clinical factors [24]. These findings are consistent with data from the EU-PACT trial, which demonstrated greater time in the therapeutic INR range with genotype-guided dosing compared with a traditional dosing approach [23]. In contrast, the Classification of Optimal Anticoagulation Through Genetics (COAG) trial, which included a more racially diverse population than either the EU-PACT trial or GIFT, found no difference in time in therapeutic INR range between genotype-guided dosing versus clinically guided dosing [22]. In the subset of African Americans, genotype-guided dosing led to lower time in therapeutic range compared with clinical dosing, which is probably because the study did not genotype for many of the

TABLE 1
Examples of Randomized Controlled Trials of Genotype-Guided Therapies

Gene-Drug Pair	Trial Acronym	Patient Population	Summary of Results
*HLA-B*57:01*-Abacavir	PREDICT-1 [17]	1956 patients with HIV randomized to prospective genetic screening with avoidance of abacavir in patients screening positive or to abacavir use without screening	Immunologically confirmed hypersensitivity occurred in 0% of patients in the prospective-screening group vs 2.7% of controls, *P*<.001
TPMT-Thiopurines	TOPIC [20]	783 patients with inflammatory bowel disease randomized to pretreatment screening with thiopurine dose reduction in carriers of a variant allele according to DPWG guidelines or to usual thiopurine dosing without screening	Adverse hematologic reactions did not differ between genotype vs control patients in the population overall, but were less common in *TPMT* variant allele carriers in the genotype vs control group (2.6% vs 22.9%, RR, 0.11, 95% CI 0.01–0.85)
CYP2C9/ VKORC1-warfarin	COAG [22]	1015 patients randomized to genotype-guided dosing or clinically guided dosing	Mean percent of time in therapeutic range in the first 4 wk was similar between the genotype- and clinically guided groups (45.2% and 45.4%) for the population overall. Among Blacks, the mean time in range was lower with genotype- vs clinically guided dosing (35.2% vs 43.5%, *P* = .01)
	EU-PACT [23]	455 patients randomized to genotype-guided dosing or fixed dosing (5–10 mg day 1, then 5 mg/d days 2–3, then adjustment based on INR)	Mean percent of time in therapeutic range in the initial 12 wk was lower in the control group vs the genotype group (60.3% vs 67.4%, *P*<.001)
	GIFT [24]	1650 older patients (≥65 y) undergoing elective hip or knee arthroplasty randomized to genotype-guided dosing or clinically guided dosing	The rate of the composite outcome of death, venous thromboembolism, major bleeding, or INR ≥4 during the initial 4–6 wk was 10.8% in the genotype-guided arm and 14.7% in the clinically guided arm, representing a 27% relative rate reduction in the primary endpoint
CYP3A5-Tacrolimus	Not available	280 renal transplant recipients randomized to *CYP3A5*-guided tacrolimus dosing or standard dosing [60]	A higher proportion of patients in the genotype-guided group achieved therapeutic tacrolimus levels at day 10 post-transplant compared with those in the standard dosing group (43.2% vs 29.1%, *P* = .03).
CYP2C19-clopidogrel	TAILOR-PCI (ClinicalTrials.gov ID NCT01742117)	5270 patients undergoing PCI for an acute coronary syndrome or stable coronary disease randomized to *CYP2C19* genotype–guided antiplatelet therapy, with clopidogrel avoided in carriers of a nonfunctional allele, or to routine clopidogrel	Estimated to be completed in 2020. The primary outcome is the occurrence of a major adverse cardiovascular event, defined as nonfatal myocardial infarction, nonfatal stroke, cardiovascular mortality, severe recurrent ischemia, and stent thrombosis at 1 year

(*continued on next page*)

TABLE 1
(continued)

Gene-Drug Pair	Trial Acronym	Patient Population	Summary of Results
	POPular Genetics (ClinicalTrials.gov ID NCT01761786) [44]	2700 patients with ST-segment elevation myocardial infarction undergoing PCI randomized to *CYP2C19* genotype–guided antiplatelet therapy, with clopidogrel avoided in carriers of a nonfunctional allele, or to routine ticagrelor or prasugrel	Estimated to be completed in 2019. The primary endpoint is the composite of death, myocardial infarction, stent thrombosis, stroke, and major bleeding at 1 year

Abbreviations: CI, confidence interval; DPWG, Dutch Pharmacogenetics Working Group; HIV, human immunodeficiency virus; INR, international normalized ratio; PCI, percutaneous coronary intervention; RR, relative risk.

variants influencing warfarin dose requirements in African Americans [25]. Other factors that may have contributed to disparate findings across studies are summarized elsewhere [26,27].

CPIC guidelines for genotype-guided warfarin dosing were originally published in 2011 before the release of data from large RCTs [28]. Even so, the guidelines strongly recommended using genotype data to dose warfarin when such data are available based on the strong and consistent evidence that genotype influences dose requirements. The guidelines were updated in 2017 to emphasize the importance of genotyping persons of African ancestry for variants important in this population [29]. However, based on the disparate results of the EU-PACT and COAG trials and controversy generated, there are few examples of genotype-guided warfarin dosing in practice, and most of these involve pharmacogenomic panel-based testing where warfarin-related genotypes are included among numerous other genotypes with implications for other drug responses [2,6,8,30].

Alternative Methods of Evidence Generation

With the rapidly growing number of discoveries in pharmacogenomics, conducting an RCT for each gene-drug pair is impractical from a time and cost perspective, and a more efficient approach is needed to generate evidence to support translation into patient care. Pharmacogenomic clinical trials are especially challenging because for any given gene-drug pair only a small portion of the population carries a variant allele associated with drug toxicity or ineffectiveness. Otherwise the drug would never have reached the market. In this regard, pharmacogenomics is a study of outliers, and very large study populations may be needed to detect significant effects. An RCT may also be unethical when the consequences of drug exposure in a genetically predisposed patient can be life-threatening. Such is the case with the *HLA-B*15:02* allele, which is found most often in persons of southeastern Asian ancestry and significantly increases the risk for carbamazepine-induced Stevens–Johnson syndrome and toxic epidermal necrolysis. In lieu of an RCT, a prospective cohort study of 4877 carbamazepine candidates was conducted and showed that, compared with historical incidence rates, genetic screening with avoidance of carbamazepine in *HLA*15:02* positive patients significantly reduced the occurrence of severe cutaneous reactions [31]. The FDA-approved carbamazepine labeling includes a boxed warning about the risk for severe cutaneous reactions in individuals with the *HLA-B*15:02* allele and states that genotyping should be done before carbamazepine use in at-risk populations (ie, southeast Asian populations). Similar data exist with *HLA-B*58:01* screening to predict risk for severe cutaneous adverse reactions to allopurinol [32]. Guidelines by both CPIC and the Canadian Pharmacogenomics Network for Drug Safety address risk associated with the *HLA-B* genotype for carbamazepine, and CPIC provides additional guidelines for allopurinol [33–35].

One alternative approach to an RCT is to gather evidence as part of continuing clinical care in a learning health system model through practice-based pragmatic studies [36,37]. Unlike RCTs, pragmatic studies are conducted in the context of clinical practice and reflect the effectiveness of an intervention in a real-world setting [38]. As such, an advantage of pragmatic study results is that they are more generalizable than those from RCTs, which often have strict eligibility criteria and are conducted in controlled settings to minimize selection bias and confounding and maximize internal validity [39]. Pragmatic studies are also less rigorous by nature and thus more efficient to conduct. On the other hand, the major limitation with pragmatic studies is that there is less control for sources of bias creating greater uncertainty and necessitating statistical techniques such as propensity score matching to account for differences between treatment groups [39].

Pragmatic and Observational Studies of *CYP2C19*-Guided Antiplatelet Prescribing

CYP2C19-clopidogrel is an example of a gene-drug pair with evidence of benefit from pragmatic studies. Clopidogrel is a prodrug, and the CYP2C19 enzyme has a critical role in clopidogrel bioactivation. Approximately 30% of Whites and African Americans and up to 60% of Asians carry a nonfunctional *CYP2C19* allele leading to impaired clopidogrel bioactivation and lesser clopidogrel-mediated effects, the consequences of which are greatest for patients undergoing percutaneous coronary intervention (PCI) [40–42]. Specifically, numerous studies have demonstrated an increased risk for adverse cardiovascular events after PCI in clopidogrel-treated patients with a nonfunctional allele compared with similarly treated patients with normal or increased function alleles [41,43]. Two RCTs investigating the clinical utility of *CYP2C19*-guided clopidogrel prescribing after PCI are ongoing but not expected to be completed until 2019 to 2020 (ClinicalTrials.gov Identifier: NCT01742117 and NCT01761786) [44].

Several institutions have clinically implemented *CYP2C19* testing to guide post-PCI antiplatelet therapy ahead of clinical trial results [45]. In fact, *CYP2C19*-clopidogrel is one of the most common gene-drug pairs implemented in practice [8]. As part of the National Institutes of Health–funded Implementing GeNomics In pracTicE (IGNITE) Network Pharmacogenomics Working Group, 7 US institutions pooled data for 1815 patients who were genotyped for *CYP2C19* variants at the time of emergent or elective PCI, with genotype results placed in the electronic health record [8,46,47]. Consistent with a pragmatic study design, alternative antiplatelet therapy (eg, prasugrel or ticagrelor) was recommended in patients with 1 or 2 nonfunctional alleles (ie, intermediate or poor metabolizers), but the ultimate prescribing decision was left to the discretion of the physician. Thirty-one percent of patients had a nonfunctional allele, and alternative therapy was prescribed in 61% of these patients, whereas the remainders were treated with clopidogrel. In contrast, only 15.5% of patients without a nonfunctional allele were prescribed prasugrel or ticagrelor. After propensity scoring to account for differences between groups, the risk for major adverse cardiovascular events (defined as the composite outcome of death, myocardial infarction, and ischemic stroke) over a median follow-up of approximately 5 months was significantly higher in carriers of a nonfunctional allele who were prescribed clopidogrel versus alternative therapy (adjusted hazard ratio 2.26, 95% confidence interval 1.18–4.32). There was no difference in risk for cardiovascular events between carriers of a nonfunctional allele prescribed alternative therapy and those without a nonfunctional allele. The group is currently conducting a cost-effectiveness study based on these data.

These data are consistent with findings from a Dutch study of patients genotyped at the time of elective PCI [9]. In contrast to the US study, alternative antiplatelet therapy was only recommended in poor metabolizers (with 2 nonfunctional alleles). Over an 18-month follow-up period, there were significantly more adverse cardiovascular events in poor metabolizers treated with clopidogrel versus alternative antiplatelet therapy. An additional study, conducted in Spain, compared outcomes between patients who received genotype-guided antiplatelet therapy after PCI and historical controls who were mostly treated with clopidogrel [10]. Both *CYP2C19* and *ABCB1* genotypes were determined, and alternative therapy was prescribed to patients with either a *CYP2C19* nonfunctional allele or the *ABCB1* rs1045642 TT genotype. Compared with controls who underwent PCI before genotype implementation, there were significantly fewer cardiovascular events in the genotype group.

Pragmatic Trials of Pharmacogenomic-Guided Treatment of Depression and Anxiety

Both the *CYP2D6* and *CYP2C19* genes influence the pharmacokinetics and response to multiple antidepressants, and there are other genes in the serotonergic pathway with potential effects on antidepressant drug response [48,49]. The clinical effectiveness of genotype-guided management of depression and anxiety has been the subject of several pragmatic clinical trials and observational studies [50–52]. In a recent multicenter study, 685 patients with depression and/or anxiety, who were either new to treatment or had inadequately controlled symptoms, were randomized to a genotype-guided approach to therapy or usual care [50]. Patients were blinded to treatment assignment. Patients in the genotype group were tested using a commercially available panel of 10 genes, including *CYP2D6* and *CYP2C19*. Genotype results were provided to the physician to consider when making drug prescribing decisions. Patients in the genotype arm reported greater response rates for both depression and anxiety at 8 and 12 weeks compared with those in the control group. A smaller pragmatic trial [52] and observational study [51] also showed favorable effects with a genotype-guided strategy of antidepressant prescribing.

Pragmatic Trials of Panel-Based Pharmacogenomic Testing

The examples discussed earlier focus on individual drugs or drug classes. As of early 2018, CPIC and DPWG guidelines are available for at least 19 gene-drug pairs. Thus, a panel-based approach to testing whereby multiple variants with implications for multiple drugs are tested at once has been proposed as a more practical approach to pharmacogenomic testing than testing genes one at a time. More than 90% of the population is estimated to have at least one variant associated with reduced drug response or increased risk for toxicity, supporting a panel-based approach done preemptively so that genotype data are readily available to inform prescribing decisions across a person's lifetime [53].

Initial efforts have established the feasibility of incorporating multiple genotypes from panel-based testing into clinical care [2,3,5]. This includes the Mayo Clinic Right Drug, Right Dose, Right Time-Using Genomic Data to Individualize Treatment (RIGHT) pilot project, whereby actionable variants in 4 genes from a next-generation sequencing panel plus *CYP2D6* genotype were integrated into the electronic health records for more than 1000 patients along with point-of-care clinical decision support [54]. An expansion of the project is underway, with preemptive testing of 13 pharmacogenes in 10,000 patients who receive care at Mayo Clinic with the goal of examining the clinical and economic impact of this approach in addition to providing genetic data for discovery purposes.

Pragmatic trials are examining the clinical utility of panel-based testing [6,11]. The INdiana GENomics Implementation: an Opportunity for the UnderServed (INGENIOUS) trial, funded by NHGRI, is examining the economic impact of genotyping for 43 variants in 14 pharmacogenes on the incidence of adverse events and health care cost [6]. The Ubiquitous Pharmacogenomics Consortium, funded by the European Commission's Horizon-2929 program, is examining similar outcomes with panel-based pharmacogenomic testing in the PREemptive Pharmacogenomics testing for prevention of Adverse drug REactions (PREPARE) trial [11]. The trial is being conducted in 7 European countries using a block-randomized design. Participating countries are randomized to an 18-month block of pharmacogenomics-guided prescribing or standard of care, after which they switch to the opposite strategy for a second 18-month block. The trial is targeting enrollment of 4050 total patients during each block. The pharmacogenomics panel includes 50 variants in 13 genes, and drug therapy recommendations are provided according to DPWG guidelines.

REIMBURSEMENT FOR PHARMACOGENETIC TESTING

Reimbursement for pharmacogenomics testing involves many constantly moving parts. First, there must be evidence (ie, clinical validity) to obtain a Current Procedural Terminology (CPT) code. Once a CPT code is obtained, such as a catalog number, a value must be assigned to it. Then payers, whether governmental or private, decide whether or not to reimburse the pharmacogenomics test (or panel). This section provides an overview of evidence needed for reimbursement for pharmacogenomics.

Billing and reimbursement for medical services including pharmacogenetics testing are codified by a code set that is maintained and administered by the American Medical Association (AMA). CPT codes are considered level 1 Healthcare Common Procedure Coding System (HCPCS, pronounced as "hickspicks"), which is overseen by the Centers for Medicare and Medicaid Services (CMS). To obtain a CPT code, the medical service must demonstrate clinical validity (Fig. 2). CPT codes are assigned categories. Category I include procedures that are consistent with contemporary medical practice and are widely performed. Category III include temporary codes for emerging technology, services, and procedures. For molecular pathology procedures in which pharmacogenomics falls, the AMA created additional criteria to help guide category I status as follows [55].

- For Mendelian and somatic disorders, there is a demonstrated relationship between biomarker and phenotype (ie, clinical validity).
- Biomarkers (eg, SNPs) that have an association but not a proven causative effect to a known clinical phenotype should have demonstrated clinical usefulness (eg, high positive predictive value, high negative predictive value, directing therapy/management).

The US government, through programs such as CMS, pays for approximately half of the country's health

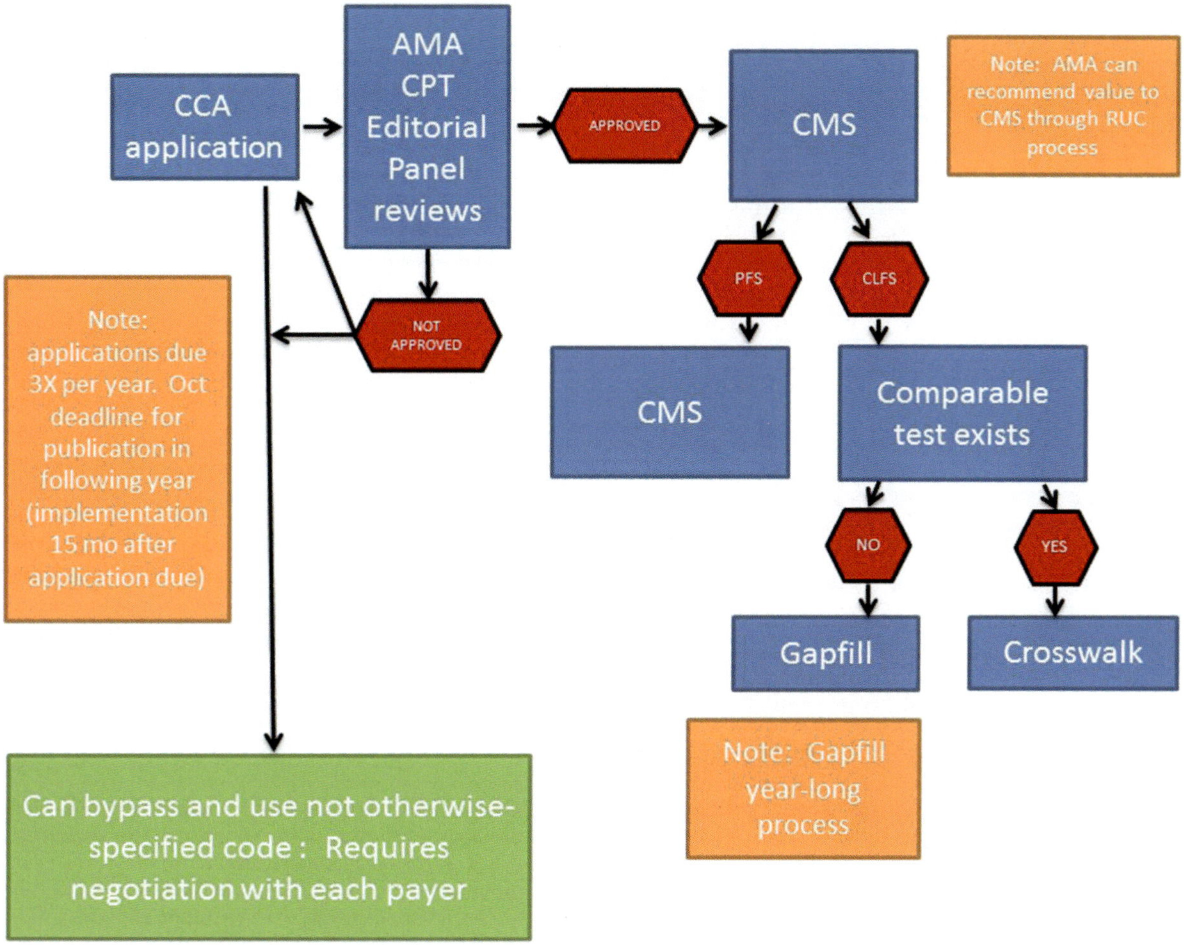

FIG. 2 The process map for requesting a new CPT from the American Medical Association (AMA) with how the US governmental payer determines a reimbursement value. CCA, coding change application; CLFS, clinical lab fee schedule; CMS, Centers for Medicare and Medicaid Services; PFS, physician fee schedule; RUC, specialty society relative value scale update committee or relative value update committee (pronounced "ruck").

care [56]. CMS uses Medicare Administrative Contractors (MACs), who are private health care insurers, to administer the Medicare program. The MACs are responsible for various geographic jurisdictions to process Medicare Part A and Part B (A/B) medical claims such as pharmacogenomic testing for Medicare fee-for-service beneficiaries. Medicare Part A is hospital insurance, which includes, but is not limited to, inpatient care in hospitals, nursing homes, skilled nursing facilities, and critical access hospitals. Medicare Part B covers 2 types of services: (1) medically necessary services that are needed to diagnose or treat a medical condition and that meet accepted standards of medical practice and (2) preventive services. Pharmacogenomics testing can occur in both inpatient and outpatient settings and would be covered in Part A/B. Title XVIII of the Social Security Act, Section 1862(a) (1) (A) prohibits Medicare payment "...for items or services which are not reasonable and necessary (often equated to clinical validity) for the diagnosis and treatment of illness or injury...." with certain exceptions. The MACs use a process called Local Coverage Determinations (LCDs) to determine whether they will cover a particular service on a MAC-wide basis. National Coverage Decisions (NCDs) are issued by CMS for the entire country.

Most, if not all, MACs have issued LCDs limiting pharmacogenomics testing reimbursement to few medications and associated gene testing [57]. For a medical test, the MACs are using the concept of reasonable and necessary to equate to clinical utility. Although there is no standardized definition for clinical utility, in its simplest form, it is equated to a change in medical management. Testing for pharmacogenomic variants can determine if a medication is predicted to be effective at current dosage, should be discontinued, or if a dosing change is needed, which should equate to a change in medical management of a patient.

Government reimbursement has an impact on private insurance. Often when the MACs or CMS make LCDs or NCDs to limit coverage on services such as pharmacogenomics testing due to not being reasonable or necessary, private insurance companies follow these same decisions. This is usually determined by the employer's contract with the private insurance companies. In some instances, employers have determined that covering a service may make them a differentiator and save them money in the long term. In addition, because reimbursements from government programs such as Medicare and Medicaid are lower than the average cost of serving those patients, laboratories or other providers may charge privately insured patients higher rates in order to recoup their costs. This increase in private sector prices to adjust for government payment levels is called "cost-shifting" and is a controversial concept.

CPIC evaluates both clinical and research studies of pharmacogenes and administered medications and publishes the drug-gene pair clinical validity [12]. The stance of CPIC is to guide medication dosing or selection if the pharmacogenomic results are already present in the medical record. They do not make statements on whether or not pharmacogenomics testing should be performed before or concurrently with medication administration. This is left to the US FDA in the package insert for a medication and to the prescriber to follow. The FDA can also make determinations of a boxed warning, commonly referred to as a "black box" warning, for prescribers about serious adverse reactions. It is still up to the medical practice of the prescriber based on their knowledge of the patient to follow (or not) boxed warnings. Even with a boxed warning for pharmacogenomic testing, there is no requirement for testing to be performed. As such, payers would prefer that CPIC support preemptive testing in their guidelines [58].

PRESENT RELEVANCE AND FUTURE AVENUES TO CONSIDER OR TO INVESTIGATE

Data from a limited number of RCTs and prospective cohort and pragmatic studies provide support for clinical implementation of various gene-drug pairs. Research projects such as the National Institutes of Health–sponsored IGNITE Network and the Ubiquitous Pharmacogenomics Consortium PREPARE trial are using pragmatic trial designs to build further evidence of clinical utility of pharmacogenomics as well as other genomics. Although the IGNITE network as a whole aims to identify and address barriers to implementing genomics, the Pharmacogenetics Working Group is examining outcomes with pharmacogenomic testing across network sites. In addition, the IGNITE INGenious project when completed will look at the economic value of panel-based pharmacogenomics testing [59]. Similarly, outcomes and cost-effectiveness data are expected from the PREPARE trial. Together, these data may demonstrate improved patient outcomes and cost savings to the health care system with pharmacogenomic testing and further drive the field forward.

SUMMARY

Pharmacogenomic research and implementation continues to be an active area in molecular medicine. In some cases such as with abacavir and *HLA-B*57:01*, pharmacogenomics can help reduce the frequency of adverse drug reactions by allowing preemptive identification of at-risk individuals in whom the drug can be avoided. In other cases, such as with clopidogrel and *CYP2C19* testing, pharmacogenomics allows for predicting patients unlikely to respond in whom alternative therapy may be initiated. Together, such examples can have a tremendously positive impact on morbidity and mortality of patients. The trial-and-error approach to prescribing where one-drug-fits-all that is current practice, all too often results in a medication being ineffective, thus causing wasted treatment time, high health care and drug costs, and, most importantly, therapeutic failures or alternatively in a medication causing toxicity, also causing significant medical expenditure and threatening patient life and well-being. As additional evidence is gained for the clinical benefit of genotype-guided therapy, it is expected that reimbursement for pharmacogenomic testing will follow of which both are critical to support broader adoption and sustainability of pharmacogenomics in practice.

REFERENCES

[1] Collins FS, Varmus H. A new initiative on precision medicine. N Engl J Med 2015;372:793–5.

[2] O'Donnell PH, Wadhwa N, Danahey K, et al. Pharmacogenomics-based point-of-care clinical decision support

significantly alters drug prescribing. Clin Pharmacol Ther 2017;102:859–69.

[3] Hoffman JM, Haidar CE, Wilkinson MR, et al. PG4KDS: a model for the clinical implementation of pre-emptive pharmacogenetics. Am J Med Genet C Semin Med Genet 2014;166C:45–55.

[4] Peterson JF, Field JR, Unertl KM, et al. Physician response to implementation of genotype-tailored antiplatelet therapy. Clin Pharmacol Ther 2016;100:67–74.

[5] Pulley JM, Denny JC, Peterson JF, et al. Operational implementation of prospective genotyping for personalized medicine: the design of the vanderbilt PREDICT project. Clin Pharmacol Ther 2012;92:87–95.

[6] Eadon MT, Desta Z, Levy KD, et al. Implementation of a pharmacogenomics consult service to support the INGENIOUS trial. Clin Pharmacol Ther 2016;100:63–6.

[7] Hicks JK, Stowe D, Willner MA, et al. Implementation of clinical pharmacogenomics within a large health system: from electronic health record decision support to consultation services. Pharmacotherapy 2016;36:940–8.

[8] Cavallari LH, Beitelshees AL, Blake KV, et al. The IGNITE pharmacogenetics working group: an opportunity for building evidence with pharmacogenetic implementation in a real-world setting. Clin Transl Sci 2017;10:143–6.

[9] Deiman BA, Tonino PA, Kouhestani K, et al. Reduced number of cardiovascular events and increased cost-effectiveness by genotype-guided antiplatelet therapy in patients undergoing percutaneous coronary interventions in the Netherlands. Neth Heart J 2016;24:589–99.

[10] Sanchez-Ramos J, Davila-Fajardo CL, Toledo Frias P, et al. Results of genotype-guided antiplatelet therapy in patients who undergone percutaneous coronary intervention with stent. Int J Cardiol 2016;225:289–95.

[11] van der Wouden CH, Cambon-Thomsen A, Cecchin E, et al. Implementing pharmacogenomics in Europe: design and implementation strategy of the ubiquitous pharmacogenomics consortium. Clin Pharmacol Ther 2017;101:341–58.

[12] Relling MV, Klein TE. CPIC: clinical pharmacogenetics implementation consortium of the pharmacogenomics research network. Clin Pharmacol Ther 2011;89:464–7.

[13] Swen JJ, Nijenhuis M, de Boer A, et al. Pharmacogenetics: from bench to byte–an update of guidelines. Clin Pharmacol Ther 2011;89:662–73.

[14] Relling MV, Altman RB, Goetz MP, et al. Clinical implementation of pharmacogenomics: overcoming genetic exceptionalism. Lancet Oncol 2010;11:507–9.

[15] Khoury MJ. Dealing with the evidence dilemma in genomics and personalized medicine. Clin Pharmacol Ther 2010;87:635–8.

[16] van der Wouden CH, Swen JJ, Samwald M, et al. A brighter future for the implementation of pharmacogenomic testing. Eur J Hum Genet 2016;24:1658–60.

[17] Mallal S, Phillips E, Carosi G, et al. HLA-B*5701 screening for hypersensitivity to abacavir. N Engl J Med 2008;358:568–79.

[18] Guidelines for the use of antiretroviral agents in adults and adolescents living with HIV. Department of Health and Human Services. Panel on antiretroviral guidelines for adults and adolescents. Available at: http://www.aidsinfo.nih.gov/ContentFiles/AdultandAdolescentGL.pdf. Accessed February 28, 2018.

[19] Relling MV, Gardner EE, Sandborn WJ, et al. Clinical Pharmacogenetics Implementation Consortium guidelines for thiopurine methyltransferase genotype and thiopurine dosing. Clin Pharmacol Ther 2011;89:387–91.

[20] Coenen MJ, de Jong DJ, van Marrewijk CJ, et al. Identification of patients with variants in TPMT and dose reduction reduces hematologic events during thiopurine treatment of inflammatory bowel disease. Gastroenterology 2015;149:907–17.e7.

[21] Weitzel KW, Smith DM, Elsey AR, et al. Implementation of standardized clinical processes for TPMT testing in a diverse multidisciplinary population: challenges and lessons learned. Clin Transl Sci 2018;11(2):175–81.

[22] Kimmel SE, French B, Kasner SE, et al. A pharmacogenetic versus a clinical algorithm for warfarin dosing. N Engl J Med 2013;369:2283–93.

[23] Pirmohamed M, Burnside G, Eriksson N, et al. A randomized trial of genotype-guided dosing of warfarin. N Engl J Med 2013;369:2294–303.

[24] Gage BF, Bass AR, Lin H, et al. Effect of genotype-guided warfarin dosing on clinical events and anticoagulation control among patients undergoing hip or knee arthroplasty: the GIFT randomized clinical trial. JAMA 2017;318:1115–24.

[25] Drozda K, Wong S, Patel SR, et al. Poor warfarin dose prediction with pharmacogenetic algorithms that exclude genotypes important for African Americans. Pharmacogenet Genomics 2015;25:73–81.

[26] Cavallari LH. Time to revisit warfarin pharmacogenetics. Future Cardiol 2017;13:511–3.

[27] Johnson JA, Cavallari LH. Warfarin pharmacogenetics. Trends Cardiovasc Med 2015;25:33–41.

[28] Johnson JA, Gong L, Whirl-Carrillo M, et al. Clinical pharmacogenetics implementation consortium guidelines for CYP2C9 and VKORC1 genotypes and warfarin dosing. Clin Pharmacol Ther 2011;90:625–9.

[29] Johnson JA, Caudle KE, Gong L, et al. Clinical Pharmacogenetics Implementation Consortium (CPIC) guideline for pharmacogenetics-guided warfarin dosing: 2017 update. Clin Pharmacol Ther 2017;102:397–404.

[30] Nutescu EA, Drozda K, Bress AP, et al. Feasibility of implementing a comprehensive warfarin pharmacogenetics service. Pharmacotherapy 2013;33:1156–64.

[31] Chen P, Lin JJ, Lu CS, et al. Carbamazepine-induced toxic effects and HLA-B*1502 screening in Taiwan. N Engl J Med 2011;364:1126–33.

[32] Ko TM, Tsai CY, Chen SY, et al. Use of HLA-B*58:01 genotyping to prevent allopurinol induced severe cutaneous adverse reactions in Taiwan: national prospective cohort study. BMJ 2015;351:h4848.

[33] Phillips EJ, Sukasem C, Whirl-Carrillo M, et al. Clinical pharmacogenetics implementation consortium guideline

for HLA genotype and use of carbamazepine and oxcarbazepine: 2017 update. Clin Pharmacol Ther 2018; 103(4):574–81.

[34] Saito Y, Stamp LK, Caudle KE, et al, Clinical Pharmacogenetics Implementation Consortium. Clinical Pharmacogenetics Implementation Consortium (CPIC) guidelines for human leukocyte antigen B (HLA-B) genotype and allopurinol dosing: 2015 update. Clin Pharmacol Ther 2016;99:36–7.

[35] Amstutz U, Shear NH, Rieder MJ, et al, CPNDS clinical recommendation group. Recommendations for HLA-B*15:02 and HLA-A*31:01 genetic testing to reduce the risk of carbamazepine-induced hypersensitivity reactions. Epilepsia 2014;55:496–506.

[36] Ginsburg G. Medical genomics: gather and use genetic data in health care. Nature 2014;508:451–3.

[37] Rosenthal GE. The role of pragmatic clinical trials in the evolution of learning health systems. Trans Am Clin Climatol Assoc 2014;125:204–16 [discussion: 17–8].

[38] Patsopoulos NA. A pragmatic view on pragmatic trials. Dialogues Clin Neurosci 2011;13:217–24.

[39] Terry SF. An evidence framework for genetic testing. Genet Test Mol Biomarkers 2017;21:407–8.

[40] Mega JL, Close SL, Wiviott SD, et al. Cytochrome p-450 polymorphisms and response to clopidogrel. N Engl J Med 2009;360:354–62.

[41] Scott SA, Sangkuhl K, Stein CM, et al. Clinical Pharmacogenetics Implementation Consortium guidelines for CYP2C19 genotype and clopidogrel therapy: 2013 update. Clin Pharmacol Ther 2013;94:317–23.

[42] Sorich MJ, Rowland A, McKinnon RA, et al. CYP2C19 genotype has a greater effect on adverse cardiovascular outcomes following percutaneous coronary intervention and in Asian populations treated with clopidogrel: a meta-analysis. Circ Cardiovasc Genet 2014;7:895–902.

[43] Mega JL, Simon T, Collet JP, et al. Reduced-function CYP2C19 genotype and risk of adverse clinical outcomes among patients treated with clopidogrel predominantly for PCI: a meta-analysis. JAMA 2010;304:1821–30.

[44] Bergmeijer TO, Janssen PW, Schipper JC, et al. CYP2C19 genotype-guided antiplatelet therapy in ST-segment elevation myocardial infarction patients-Rationale and design of the Patient Outcome after primary PCI (POPular) Genetics study. Am Heart J 2014;168:16–22 e1.

[45] Empey PE, Stevenson JM, Tuteja S, et al, IGNITE Network. Multisite investigation of strategies for the implementation of CYP2C19 genotype-guided antiplatelet therapy. Clin Pharmacol Ther 2017. [Epub ahead of print].

[46] Weitzel KW, Alexander M, Bernhardt BA, et al. The IGNITE network: a model for genomic medicine implementation and research. BMC Med Genomics 2016;9:1.

[47] Cavallari LH, Lee CR, Beitelshees AL, et al, IGNITE Network. Multisite investigation of outcomes with implementation of CYP2C19 genotype-guided antiplatelet therapy after percutaneous coronary intervention. JACC Cardiovasc Interv 2018;11:181–91.

[48] Hicks JK, Bishop JR, Sangkuhl K, et al, Clinical Pharmacogenetics Implementation Consortium. Clinical Pharmacogenetics Implementation Consortium (CPIC) guideline for CYP2D6 and CYP2C19 genotypes and dosing of selective serotonin reuptake inhibitors. Clin Pharmacol Ther 2015;98:127–34.

[49] Hicks JK, Sangkuhl K, Swen JJ, et al. Clinical pharmacogenetics implementation consortium guideline (CPIC) for CYP2D6 and CYP2C19 genotypes and dosing of tricyclic antidepressants: 2016 update. Clin Pharmacol Ther 2016. [Epub ahead of print].

[50] Bradley P, Shiekh M, Mehra V, et al. Improved efficacy with targeted pharmacogenetic-guided treatment of patients with depression and anxiety: a randomized clinical trial demonstrating clinical utility. J Psychiatr Res 2018;96:100–7.

[51] Brennan FX, Gardner KR, Lombard J, et al. A naturalistic study of the effectiveness of pharmacogenetic testing to guide treatment in psychiatric patients with mood and anxiety disorders. Prim Care Companion CNS Disord 2015;17.

[52] Perez V, Salavert A, Espadaler J, et al. Efficacy of prospective pharmacogenetic testing in the treatment of major depressive disorder: results of a randomized, double-blind clinical trial. BMC Psychiatry 2017;17:250.

[53] Van Driest SL, Shi Y, Bowton EA, et al. Clinically actionable genotypes among 10,000 patients with preemptive pharmacogenomic testing. Clin Pharmacol Ther 2014;95:423–31.

[54] Ji Y, Skierka JM, Blommel JH, et al. Preemptive pharmacogenomic testing for precision medicine: a comprehensive analysis of five actionable pharmacogenomic genes using next-generation DNA sequencing and a customized CYP2D6 genotyping cascade. J Mol Diagn 2016;18:438–45.

[55] CPT Code Application. American Medical Association. Available at: https://www.ama-assn.org/practice-management/applying-cpt-codes. Accessed February 25, 2018.

[56] NHE Fact Sheet. Center for medicare & medicaid services. Available at: https://www.cms.gov/research-statistics-data-and-systems/statistics-trends-and-reports/nationalhealthexpenddata/nhe-fact-sheet.html. Accessed February 25, 2018.

[57] Medicare Coverage Database. Center for medicare & medicaid services. Available at: https://www.cms.gov/medicare-coverage-database. Accessed February 25, 2018.

[58] Keeling NJ, Rosenthal MM, West-Strum D, et al. Preemptive pharmacogenetic testing: exploring the knowledge and perspectives of US payers. Genet Med 2017. [Epub ahead of print].

[59] Rosenman MB, Decker B, Levy KD, et al. Lessons learned when introducing pharmacogenomic panel testing into clinical practice. Value Health 2017;20:54–9.

[60] Thervet E, Loriot MA, Barbier S, et al. Optimization of initial tacrolimus dose using pharmacogenetic testing. Clin Pharmacol Ther 2010;87:721–6.

Informatics

Advances in Molecular Pathology 1 (2018) 135–148
ADVANCES IN MOLECULAR PATHOLOGY

Large-Scale Data Sharing Initiatives in Genomic Oncology

Jorge Andrade, PhD[a], Suzanne M. Cox, PhD, MPH[b], Samuel L. Volchenboum, MD, PhD[a,*]
[a]Knapp Center for Biomedical Discovery, Center for Research Informatics and Department of Pediatrics, University of Chicago, 900 East 57th Street, Chicago, IL 60637, USA; [b]Graham School of Continuing Liberal and Professional Studies, University of Chicago, 1427 East 60th Street, Suite 200, Chicago, IL 60637, USA

KEYWORDS
• Data sharing • Oncology • Genomics • Translational science • Pathology

KEY POINTS

- Large-scale genomic data sharing initiatives offer researchers the ability to centralize data, processing power, and tools used in discovery in genomic oncology.
- A variety of sharing data sources are described that will be useful to molecular pathologists and other genomic researchers.
- Privacy, data standards, and accessibility are all key issues for the research community, funders, and organizers to address as these initiatives continue to develop.
- By increasing the volume of data (types and subtypes of cancers, as well as the diversity of populations) and access to the data, potential discovery and translational science opportunities are increased through data sharing.

INTRODUCTION

The volume of existing genomic data is enormous and increasing quickly. To manage this growing complexity, researchers and physicians require new computational and analytics paradigms to enable the accumulation, harmonization, and sharing of heterogeneous data in oncology, from the characterization of tumor biology to the associated clinical information, via secure and compliant large-scale centralized platforms. The goal is to improve understanding of cancer biology, to enable researchers to ask complex questions and identify new knowledge in existing data, and for clinicians and oncologists to use this information to help diagnose and manage patients with cancer. Accumulation of data beyond DNA via application and integration of "multi-omics" approaches, including transcriptomics, proteomics, and epigenomics, are expanding the understanding of the biology of cancers while adding substantial complexity to the data and its analysis. However, this explosion of data has tantalizing potential for driving many important discoveries, provided the practical considerations surrounding these large data sets are properly addressed.

Advances in molecular pathologic condition continue to enable novel approaches to diagnosis and treatment, and multi-omics methodologies have been instrumental

Disclosure: Dr. J. Andrade has nothing to disclose. Dr. S. M. Cox serves as consulting or advisory role at Litmus Health. Dr. S.L. Volchenboum serves as stock and other ownership interests at Litmus Health and also as consulting or advisory role at Accordant Health Services, a CVS Caremark Company; Baxter Travel, Accommodations, Expenses, Marcus Evans. The Center for Research Informatics is funded by the Biological Sciences Division at the University of Chicago with additional funding provided by the Institute for Translational Medicine NIH CTSA grant number UL1 TR000430.

*Corresponding author, *E-mail address:* svolchen@peds.bsd.uchicago.edu

https://doi.org/10.1016/j.yamp.2018.06.009
2589-4080/18/

in teasing out previously unseen biological and clinical diversity in many cancer types. In breast cancer, 5 major molecular subtypes have been identified, including luminal A, luminal B, triple negative/basal-like, HER2 overexpression, and basal-normal-like [1]. Each molecular subtype is associated with a distinct outcome and a specific therapeutic approach. Similar gains have been made in colorectal cancer, with several important molecular subtypes characterized and associated with diverse outcomes and drug responses. *Ras* gene mutation status is now a key determinant for anti-epidermal growth factor receptor–based therapeutics, and hypermutation status (due to either microsatellite instability or polymerase gene mutations) is now a critical factor in the decision process for newer immunotherapies [2]. In addition, numerous advances have been made in the characterization of biological subtypes of acute myeloid leukemia (AML) and acute lymphoblastic leukemia [3,4]. A large variety of genetic alterations are now key to risk stratification and therapeutic decisions in these diseases. Proper diagnosis of AML is now directed by the genetics, including the presence of any of a variety of recurrent gene fusions or biallelic *CEBPA* mutations, whereas anomalies in other genes can guide prognosis (*FLT3*, *NPM1*, *ASXL1*) and therapy (*FLT3*/*IDH1*/*IDH2*) [5]. This wide array of actionable targets has driven an accelerated adoption of large-scale omics technologies into clinical laboratories, particularly next-generation sequencing (NGS) [6].

Despite the astounding progress in this field over the past decade driven by these new technologies, it is clear that the field is still nascent with clinical sequencing certain to expand greatly in the coming years to cover not just more genes but also additional areas of genomics, including RNA analysis and epigenetics. Although this progress and increased scale of data collection will create unprecedented difficulties in data aggregation and analysis, perhaps the most pressing challenges will be related to multimodality integration and analysis. An important issue limiting the utility of genomic information is the paucity of clinical data available for analysis. Many critical molecular subtypes may not be apparent unless analysis is performed with shared patient characteristics, including diagnostic data, outcome information, and information about therapeutic response. The successful analysis and clinical application of large data "-omics" require the facility to process data at scale but also to abstract, quantify, and to cross-compare it against clinical data, including structured clinical information, such as vital signs, medications, and laboratory data, as well as unstructured data from notes and reports. Beyond the obvious potential for a wealth of basic discoveries related to the biology and genetics of cancer, it is efforts like this that will be key to guiding the development of the next generation of oncology diagnostics assays and for providing the necessary genetic/clinical correlates in order to support their interpretation and reporting by pathologists. Continued research, data sharing, and interinstitutional collaboration will be necessary to increase the rate and success of these efforts.

Several large-scale "multi-omics" data collection and integration initiatives are available for oncology research. Here the authors present a compendium of some of the most important large-scale data-sharing initiatives in genomic oncology to provide a review of the current landscape for advanced molecular pathologic condition and to propose critical next steps as these resources develop.

REVIEW OF CURRENT DATA-SHARING INITIATIVES IN GENOMIC ONCOLOGY

Across biomedical disciplines, communities have acknowledged the need to "eliminate data silos and promote data sharing" [7,8]. The concept of collective research that led to the success of the human genome project exemplifies how open, rapid sharing of data can accelerate discovery. In oncology, researchers sometimes use local databases and repositories for their research. However, given the need for larger cohort sizes to characterize rare molecular subtypes, oncology research is better enabled through the use of data commons: large collections of genomic data in a cloud-based environment. Data commons should also contain shared analysis tools, allowing researchers to conduct their work in a cloud environment without having to download the data [9]. Finally, data in a commons must adhere to FAIR data practices (findable, accessible, interoperable, reusable) [10]. The authors have profiled some of the largest genomic data commons initiatives for use in genomic oncology. Table 1 summarizes key aspects of each data source.

The Genomic Data Commons

The Genomic Data Commons (GDC) is an initiative of the National Cancer Institute (NCI), developed and operated by the University of Chicago, under a subcontract from Leidos Biomedical Research at the Frederick National Laboratory for Cancer Research, in collaboration with the Ontario Institute for Cancer Research [12,13]. The goal of the GDC is to centralize, standardize, and make accessible data from large-scale NCI programs, including The Cancer Genome Atlas (TCGA); Therapeutically Applicable Research to Generate Effective Treatments (TARGET); Foundation Medicine, an oncology genetic diagnostics company;

TABLE 1
Key Elements of Data Sources/Sharing Platforms

Data Source	Description	Approximate Number	Programmatic Access	Data	Access Level	Analytical/ Visualization Tools Available
Genomics data commons	33 cancer types and subtypes; hard-to-treat childhood cancers; CCLE (available on the Legacy archive)	Projects: 40; primary sites: 61; cases: 32,555 Files: 310,859; genes: 22,147; mutations: 3,142,246	Yes, the GDC API	Whole genome seq; whole exome seq; RNA-seq; genotyping array; target sequencing; miRNA-seq; methylation array	Open access and controlled access	Yes
TCGA	33 cancer types and subtypes	Projects: 40; primary sites: 61; cases: 32,555 Files: 310,859; genes: 22,147; mutations: 3,142,246	Yes, the GDC API	Whole genome seq; whole exome seq; RNA-seq; genotyping array; target sequencing; miRNA-seq; methylation array	Open access and controlled access	Yes
TARGET	Hard-to-treat childhood cancers	Cases: 3236	Yes, the GDC API	Whole genome seq; SNP array; mRNA-seq; miRNA-seq target resequencing; copy number; ChIP-seq	Open access and controlled access	Yes
Seven Bridges	Same as TCGA	Same as TCGA	Yes, the Seven Bridges Software Development Kit and API	Whole genome seq; whole exome seq; RNA-seq; genotyping array; target sequencing; miRNA-seq; methylation array	Open access and controlled access	Yes
ISB-CGC	Same as TCGA	Same as TCGA	Yes, the ISB-CGC Google cloud platform	Same as TCGA	Open access and controlled access	Yes

(continued on next page)

TABLE 1
(continued)

Data Source	Description	Approximate Number	Programmatic Access	Data	Access Level	Analytical/ Visualization Tools Available
COSMIC	Expert-curated database of somatic mutations	Samples: 1,358,288; coding mutations: 5,448,850; whole genomes: 33,291; copy number variants: 1,195,556; gene expression variants: 9,176,464; differentially methylated CPGs: 7,879,142; noncoding variants: 18,056,654	No, database can be downloaded	Targeted gene-screening panels; >25,000 peer reviewed papers; metadata (environmental factors and patient history); >32,000 genomes (peer-reviewed large-scale genome screening data); genome-level profiling of diseases	Open access	No
ICGC	Members from 16 countries contribute multiple genomic mutation data from cancer subtypes	Projects: 84; donors: 24,077; somatic mutations: 77,462,290	Yes, ICGC API is a set of RESTful endpoints, programmable interfaces over the Web that allows third-party developers to build automation scripts and apps	Patient characteristics; cancer subtype; and somatic mutations	Open access and controlled access	Yes
CCLE	Database of cancer cell lines genomic profiles and mutations	Cell lines: 1457; genes: 84,434; unique data sets: 136,488; mutation entries: 1,159,663; distribution scores: 118,661,636; methylation scores: 411,948,577	No	Cell lines, annotated genes, mutation entries, distribution scores, methylation scores	Open access	Yes, several tools available for specific analysis

cBioPortal	Same as TCGA	213 cancer studies	Yes, Web API; the cBioPortal software is available via GitHub	DNA copy number, mRNA and miRNA expression, nonsynonymous mutations, protein level, and phosphoprotein level (RPPA), DNA methylation and limited deidentified clinical data	Open access	Yes
GEO	Functional genomics data repository	Samples: 2,457,235; data sets: 4348	Yes, the Entrez Programming Utilities (E-Utils)	Curated gene expression data sets	Open access	Yes
Gabriella Miller Kids First	To include genomic data from children with cancer and structural birth defects	Initial sequencing projects funded via the X01 mechanism https://commonfund.nih.gov/kidsfirst/X01Projects	To be announced	Mostly WGS	Open and controlled access	Yes, details yet to be announced
St. Jude Cloud	Pediatric Cancer Genome Project, St. Jude LIFE; Genomes 4 Kids; clinical pilot	St. Jude LIFE: 3332 subjects; Pediatric Cancer Genome Project (PCGP): 1626 subjects; PCGP: 299 subjects; clinical pilot: 78 subjects	No	RNA-seq; whole genome seq; whole exome seq	Open access	Yes
Tempus	Targeted panels of 595 and 1714 genes and WES	Unknown	No	Targeted gene sequencing and WES	NA	No
Foundation Medicine	Targeted panels for a variety of tumors and heme malignancies as well as companion diagnostic assays	>180,000 profiles over 150 cancer subtypes	No	Targeted gene sequencing	Open and controlled access via GDC and a pediatric portal [11]	No

(continued on next page)

TABLE 1
(continued)

Data Source	Description	Approximate Number	Programmatic Access	Data	Access Level	Analytical/ Visualization Tools Available
GENIE	60 major cancer types	6000 patients with lung cancer; 4500 patients with breast cancer; 4300 patients with colorectal cancer	No	Existing CLIA-/ISO-certified genomic data obtained during the course of routine practice	Open via cBioPortal or Sage Bionetworks	Yes, via cBioPortal
ORIEN	~20 types of cancer biospecimens, genomic data, and linked clinical data	>150,000 patients	No	WES and RNA sequencing on tumors and WES on germline tissue	Controlled access	Unknown
Flatiron Health	Clinico-Genomic Database has linked sequencing data and clinical data on 9 cancers (non–small cell lung, breast, colorectal, ovarian, pancreatic, melanoma, prostate, renal cell carcinoma, multiple myeloma)	2 million EHRs; ~6500 in Clinico-Genomic Database (June 2017)	No	Molecular alterations across 300+ genes; clinical interpretation and recommended therapies; tumor mutation burden; microsatellite instability plus clinical data	Controlled access	Unknown

Abbreviations: CLIA, Clinical Laboratory Improvement Amendments; ISO, International Organization for Standardization.

and the Multiple Myeloma Research Foundation, a nonprofit advocacy organization [14]. The TCGA offers complete genomic data, including molecular data, from multiple types of analyses. Multiple samples from each patient were analyzed using multiple approaches, including the methodology and data in Table 2.

The research community can access the GDC through an interactive portal; computer systems can interact with the GDC using an application programming interface (API) [15], and developers can suggest new features based on GDC open-source code [16]. The GDC makes more than 2.5 PB of cancer genomics data available to the research community; the latest release (December 21, 2017) contains data from 40 projects, 60 primary sites, 32,555 cases in 310,859 files, more than 22,147 genes, and 3,142,246 mutations.

TABLE 2
Multi-Omic Data in the Cancer Genome Atlas

Method	Data
DNA sequencing	WGS; WES; sequence traces; mutations, including coding, splice site, germline, and noncoding somatic variants
RNA sequencing	miRNA sequences (calculated expression per miRNA and isoform); mRNA sequences (calculated expression per gene, exon, splice junction, isoform); total RNA sequences (calculated expression per gene, exon, splice junction, isoform); expression signals per gene, exon, splice junction, miRNA, and isoforms
Copy number	Arrays (raw, unnormalized, normalized); low-pass DNA sequencing (whole genomes sequences, variants, coverage)
Array-based expression	Gene expression (raw, normalized, calls); exon expression (raw, normalized, calls); miRNA expression (raw, normalized, calls)
DNA methylation	Bisulfite sequencing (whole genome sequence, methylation, and mutation calls); array-based methylation (raw signal intensity, calculated beta values)
Others	Protein expression (high-resolution images of protein arrays, raw signals, normalized expression); microsatellite instability (markers, classifications)

From National Cancer Institute. Data levels and types. The Cancer Genome Atlas. Available at: https://cancergenome.nih.gov/abouttcga/aboutdata/datalevelstypes. Accessed April 16, 2018.

The TCGA data are accessible in 2 tiers: the *Open Access* tier includes deidentified clinical and demographic data, gene expression data, copy number alterations, epigenetic data, compiled summaries, and anonymized single amplicon DNA sequence data. The *Controlled Access* tier consists of data that can be unique to individuals, and these data include primary sequence data, SNP array data, exon array data, variant call format data, and certain information from minor allele frequencies. The *Controlled Access* tier requires user authentication through the Database of Genotypes and Phenotypes (dbGaP) system. The National Center for Biotechnology Information hosts dbGaP, which contains a collection of studies focused on the interaction of genotype and phenotype in humans [17]. To protect the privacy of research participants and to support data integrity, the GDC requires user authorization and authentication for downloading controlled-access data and for submitting data to the GDC. To perform these functions, GDC users must first obtain appropriate authorization via dbGaP and then authenticate via electronic Research Administration (eRA) Commons. The GDC sets user permissions at the project level according to dbGaP authorizations.

The Cancer Genomics Cloud pilots

In 2014, the NCI selected 3 groups to explore the paradigm of colocalizing massive genomics data sets, alongside secure and scalable computational resources to analyze them. The 3 groups selected to develop these pilot systems are the Broad Institute, the Institute for Systems Biology (in collaboration with Google), and Seven Bridges Genomics. By colocating the data set and the computational resources needed to process and analyze the data in a cloud environment, researchers across institutions will be able to process the data with standard analytical methods and tools in an efficient and cost-effective manner, thereby promoting democratization or resources and collaboration across the cancer genomics community [18].

The Seven Bridges Cancer Genomics Cloud

Built on Amazon Web Services enterprise-level cloud services, the Seven Bridges Cancer Genomics Cloud enables secure on-demand access to genomic data (including the TCGA), colocated with elastic compute, analytical tools, and workflows [19,20]. Researchers from diverse backgrounds can easily visualize, query, and explore cancer genomic data sets. Data of interest can be analyzed in the cloud using more than 200 preinstalled bioinformatics tools and workflows, including pipelines for variant calling on whole genome and exome sequencing data, differential expression analysis on RNA sequencing data, and complex data visualization. Tools are continually revised, updated, and packaged using docker containers [21]. A container is a lightweight software virtualization technology that enables the creation of stand-alone, executable package software that includes everything needed to run it: code, runtime, system tools, system libraries, and settings. Researchers can also extend the functionality of the platform by adding their own data and tools via an intuitive software development kit.

In collaboration with the United Kingdom's 100,000 Genomes Project, Seven Bridges developed Graph Genome technology. Graph Genome Suite is a set of bioinformatics tools for highly accurate analysis of whole genome sequencing (WGS) data. This tool kit leverages vast databases of genomic variants and uses innovative algorithms to deliver the most accurate variant calling. The Graph Genome is a self-improving system for representing and analyzing genomic information using graphs rather than strings of bases. It allows scientists to heavily compress data and thus operate at unprecedented scale. It is an extremely accurate way to detect individual genetic variation, and this accuracy improves with every new sequence added to the graph. It also offers anonymity for individual genomic sequences. A semantic Web approach is used to link more than 140 clinical, biospecimen, and analysis metadata properties, enabling researchers to build and visualize complex queries and explore data sets of interest. The colocalization of resources in the cloud enables fast, on-demand, reproducible, and scalable analyses. To access the Seven Bridges cloud, researchers from around the world can create a free profile online or log in using their eRA Commons or National Institutes of Health (NIH) Center for Information Technology account.

The Institute for Systems Biology Cancer Genomics Cloud

The Institute for Systems Biology Cancer Genomics Cloud (ISB-CGC) provides interactive Web-based systems and applications to access and explore the TCGA, TARGET, the Cancer Cell Line Encyclopedia (CCLE), and the Catalogue Of Somatic Mutations In Cancer (COSMIC) data sets. The ISB-CGC focus is to serve a broad range of nonprogrammer cancer researchers, who prefer the use of interactive Web-based applications rather than command line tools or frameworks to access and explore cancer genomics data. For skilled bioinformaticians, as well as computational scientists who want to write their own custom scripts, an API is available for languages like R or Python. Developers can instantiate on-demand virtual machines (VMs) to analyze sequence data of virtually any size.

The ISB-CGC provides interactive and programmatic access to all data hosted by the GDC and the Wellcome Trust Sanger Institute. The ISB-CGC uses Google Cloud Platform and technologies, including BigQuery, Compute Engine, App Engine, Cloud Datalab, and Google Genomics. Low-level DNA and RNA-Seq data, as well as TCGA proteomics, TCGA radiology, and tissue images, are stored in Google Cloud Storage. High-level clinical, biospecimen, and molecular data are available as curated data sets and tables available for analysis using the Google BigQuery engine. Controlled-access DNA and RNA sequence data are available to dbGaP-authorized users in the original BAM and FASTQ file formats for TCGA and TARGET.

The ISB-CGC Web application functionality is accessed via a freely available Google account. After sign in, the user is presented with a personal dashboard, where analyses can be conducted. Multiple sample analyses can be aggregated into workbooks and saved for later use, editing, and sharing. Users can create different workbooks for each project, and these workbooks can be shared with other users. To access controlled data, users must first link the Google identity with the NIH credentials in dbGaP (either an eRA account ID or an NIH account User ID).

All the data that are available via the Web interface can be accessed programmatically through a combination of ISB-CGC APIs and Google APIs. Most of the ISB-CGC data in BigQuery tables and in Google Cloud Storage are accessed directly via Google Cloud tools and interfaces. The programmatic API also enables access to metadata and user data, such as cohort definitions. A growing set of tutorials and examples is publically available at the ISB-CGC's GitHub repository for users who want to perform custom analyses using R or Python scripts [22]. These tutorials illustrate how one can work with the hosted data using Google Compute Engine VMs and the Google Genomics Pipelines.

The Broad Institute Genomics Cloud

The Broad Institute of Massachusetts Institute of Technology and Harvard University teamed up with Google Genomics to leverage the power, security, and scalability of Google Cloud with the Broad Institute's expertise in scientific analyses. The first product of this collaboration is the Broad Institute Genome Analysis Toolkit (GATK) on Google Cloud. GATK best practices are the de facto standard adopted by the community for variant discovery in human WGS data. By running the GATK pipeline as a service through Google Genomics, scientists can be more confident that they are processing their data according to community best practices, without worrying about managing the information technology infrastructure. The workflow is written in the Broad's Workflow Definition Language (WDL) and executed with a WDL runner called Cromwell. By running GATK on the Google Cloud Platform, users will incur Google Cloud Platform charges for the use of Google Compute VMs, disk storage, and data transfer. Users are responsible for complying with the terms of the GATK End User License Agreement, including the attribution requirement. Google Cloud offers a step-by-step tutorial on how to run GATK [23].

The Catalogue of Somatic Mutations in Cancer

The Wellcome Trust Sanger Institute COSMIC database is the world's largest source of expert manually curated somatic mutation information relating to human cancers [19]. The COSMIC database combines 2 main types of data: (1) genome-wide screen data consisting of more than 32,000 genomes, including large-scale genome screening and other databases like the TCGA and the International Cancer Genome Consortium (ICGC); and (2) the expert-curated knowledge database that includes targeted gene panels, more than 25,000 peer-reviewed papers, and the corresponding metadata (patient history, environmental factors, and so forth). The knowledge database is focused on known and suspected cancer genes and mutations and includes full details on the curation process and data captured [24].

The database is updated every 2 months; the release of v84 February 2018 integrates 1,358,288 samples; 5,448,850 coding mutations; 25,807 papers; 18,926 fusions; 33,291 whole genomes; 1,195,556 copy number variants; 9,176,464 gene expression variants; 7,879,142 differentially methylated CPGs (cytosine and guanine separated by only one phosphate group); and 18,056,654 noncoding variants.

Together, this compilation of data provides extensive coverage of the cancer genomic landscape. New and potentially significant data are continually captured and made available through 4 significant updates to COSMIC each year. Access to the COSMIC database is free for academic use, whereas commercial use requires a paid license.

International Cancer Genome Consortium

The ICGC was founded in 2007 to create a catalog of mutations in cancer through an international effort to harmonize the large number of projects [25]. The ICGC documents genomic alterations in 50 cancer subtypes and makes these data points available to researchers by request. The ICGC also publishes information on the methods used to produce, analyze, and integrate large genomic data sets. The international membership allows communication and collaboration as well as the opportunity for researchers to compare molecular differences in specific cancer subtypes across geographic areas. In 2016, the ICGC published a white paper describing how the research achievements of the ICGC "can be linked to clinical data to accelerate the development and implementation of effective cancer control measures and treatments" [26].

Cancer Cell Line Encyclopedia

The CCLE is a collaboration between the Broad Institute and the Novartis Institutes for Biomedical Research. It is an effort to conduct a detailed genetic characterization of a large panel of human cancer cell lines [27]. As of April 2018, the CCLE contains 1457 cancer cell lines; 136,488 unique data sets; 1,159,663 mutation entries. The CCLE provides public access analysis and visualization of DNA copy number, messenger RNA (mRNA) expression, mutation data, and more.

The CCLE aims to develop integrated computational analyses that link distinct pharmacologic vulnerabilities to genomic features and to translate cell line integrative genomics into patients with cancer. The 5 major data set types available are copy number, mRNA expression (Affymetrix), reverse phase protein array (RPPA), reduced representation bisulfite sequencing, and mRNA expression (RNA-seq). Four different visualizations are available for genes: box plots, scatter plots, mutation data, and a bubble map. Each gene has multiple data sets and data identifiers. Mutation data for individual cell lines are viewable and downloadable.

cBioPortal

The cBioPortal for Cancer Genomics was originally developed at Memorial Sloan Kettering Cancer Center (MSKCC) [19]. The cBioPortal software and its database are now developed and maintained by a multi-institutional consortium, consisting of MSKCC, the Dana-Farber Cancer Institute, Princess Margaret Cancer Centre in Toronto, Children's Hospital of Philadelphia, The Hyve in the Netherlands, and Bilkent University in Ankara, Turkey. Although the portal contains 171 cancer studies, the number of available samples, assays, and technologies varies per study. They include DNA-Seq (whole genome and whole exome), RNA-Seq, and copy number alterations. Some studies also include microarray-based tumor mRNA profiling, tumor micro-RNA (miRNA), and methylation data.

The Gene Expression Omnibus

The Gene Expression Omnibus (GEO) is a public functional genomics data repository supporting the minimum information about a microarray experiment standards for microarray data [28]. GEO contains array and sequence-based data and aims to provide the community with a robust and efficient genomics data repository with a simple submission procedure and a user-friendly mechanism for users to query and download gene expression profiles [27]. The GEO data sets can be searched using many different attributes, including keywords, organism, type, and authors. In addition, the GEO provides a set of data analysis tools, including visualization of expression profiles in cluster heat maps supporting a full range of cluster types, including unsupervised hierarchical clusters, K-means/K-median clusters, and heat maps organized by location of genes on the chromosome. GEO's experimental design and value distribution tools enable the visualization of the distribution of expression values of each sample within a data set. As of April 2018, the GEO contains a total of 2,447,097 samples in 4348 data sets. A list of all submitters and the summary of their contributions are available at the GEO repository [29].

Genomics Evidence Neoplasia Information Exchange

The Genomics Evidence Neoplasia Information Exchange (GENIE) is an American Association of Cancer Research project and is a multiphase, multiyear effort aimed at facilitating precision oncology by linking deep phenotype data with regulatory-grade genomic data from tens of thousands of patients [30]. Because many single-institution studies lack the statistical power to study rare cancers and/or rare variants, the GENIE project aims to provide many more patients to study in the context of associated abstracted clinical information. After a predefined embargo period, genomic data are shared with the global research community through the cBioPortal and Synapse platforms. However, therapeutic response data are not shared until the corresponding publications are released. Because the registry contains data collected from patients seen at participating institutions, a large variety of cancer types are represented, approximating "real world" data. Although the original pilot phase included 8 institutions, a second round of participating centers have recently joined the consortium. GENIE estimates that less than 0.1% of its genomic data also reside in the TCGA.

St. Jude Cloud

The newest addition to genomics commons is the St. Jude Cloud, billed as "the largest public repository of pediatric cancer genomics data." At launch in April 2018, the platform includes data on 5000 whole-genome (WGS), 5000 whole-exome (WES), and 1200 RNA-Seq data sets from more than 5000 pediatric patients with cancer and survivors [31]. The data were generated through 3 large St. Jude–supported genomics initiatives. Analysis and visualization tools are provided on the cloud-based environment [32].

Gabriella-Miller Kids First

The NIH Common Fund's Gabriella Miller Kids First Pediatric Research Program ("Kids First") will be a large-scale data resource for genomic and clinical data from children with cancer and structural birth defects [33]. The Kids First Data Resource will be a centralized database of well-curated genetic, genomic, and phenotype data from thousands of children and their families. Cloud-based analysis tools will allow researchers to study the genetic pathways underlying childhood cancer and structural birth defects. This platform will leverage technology developed for the GDC, and one of the unique features is requiring that genomic data be made quickly available on the platform for the research community.

COMMERCIAL GENOMICS COMPANIES

Several for-profit companies are endeavoring to collect large amounts of patient samples and corresponding clinical data, and in some cases, make those data available to researchers. Working in conjunction with academic and nonprofit institutions, these commercial entities offer varying degrees of access to the raw and analyzed data and may require permanent access to and use of deidentified patient information for monetization.

Tempus

Tempus is a Chicago-based company founded in 2015 [34]. Tempus bills itself as a technology company focused on collecting and analyzing large volumes of molecular and clinical data. The company provides genomic sequencing services and analyzes the molecular and clinical data in order to feed-back results and recommendations to physicians. As of April 2018, Tempus advertises 3 tests on their Web site, including Tempus|xT, a targeted panel of 595 genes; Tempus|xO, an Onco-seq panel of 1714 genes; and Tempus|xE, whole exome sequencing.

Foundation Medicine

Founded in 2013, Foundation Medicine develops, makes, and sells genomic analysis diagnostics for cancer. As of May 2018, the company advertises 5 tests on their Web site, including their original FoundationOne and FoundationOne Heme tests, a recently US Food and Drug Administration–approved test (Foundation One CDx), and a new plasma DNA test (Foundation ACT) [35,36]. Most (>60%) of the company's revenue derives from partnerships with pharmaceutical companies. Foundation Medicine's Web site contains extensive documentation on their testing and validation. Shortly after the launch of the GDC in 2016, Foundation Medicine announced that it would be contributing 18,000 additional cases to the commons.

Oncology Research Information Exchange Network

The Oncology Research Information Exchange Network (ORIEN) is a research partnership among cancer centers in North America to leverage multiple data sources and match patients to treatments. The founding centers are the Moffitt Cancer Center in Tampa and The Ohio State University Comprehensive Cancer Center–Arthur G. James Cancer Hospital and Richard J. Solove Research Institute in Columbus, Ohio. ORIEN partners use the Total Cancer Care common protocol, developed by Moffitt in 2006, for tracking a patient's molecular, clinical, and epidemiologic data. ORIEN partners have access to clinically annotated tissue repository data on more than 150,000 research subjects [37,38]. Moffitt launched M2Gen, an informatics company that manages the data management and infrastructure needed for research, and the biopharmaceutical company AbbVie joined the network in March 2017 [37]. ORIEN provides a data-sharing and tissue-sharing federated effort, which transparently maps multiple autonomous database systems into a single federated database [38].

Flatiron

Founded in 2012, Flatiron Health aims to connect the electronic health records of patients with cancer to clinical trial data in order to link real-world clinical data to research data. The company Web site currently lists that they have 2 million active patient records, more than 265 community oncology clinics participating, 55 community oncology practices across 20 states, 6 major academic research center partners, and more than 2500 clinician users [39]. Details on the Clinico-Genomic Database, which was created in partnership with Foundation Medicine, is also available on the company Web site. The Clinico-Genomic Database integrates tumor sequencing data with longitudinal treatment and outcomes data captured from the electronic health record [40]. In February 2018, Flatiron Health was acquired by the pharmaceutical company, Roche [41]. Despite the acquisition, Flatiron Health asserted that it would continue to partner with other drug companies; a 3-year partnership with Bristol-Myers Squibb was announced on May 2, 2018 [42].

IMPORTANT CONSIDERATIONS FOR LARGE-SCALE GENOMICS DATA SHARING

Large-scale genomics data-sharing repositories could lead to important breakthroughs and novel discoveries in oncology research but also require the funders, hosts, and community of researchers to address several important considerations, chief among them data *privacy*. The NIH has established a Genomic Data Sharing (GDS) policy outlining the "expectations that ensure the broad and responsible sharing of genomic research data" [26]. The GDS policy specifies that investigators should comply with Health and Human Services regulations for the Protection of Human Subjects and the HIPAA Privacy Rule. This means that human genomic data submitted to NIH-designated data repositories have to meet human subjects' research as well as clinical privacy standards.

Despite these policies, there have been several reported cases where links between deidentified genomic data and named individuals could be reestablished [27,43]. These academic and proof-of-concept reidentification efforts appear to be motivated by curiosity and academic advancement rather than by criminal self-interest; nevertheless, they have motivated the community to create and adopt ad hoc mechanisms and sharing practices that run the risk of inflicting unnecessary burden or even impeding data sharing. To address these concerns, host organizations are starting to rely on formal legal instruments that often carry penalties for attempted reidentification of participants. Importantly, the community is now considering the use of obfuscation and game theory algorithms to develop effective protections for GDS [44]. Ultimately, tradeoffs between risk and scientific utility should be reached as large-scale genomic data are released to the research community.

The NIH encourages the use of *data standards* in order to improve data quality and to enable the comparison and harmonization of data from multiple studies. The NIH funds several genomic data standards initiatives and various community resources. Starting in 2013, the NIH funded an initiative to develop standard formats for gathering and depositing genomic variants in publically accessible common repositories. One example of NIH efforts toward data standardization is ClinVar, an initiative that aggregates information about genomic variation and its relationship to human health [45].

ClinVar is a public archive of reports of the relationships between known human variations and phenotypes with supporting evidence. ClinVar thus is an evidence-based knowledge database for human variation and observed health status, together with the history of that interpretation. The information archived in ClinVar is freely available to users and organizations to ensure the broadest utility to the medical genetics community. To that end, ClinVar uses data structures that are designed to facilitate data exchange.

Large-scale data sharing initiatives or data commons share 4 requirements. First, storage and compute resources must be available for cloud-based analysis of data. Until recently, the most efficient and cost-effective storage was local, on premises, managed arrays of hard drives. The availability of cheap, reliable cloud-based storage obviates researchers to purchase and manage their own storage or compute clusters. The increasing willingness of third-party cloud-service providers to engage in business associate agreements with covered entities is helping propel the use of these resources for academic research. Second, a data commons must contain data that are publicly accessible, such as data from NCI-controlled resources like dbGaP and TARGET. Note that "publicly available" means that the data can be obtained through a transparent application process and does not necessarily mean "freely available" to anyone (see Table 1). For example, whole exome or whole genome data deposited in dbGaP or TARGET is only available after the investigator completes an application and once their sponsoring institution completes the necessary materials transfer agreement. Third, a data commons must contain software services and tools to enable cloud-based analysis of the data. Increasingly, researchers do not have the means or expertise to provision their own servers and tools or keep up with updates and new versions. Centralized access to tools facilitates a common platform for analysis across data sets. Fourth, data must conform to the FAIR digital compliance model [18,46].

To be *Findable*, data must contain sufficient metadata to be persistently identifiable and distinguishable from other objects. For example, a genomic sequence should contain machine-readable metadata that ties it back to the original source in a unique and persistent way. *Accessible* data are defined as requiring appropriate authorization via a well-defined protocol. For instance, individual-level genomic data stored in the genomic data commons are accessed once the user receives authorization via the dbGaP system. The GDC authenticates users to access these data based on information passed through from dbGaP. *Interoperability* is key to building a successful data commons, and key components are shared vocabularies and ontologies. Furthermore, the data must be machine-actionable. By being both syntactically parsable and semantically machine-accessible, data can be shared between systems, facilitating a degree of sharing and interoperability that is currently a rare commodity. If these 3 criteria are met, findability, accessibility, and interoperability, the data can be *reusable,* if the metadata and other descriptors are sufficiently rich that the data can be linked to other sources. Furthermore, these descriptors should allow linkage back to the original source. Increasingly, documentation of data lineage is being required for publication, and observation of these FAIR principles will help to ensure sufficient data provenance [47].

FUTURE DIRECTIONS

By increasing sharing of data, the speed of discovery can be accelerated. More data from a wider range of individuals and communities will facilitate enormous increases in analytical power. Increasing access to data and analytical tools will enable researchers from previously excluded institutions to participate in collaborative research as well as to contribute unique findings.

As an illustrative example, Thorsson and colleagues [47] used TCGA data to perform an extensive immunogenomics analysis of more than 10,000 tumors comprising 33 diverse cancer types. Because of this data-sharing initiative, they were able to identify 6 immune subtypes—wound healing, IFN-γ dominant, inflammatory, lymphocyte depleted, immunologically quiet, and TGF-β dominant—across 33 cancers. The immunogenomics pipeline that was created for this study can now serve as a resource for additional studies that will advance immunotherapy treatments, such as those that been already discovered, such as antibodies against CTLA-4, PD-1, and PD-L1, which are effective in treating a variety of malignancies [47].

Initiatives to centralize genomic data, processing power, and tools present a valuable opportunity to share resources and thus increase the efficiency, power, and impact of research. In time, the speed and level of discovery enabled by these large-scale GDS initiatives hold great promise to continue to advance diagnosis and treatment in genomic oncology.

REFERENCES

[1] Dai X, Li T, Bai Z, et al. Breast cancer intrinsic subtype classification, clinical use and future trends. Am J Cancer Res 2015;5(10):2929–43.

[2] Schmiegel W, Scott RJ, Dooley S, et al. Blood-based detection of RAS mutations to guide anti-epidermal growth factor receptor therapy in colorectal cancer patients: concordance of results from circulating tumor DNA and tissue-based RAS testing. Mol Oncol 2017;11(2):208–19.
[3] Bacher U, Schnittger S, Haferlach C, et al. Molecular diagnostics in acute leukemias. Clin Chem Lab Med 2009;47(11):1333–41.
[4] Kohlmann A, Bacher U, Schnittger S, et al. Perspective on how to approach molecular diagnostics in acute myeloid leukemia and myelodysplastic syndromes in the era of next-generation sequencing. Leuk Lymphoma 2014;55(8):1725–34.
[5] Arber DA, Orazi A, Hasserjian R, et al. The 2016 revision to the World Health Organization classification of myeloid neoplasms and acute leukemia. Blood 2016;127(20):2391–405.
[6] Lin P-H, Li H-Y, Fan S-C, et al. A targeted next-generation sequencing in the molecular risk stratification of adult acute myeloid leukemia: implications for clinical practice. Cancer Med 2017;6(2):349–60.
[7] Delaney SK, Hultner ML, Jacob HJ, et al. Toward clinical genomics in everyday medicine: perspectives and recommendations. Expert Rev Mol Diagn 2016;16(5):521–32.
[8] Rehm HL, Berg JS, Brooks LD, et al. ClinGen — the clinical genome resource. N Engl J Med 2015;372(23):2235–42.
[9] Data Commons | NIH Common Fund. Available at: https://commonfund.nih.gov/commons. Accessed April 15, 2018.
[10] Admin F. Guiding principles for findable, accessible, interoperable and re-usable data publishing version b1.0. FORCE11. 2014. Available at: https://www.force11.org/fairprinciples. Accessed April 15, 2018.
[11] Website. Available at: https://pediatric-data.foundationmedicine.com. Accessed May 7, 2018.
[12] Volchenboum SL, Cox SM, Heath A, et al. Data commons to support pediatric cancer research. Am Soc Clin Oncol Educ Book 2017;37:746–52.
[13] Grossman RL, Heath AP, Ferretti V, et al. Toward a shared vision for cancer genomic data. N Engl J Med 2016;375(12):1109–12.
[14] Genomic Data Commons. National Cancer Institute. Available at: https://www.cancer.gov/about-nci/organization/ccg/research/computational-genomics/gdc. Accessed April 15, 2018.
[15] GDC. Available at: https://gdc-portal.nci.nih.gov. Accessed May 7, 2018.
[16] Wilson S, Fitzsimons M, Ferguson M, et al. Developing cancer informatics applications and tools using the NCI genomic data commons API. Cancer Res 2017;77(21):e15–8.
[17] Data Levels and Types. The Cancer Genome Atlas - National Cancer Institute. Available at: https://cancergenome.nih.gov/abouttcga/aboutdata/datalevelstypes. Accessed April 16, 2018.
[18] Big Data to Knowledge | NIH Common Fund. Available at: https://datascience.nih.gov/commons. Accessed April 15, 2018.
[19] Lau JW, Lehnert E, Sethi A, et al. The cancer genomics cloud: collaborative, reproducible, and democratized-a new paradigm in large-scale computational research. Cancer Res 2017;77(21):e3–6.
[20] Home. Cancer Genomics Cloud. Available at: http://www.cancergenomicscloud.org/. Accessed May 6, 2018.
[21] Docker. Docker. Available at: https://www.docker.com/. Accessed May 6, 2018.
[22] ISB Cancer Genomics Cloud. GitHub. Available at: https://github.com/isb-cgc. Accessed May 7, 2018.
[23] Website. Available at: https://cloud.google.com/genomics/gatk. Accessed May 6, 2018.
[24] Forbes SA, Beare D, Bindal N, et al. COSMIC: high-resolution cancer genetics using the catalogue of somatic mutations in cancer. Curr Protoc Hum Genet 2016;91:10, 11.1-10.11.37.
[25] International Cancer Genome Consortium. Available at: http://icgc.org/. Accessed May 31, 2018.
[26] The International Cancer Genome Consortium for Medicine (ICGCmed) defined the opportunities for the ICGC to align closer and begin to integrate with the clinical practise of oncology. | ICGC med. Available at: http://icgcmed.org. Accessed May 31, 2018.
[27] Barretina J, Caponigro G, Stransky N, et al. The Cancer Cell Line Encyclopedia enables predictive modelling of anticancer drug sensitivity. Nature 2012;483(7391):603–7.
[28] Brazma A. Minimum information about a microarray experiment (MIAME) – successes, failures, challenges. ScientificWorldJournal 2009;9:420–3.
[29] geo. GEO Browser - GEO - NCBI. Available at: https://www.ncbi.nlm.nih.gov/geo/browse/?view=samples. Accessed May 6, 2018.
[30] AACR Project GENIE. Available at: http://www.aacr.org/Research/Research/Pages/aacr-project-genie.aspx#.WtN8C4gbPD4. Accessed April 16, 2018.
[31] St. Jude Children's Launches Cloud-Based Pediatric Cancer Genomic Database | Articles | ClinicalOMICs. 2018. Available at: https://www.clinicalomics.com/articles/st-jude-children-s-launches-cloud-based-pediatric-cancer-genomic-database/1603. Accessed May 7, 2018.
[32] St. Jude Cloud. Available at: https://stjude.cloud/. Accessed May 7, 2018.
[33] Gabriella Miller Kids First Pediatric Research Program | NIH Common Fund. Available at: https://commonfund.nih.gov/KidsFirst. Accessed April 16, 2018.
[34] Tempus (business) - Wikipedia. Available at: https://en.wikipedia.org/wiki/Tempus_(business). Accessed April 16, 2018.
[35] Foundation Medicine - Wikipedia. Available at: https://en.wikipedia.org/wiki/Foundation_Medicine. Accessed April 16, 2018.
[36] Genomic Testing. Foundation Medicine. Available at: https://www.foundationmedicine.com/genomic-testing. Accessed April 16, 2018.
[37] AbbVie and M2Gen Announce New Collaboration for the Oncology Research Information Exchange Network® (ORIEN) Avatar Research Program | AbbVie Newsroom.

Available at: https://news.abbvie.com/news/abbvie-and-m2gen-announce-new-collaboration-for-oncology-research-information-exchange-network-orien-avatar-research-program.htm. Accessed May 4, 2018.

[38] AACI. Available at: http://www.aaci-cancer.org/commentary2015_03.asp. Accessed May 4, 2018.

[39] Flatiron Health. Flatiron Health. Available at: https://flatiron.com/. Accessed May 6, 2018.

[40] Development and Validation of a Real-World Clinico-Genomic Database. Paperpile. Available at: https://paperpile.com/app/p/5909f60a-53c3-0127-adc7-a3bc4cd26398. Accessed May 3, 2018.

[41] Philippidis A. Precision oncology-focused roche to acquire flatiron health for $1.9B. Clinical OMICs 2018;5(2):47. Available at: https://www.clinicalomics.com/articles/precision-oncology-focused-roche-to-acquire-flatiron-health-for-1-9b/1496.

[42] Herper M. Flatiron health, purchased by Roche, signs three-year deal with Bristol-Myers. New York: Forbes; 2018. Available at: https://www.forbes.com/sites/matthewherper/2018/05/02/flatiron-health-purchased-by-roche-signs-three-year-deal-with-bristol-myers/. Accessed May 3, 2018.

[43] Gao J, Lindsay J, Watt S, et al. Abstract 5277: the cBioPortal for cancer genomics and its application in precision oncology. Cancer Res 2016;76(14 Supplement):5277.

[44] Wang S, Jiang X, Tang H, et al. A community effort to protect genomic data sharing, collaboration and outsourcing. NPJ Genom Med 2017;2:33.

[45] Rehm HL, Harrison SM, Martin CL. ClinVar is a critical resource to advance variant interpretation. Oncologist 2017;22(12):1562.

[46] Wilkinson MD, Dumontier M, Aalbersberg IJJ, et al. The FAIR guiding principles for scientific data management and stewardship. Sci Data 2016;3:160018.

[47] Thorsson V, Gibbs DL, Brown SD, et al. The immune landscape of cancer. Immunity 2018;48(4):812–30.e14.

Advances in Molecular Pathology 1 (2018) 149–166
ADVANCES IN MOLECULAR PATHOLOGY

Advances in Next-Generation Sequencing Bioinformatics for Clinical Diagnostics

Taking Precision Oncology to the Next Level

Sabah Kadri, PhD
Division of Genomic and Molecular Pathology, Department of Pathology, The University of Chicago, Chicago, IL 60637, USA

KEYWORDS
- Somatic testing • Next-generation sequencing (NGS) • Bioinformatics • Clinical diagnostics
- Copy number detection • Structural variants • Microsatellite instability • Tumor mutation burden

KEY POINTS

- Next-generation sequencing (NGS) has transformed precision medicine in molecular pathology by development of assays that can simultaneously detect genomic anomalies of various sizes, such as single point variants, copy number abnormalities, genes fusions, and rearrangements using custom bioinformatics methods and pipelines.
- Various metrics and signatures that are predictive biomarkers in response to therapy, such as microsatellite instability, tumor mutational burden, and homologous recombination-based DNA repair deficiency, can be calculated using existing NGS panels.
- Advances in NGS technologies and computational methods have led to development of multiple low-level tests for early detection and relapse that are a few validation studies away from the clinic.

INTRODUCTION

In recent years, there has been remarkable growth in the understanding of genetic alterations that can be used to guide personalized diagnosis and care of oncology patients. Concomitantly, molecular diagnostics laboratories face enormous pressure to develop assays of ever-increasing wet-lab and bioinformatics complexity in order keep up with the torrential pace of discovery. Next-generation sequencing (NGS) technologies have transformed clinical diagnostics in molecular pathology, allowing for the replacement of multiple traditional assay types while permitting comprehensive analyses of vanishingly small specimens. Until recently, cancer genome profiling in diagnostics has been limited to targeted DNA-based panels due to lower costs of sequencing, processing, and ease of interpretation. The past 5 years have seen numerous published works on the clinical validations of targeted NGS panels for somatic variation, but with significant variability in the types and sizes of these panels. In order to aid patient care via decision support for the most up-to-date Food and Drug administration (FDA)-approved drugs or via clinical trial enrollment, laboratories are constantly striving to update NGS tests by expanding the clinical territory to cover more genomic anomalies or developing detection methods for novel therapeutic predictors. A single NGS-based assay can now simultaneously characterize multiple somatic genomic

Disclosure: The author has nothing to disclose.

E-mail address: skadriphd@gmail.com

https://doi.org/10.1016/j.yamp.2018.06.010
2589-4080/18/

markers, such as point mutations (single nucleotide variants, SNVs), structural variants including insertions/deletions (indels), gene fusion events and other structural rearrangements, copy number variations (CNVs), microsatellite instability (MSI), tumor mutational burden (TMB), or homologous recombination-based DNA repair deficiency (HRD) signatures. Such a characterization is only possible due to major advances in bioinformatics in each of these areas.

Although it is indisputable that bioinformatics is vital to NGS testing, it routinely represents a significant barrier to clinical test setup and development. Unless laboratories are part of organizations with existing secure and powerful infrastructure and expertise, onboarding talent and installing the necessary infrastructure may require enormous investment. Even with available resources, setting up optimal bioinformatics pipelines requires a detailed understanding of the available open source and commercial software for each application, and in some cases, creation of custom scripts/tools to process, summarize, or fill performance gaps. Whether the pipelines are vendor supplied or custom developed, it is imperative to perform validation as extensively as is customary for the wet-lab component. In fact, the College of American Pathologists has outlined standards for validation of bioinformatics pipelines [1], and the Association for Molecular Pathology (AMP) recently laid out recommendations for such pipeline validations [2]. Thus, it is important to understand the pros and cons of all methods used in a clinical pipeline to identify the power and limitations of detection by the assay.

In this review, the author summarizes bioinformatics strategies and tools used to build integrative computational pipelines across NGS assays of different types and sizes in clinical oncology, to simultaneously uncover somatic genomic anomalies of various sizes and types. Over the years, there have been multiple independent reviews of specific applications of NGS technologies but none that cover all current applications of NGS in the clinic, building toward developing a single integrative and modular bioinformatics pipeline. The author hopes this comprehensive catalog of adopted and available approaches will aid new laboratories in the construction of their NGS assay pipelines. The author also reviews the latest advances in bioinformatics for detection of immunotherapy predictors and HRD signatures and discusses the future of precision medicine using circulating tumor DNA (ctDNA), minimal residual disease (MRD), gene expression, microRNAs (miRNAs), and multi-agent testing.

TARGETED DNA-BASED ASSAYS

Although whole genome sequencing and whole exome sequencing (WES) have been used extensively for research and bulk identification of cancer biomarkers [3], it is generally not currently feasible to use these methodologies for routine somatic testing in the clinic, due to inadequate sequencing depth required to detect somatic mutations at low mutant allelic frequencies (MAFs), which are common in heterogeneous tumor samples. In addition, cancer samples contain many more variants of interest than most inherited genetics tests of comparable size, necessitating increased interpretive effort. As a result, most cancer NGS assays are more targeted DNA sequencing assays restricted to a variable number of genes of interest. Targeted NGS assays are typically grouped into 2 main categories based on the type of enrichment used to investigate the regions of interest: (i) amplicon-based multiplex polymerase chain reaction (PCR), and (ii) hybridization (hybrid) capture.

From the laboratory standpoint, amplicon assays (Ion Torrent Ampliseq, Illumina TruSight, and so forth) typically covering limited territory (up to few hundred amplicons) over 1 to 100 genes, have many advantages, including capability for low DNA input, low cost, and rapid turnaround time. However, these assays are usually in terms of limited detection targets, restricted mainly to SNVs and short indels that occur between primer binding sites. Possibly because of lack of infrastructure or expertise, many laboratories initially chose vendor-supplied bioinformatics software to generate variant calls [4–6]. Software such as Torrent Suite software (Ion Torrent, Life Technologies) or Miseq Reporter (Illumina) offer limited options for software customizability and are especially weak in indel detection [4,6,7]. An example of a more advanced amplicon panel is the Oncomine Comprehensive Panel (143 genes), which is designed with noncoding probes for CNVs, whereas a separate RNA panel can detect gene fusions, all processed using the Torrent Suite software [8].

Even when panels have built custom pipelines, indel detection has proven to be an area of inconsistent and poor performance, as demonstrated by Davies and colleagues [9], who observed that 6 institutions with the same library preparation kit but distinct bioinformatics pipelines showed high concordance in SNVs but significant discordance in indel detection. Multiple solutions have been proposed; the author has previously suggested using a parallel alignment-independent method to improve indel detection (Amplicon Indel Hunter) [7], which has been clinically validated at the University of Chicago. Other software has been developed for indels, complex indels [10], and internal tandem duplication (ITD) detection in amplicon-based NGS data [11–13], although not used in clinical assays, to the author's knowledge (Table 1).

Over the last few years, as further biomarkers and predictors for therapy have been identified, laboratories started designing more powerful and larger panels targeting additional genes, using hybrid capture enrichment. Hybrid capture assays produce a fundamentally different type of data from amplicon panels, due to random fragmentation of sample DNA molecules followed by positive selection via hybridization to predesigned probes. As a result, sequencing data contains a variety of genomic start and end points, which may be used (with certain caveats, as discussed later) to define molecular uniqueness. Also, because these assays are independent of primers, nearly any type of genomic anomaly can be captured during the hybridization and may ultimately be detectable as long as the assay's bioinformatics pipelines are capable of accurately recognizing it. Hybrid capture oncology panels in use in clinical laboratories typically target 200 to 500 genes implicated in cancer biology or useful for clinical management [16–18]. Few larger panels with 1000+ genes, such as UCM-OncoPlus [19] (University of Chicago, Chicago, IL, USA) and Oncoseq1700 (University of Michigan Comprehensive Cancer Center, Ann Arbor, MI, USA) sequence data from a high number of genes but the former, for example, processes only a subset to guide clinical care. Because each assay may differ in content, size, and capabilities, hybrid-capture assays are most often processed by custom pipelines specifically developed for the assay. This customization is only possible with advanced bioinformatics methods arranged in a modular fashion to design an integrative pipeline, using a combination of customized scripts as well as commercial and publicly available software. These panels are either run as tumor-only or matched tumor-normal samples. Without delving into the pros and cons of either approach, which is decided based on laboratory-specific considerations, the author discusses the bioinformatics approaches in processing data from both methodologies in the sections below.

Fig. 1 shows a schematic of the types of analyses that can be typically performed using a single hybrid-capture assay. All pipelines contain a data preprocessing and variant-calling module, discussed briefly in later discussion, and a subset of other modules for detection of various types of alterations/biomarkers. Table 2 summarizes the main software used by some of the clinical assays reported in literature [16–19,29]. It is important to note that pipelines are constantly being updated, and thus, the information in Table 2 is based on the initial clinical validations unless more recent publications discuss the updated pipelines. The author briefly discusses the common methods used for preprocessing data and variant calling, and then outlines in detail various other bioinformatics modules that can be incrementally added to a bioinformatics pipeline to detect emerging and more complicated biomarkers in parallel with existing workflows.

DATA ALIGNMENT AND VARIANT CALLING

Cancer profiling assays used to uncover tumor genomic features of interest, either germline or somatic,

TABLE 1
Tools Developed to Specifically Aid Indel Detection in Next-Generation Sequencing Data

Software	Assay Type	Target of Detection	Mechanism	Year
Amplicon Indel Hunter [7]	Amp	Indel, ITD	De novo assembly of reads with mutant insert size	2015
ScanIndel [11]		Indel	Soft-clipped reads	2015
IndelSEEK [10]	Amp, HC	Complex indel	Scans reads for closely spaced indels, substitutions in cis	2017
Dindel [14]	Amp, HC	Short indel	Candidate alternate haplotype identification and read realignment	2011
IndelLocator [15]	Amp, HC	Indel	Uses statistics about read count and quality around indel events based on alignments	N/A
ITDseek [12]	Amp	*FLT3* ITD	Searches soft-clipping points in alignments and correlates them with any corresponding secondary alignments	2016

Abbreviations: Amp, amplicon-based; HC, hybrid-capture.

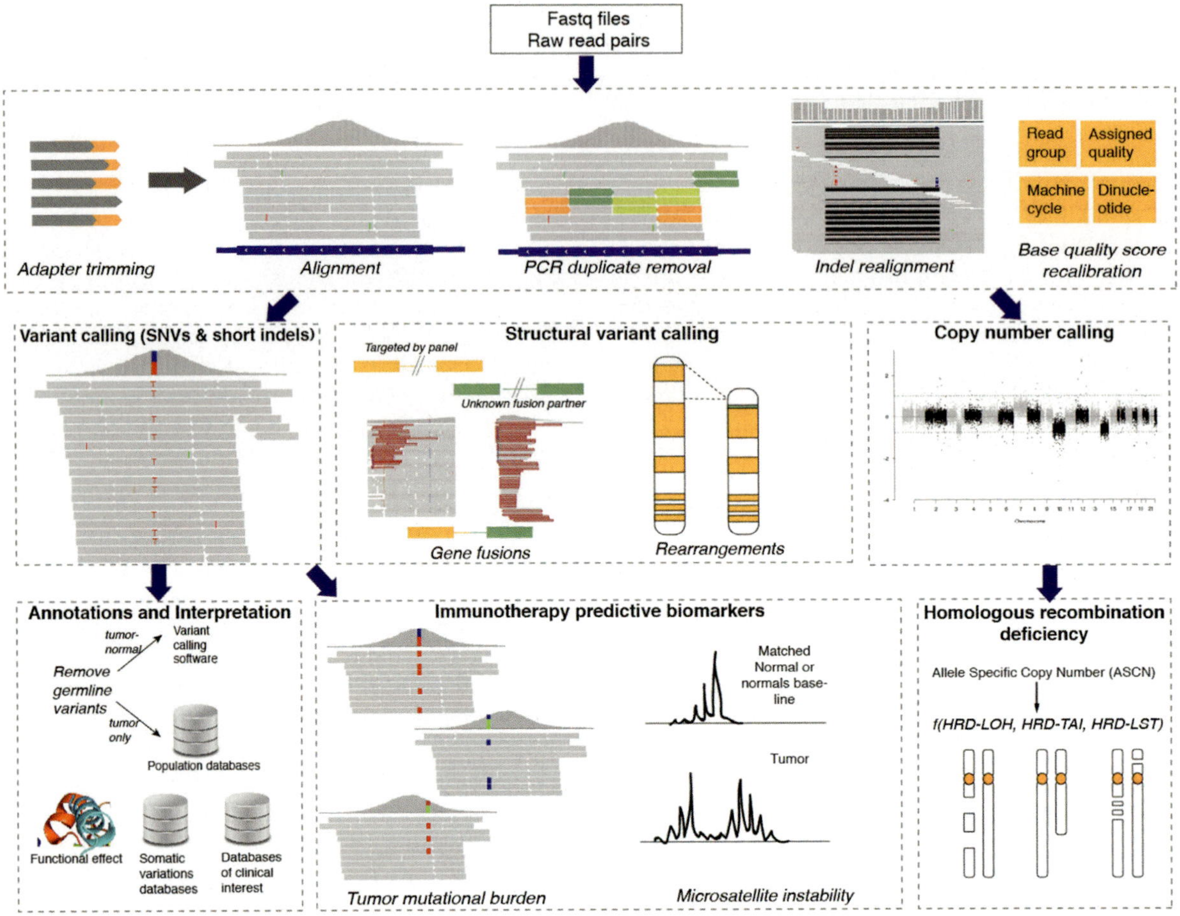

FIG. 1 Modules to build an integrative bioinformatics pipeline for an NGS hybrid-capture assay. The raw reads are first preprocessed; variant calling is performed, followed by annotation, filtering, and interpretation of somatic variants. Additional modules can be added for copy number and structural variant detection. Recently, calculations for MSI status, TMB, and HRD signatures have been proposed.

universally depend on a critical step to align sequencing reads to the reference genome sequence, which serves to organize an otherwise random assortment of sequencing reads and allow for localized genomic analysis. The dependence on mapping may serve to impair sensitivity for detection of genomic events with sequences that are highly divergent from the reference genome sequence (see Fig. 1).

- *Adapter trimming:* Typically, pipelines may first use an adapter trimming software in order to remove unwanted adapter sequences at the 3′ read ends from short library fragments using various tools such as TrimGalore (http://www.bioinformatics.babraham.ac.uk/projects/trim_galore), CutAdapt [20], and Trimmomatic [28].
- *Alignment and duplicate read removal:* Most large (100+ genes) hybrid capture panels use BWA-MEM [21] to align reads to the reference hg19 genome, whereas smaller hybrid capture panels and amplicon-based panels have used aligners such as GSNAP (http://research-pub.gene.com/gmap) and Novoalign (http://www.novocraft.com), which are potentially more accurate but slower [31]. Picard tools (http://broadinstitute.github.io/picard) are used to remove both library and potential optical duplicates from the data based on the orientation and start and end of the alignment. Some pipelines perform this step before indel realignment [16–18], whereas others realign the data first [19,29].

TABLE 2
Summary of Software Tools Used by Published Clinical Panels for Processing Hybrid-Capture Data

		Preprocessing					Variant Calling				
Panel	No. of Genes	Adapter Trimming	Alignment	Remove PCR Duplicates	Indel Realignment	Base Recalibration	SNVs	Indels	Annotation	Copy Number	Structural Variants
MSK-IMPACT [16]	341	TrimGalore, CutAdapt [20]	BWA-MEM [21]	Picard	GATK [22]	GATK	MuTect [23]	Somatic Indel Detector (GATK)	ANNOVAR [24]	Custom algorithm (uses GATK Depth OfCoverage)	DELLY [25]
OncoPanel [17]	282	N/A	BWA	Picard	GATK	GATK	MuTect	Indel Locator [15]	Oncotator	Custom R tool (VisCap [26]-Cancer) (uses GATK Depth OfCoverage)	BreaKmer [27]
Foundation Medicine [18]	287	N/A	BWA	Picard	GATK	N/A	Custom caller (Bayesian)	Custom caller (de novo local assembly)	N/A	Custom method	Custom algorithm
UCM-OncoPlus [19]	1212	Trimmomatic [28]	BWA-MEM	Picard	ABRA [32]	N/A	Custom caller (using Samtools mpileup)	Custom caller (using Samtools mpileup)	Alamut	Custom algorithm (uses GATK Depth OfCoverage)	Custom algorithm
UW-OncoPlex [29]	194	N/A	BWA	Picard	GATK	GATK	GATK, VarScan [30]	GATK, VarScan	ANNOVAR	CONTRA [58]	CREST [63]

Steps that were not mentioned in the panel literature are indicated as "N/A." The number of genes specified is at the time of publication, and most panels have increased this number since the initial validation.

- *Indel realignment for detection of insertions and deletions (indels):* Basic genome alignment should be considered adequate for detection of SNVs and indels that are small enough not to suffer from aligner mapping error (see later discussion). This threshold is aligner dependent; however, in general, aligner anomalies are likely to occur with indels larger than 10 base-pairs. Unlike amplicon data, for hybrid capture data where variant sequences can be quite complex, it is best to implement approaches that are specifically designed to leverage their power across multiple reads for more sensitive detection of anomalies with few or no initially correctly mapped reads. The most commonly used approaches begin with initially aligned reads and either perform bulk localized read realignment (eg, IndelRealigner from Genome Analysis Toolkit [GATK] [22] and ABRA [32]) or read pattern growth (eg, Pindel [33]). Panels that perform base-quality recalibration mainly used GATK for this purpose.

 Some of the hardest types of indels to detect are the ITD events in *FLT3* that are poor prognosis markers in myeloid neoplasms [34]. Tests use a variety of different methods to detect these ITDs from manual review in Integrative Genomics Browser (IGV) [42] to separate modules using a multi-software approach [19].

- *Variant (SNV and short indel) calling:* Variant calling involves detection of genomic positions that differ from the reference genome, and the exact sequence by which they differ. The selected approach depends on whether a matched normal is sequenced with the tumor sample. Box 1 lists some of the more popularly used callers along with some considerations. Clinical assays are known to use either a single or a combination of callers in parallel, either custom or publicly available (see Table 2). Multiple callers may also be used to improve sensitivity; however, the impact of this approach on specificity must be considered, and strategies must be implemented for resolution of discrepant results between callers. The quality of the results is influenced by any mapping and/or base filters used by the pipeline [18]. It is important to identify the technical limitations of variant calling during clinical validation of an assay by performing a thorough analysis of the data quality to find false positives due to the following: (i) regions affected by homologous or unclassified pseudogene sequences, (ii) repetitive regions, and (iii) recurrent false positives due to sequencing artifacts. The pipeline can then contain custom scripts or filters to remove such variants. It is also important to identify regions of inadequate coverage due to poor capture to ascertain the limitations of variant calling. Every assay and pipeline will have limitations based on some level of background noise and other considerations, such as library diversity and depth, and thus the assay should be designed with set thresholds for acceptable tumor cell purity such that expected mutations will be visible above the analytical sensitivity of the assay.

BOX 1
Variant Calling Software

Tumor-normal

MuTect [23]: Two Bayesian (log odds) classifiers to detect (i) tumor is mutated at a site, (ii) normal does not carry the mutation.

Strelka [35]: Novel Bayesian model, such that samples are modeled as a mixture of variations and calculates a joint probability score of the somatic variant. Strelka2 [36] accounts for possible tumor cell contamination in the normal sample.

VarScan2 [30]: Uses Samtools mpileup to detect variants and classify them by somatic status using a heuristic (comparison of genotypes) and statistical (Fisher's exact test applied to read counts) algorithm. Can accept tumor purity if available.

SomaticSniper [37]: Uses the genotype likelihood model of MAQ and computes a somatic score as the probability that the tumor and normal genotypes are different.

Tumor-only

Platypus [38]: A Bayesian statistical framework combining haplotype-based, multisample variant caller and local sequence assembly. Multithreading options are available.

FreeBayes [39]: Haplotype-based detector to find SNVs, indels, multinucleotide polymorphisms, and complex events.

LoFreq [40]: Infers SNVs and indels from by using base-call qualities and other sources of errors such as mapping or alignment uncertainty, and able to call variants below the average basecall quality. Multithreading options are available.

Selected custom clinical methods: Frampton and colleagues [18] used Bayesian methodology followed by strand bias (Fisher's test) and read location bias (Kolmogorov-Smirnov test) filtering. Kadri and colleagues [19] use Samtools mpileup followed by depth, base quality, MAF, and filtering of false positives characterized during validation of the clinical territory.

ANNOTATION AND INTERPRETATION

Annotation of the variants involves using a combination of software and databases to determine the putative functional impact of the variant, information about the variant across various population and mutation databases, and reported studies. Laboratories have used a variety of annotation software (see Table 2), which range from freely available solutions, such as ANNOVAR [24] and Oncotator (http://www.broadinstitute.org/oncotator), to commercial Alamut (Interactive Biosoftware, Rouen, France) and Ingenuity Variant Analysis (http://www.ingenuity.com/products/variant-analysis). It is important for the pathologist to manually review the HGVS (human genome variation society) nomenclature [41] returned by the annotation software and make any corrections if necessary. In most somatic assays, initial filtering is performed to remove germline variants:

- *Tumor-matched normal:* Either the variant calling software filters out germline variants from the tumor list (see Box 1) or custom cut-offs are set up [16].
- *Tumor-only:* Assays that do not sequence a matched normal (Box 2) rely on various population databases to filter out known germline SNPs.

Pathologists then manually review the final filtered variants using genome browsers, such as the IGV [42], to visualize the aligned BAM files at the variant locations. Detailed guidelines and standards have been provided by AMP for interpretation of somatic variants, along with relevant Web sources and databases [43]. A summary of the most commonly used databases appears in Box 2. Laboratories have developed more advanced systems, such as Clinical Genomicist Workstation [44], SeqReporter [45], and SIMPL [46], to build a knowledge base and aid more automated interpretation and reporting.

COPY NUMBER DETECTION

CNVs are extremely important somatic abnormalities in cancer that can guide patient prognosis and treatment [53]. CNV calling has been a major bioinformatics challenge in targeted NGS assays, and although many methods have been developed, it is important to choose an algorithm that can provide high accuracy for somatic CNV calling. Somatic CNV events can be either genome-wide or focal and can be complicated by factors such as tumor heterogeneity, ploidy, and purity. Targeted DNA sequencing also has systematic biases due to GC-content, mapability, hybridization, and sequencing, which must be normalized [54]. Inadequate normalization steps invariably lead to increased assay noise. The main approach for CNV calling in targeted panels involves comparison of depth of coverage of on-target, and in some algorithms, off-target regions, to one or more control samples (Design 1 in Fig. 2). Some panels add additional probes targeting SNPs across the genome for better coverage across the genome [55] (Design 2 in Fig. 2). However, the main technical difference between CNV methods lies in the normalization and segmentation methods, although the most commonly used segmentation method is circular binary segmentation (CBS) [56]. Box 3 lists specific differences between commonly used copy number calling methods.

As seen in Table 2, most clinical targeted panels use custom algorithms for CNVs with the main methodology being (i) calculation of depths of the targeted regions, (ii) normalizing the data to reduce biases, (iii) using baselines with a collection of normal samples. MSK-IMPACT [16], which performs tumor-normal sequencing, calculates the best comparator normal for each tumor sample using a sum-squared log-ratio against a set of control normal samples. Unfortunately, the biggest challenge in this area is the lack of standardization of CNV reporting across different assays, and each test reports these alterations using thresholds set during validation of the assay. Box 3 summarizes the various commonly used CNV software based on the principle approaches and only included callers that can be used for somatic calling with targeted gene panels. It is important to note that tumor purity must be considered during interpretation of copy number plots.

BOX 2
Databases to Aid Somatic Interpretation

Population databases: 1000 Genomes Project [47], ExAC (http://exac.broadinstitute.org/), dbSNP [48], Exome Variant Server (http://evs.gs.washington.edu/EVS), NHLBI ESP

Somatic variations: Catalog of Somatic Mutations in Cancer (COSMIC) [49], cBioPortal [50]

Other databases of interest: ClinVar [51], Human Gene Mutation Database (HGMD) [52]

STRUCTURAL VARIANTS DETECTION

Structural DNA variation generally includes large (>1 kb) genomic rearrangements, including novel indels, mobile-element transpositions, inversions, duplications, and translocations. Traditionally, translocations have been detected by cytogenetics, fluorescence in situ hybridization or reverse transcription-PCR. Computational methods can be added as a separate module to targeted NGS DNA panel pipelines to identify exact breakpoints

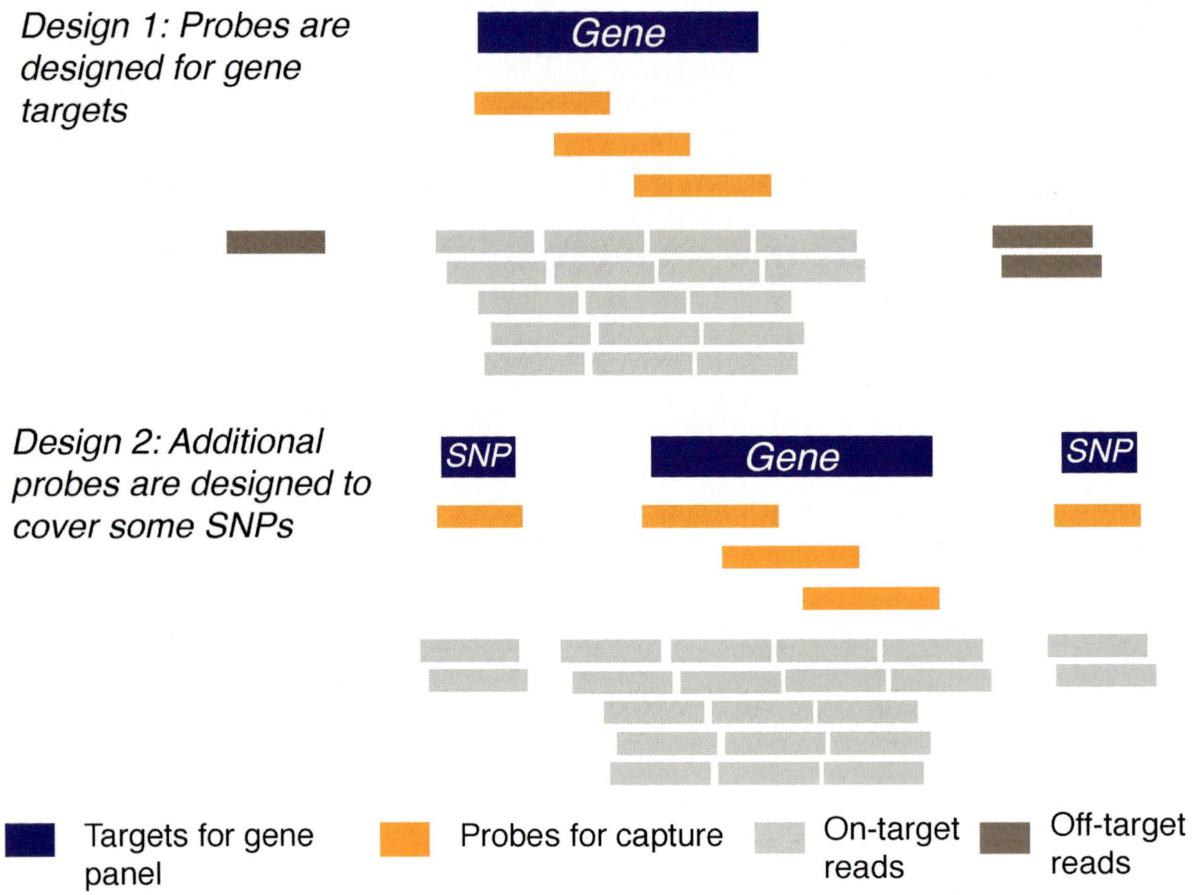

FIG. 2 General design strategies of probe design used by copy number algorithms. Approaches using the typical Design 1 of a targeted panel can either use on-target only or both on-target and off-target reads for CNVs, whereas approaches for Design 2 specifically use the SNP-targeting probes to aid in CNV calling.

and fusion partners and replace traditional methods as long as at least one of the partner genes is captured during enrichment. It is important to design the intronic probes carefully to avoid high repetitive regions, because this has been shown to compromise the specificity of detection [60]. Structural variants (SVs) are among the hardest alterations to detect due to a high rate of false positives. Despite advances in computational methods, certain SVs, such as *IGH* rearrangements testing, might still require complementary single-gene assays [17]. Thus, it is critical to recognize the limitations of detection for each assay for the various anomalies. Removal of duplicate reads is also shown to be important for a high positive predictive value for translocation software [60] (Box 4).

IMMUNOTHERAPY PREDICTIVE BIOMARKERS

Immune checkpoint inhibitors (ICIs) have quickly become the leading form of therapy for patients with various advanced cancers [64,65]. Numerous studies investigating genomic biomarkers from NGS data to predict clinical response have pointed to mismatch repair deficiency [66,67] and TMB [68–70] as "predictive" of durable clinical response, and thus, laboratories have rushed to evaluate multiple methodologies to calculate these metrics and integrate them into existing targeted panel pipelines. Cancers with high mutational loads can express more neoantigens that may prompt successful T-cell–dependent immune responses against tumors.

BOX 3
Metrics and Normalization Methods for Copy Number Calling Methods for Somatic Calling in Targeted Gene Panels

Pooled cohort: reference is pooled normals; Tumor-Normal: Matched normal is required as reference for the tumor;

VarScan2 [30]: (Tumor-*Normal*) Compare Q20 read depths between tumor and normal. Normalization is only for amount of input data, that is, unique bases mapped. Score used is the log2 of ratio of tumor depth to normal depth for each contiguous region. CBS method used for segmentation.

CNVKit [57]: (Pooled *cohort*) Uses on-target as well as nonspecific off-target reads to determine genome-wide copy number. Uses a historic baseline built with a set of normals as input. Normalizes for GC content, repetitive sequences, target size, and spacing from normals. CBS method used for segmentation.

CONTRA [58]: (Tumor-*Normal*) Calculates tumor/normal coverage ratio and uses a normal approximation to detect CNV at the exon level. Uses CBS to merge exon-level deletions/duplications into larger CNV calls.

ExomeCNV [59]: (*Tumor-Normal*) Calculates tumor/normal ratio and uses CBS along with B-allele frequency modeling to detect LOH, which is useful to verify CNV calls (deletions)

VisCap [26]: (Pooled *cohort*) R-based tool compares the fractional coverage of each exon to the median of values across all samples in a sequencing run. The tools use GATK [22] DepthOfCoverage program to calculate the coverage across each interval (GATK).

BOX 4
Structural Variant Calling Methods

DELLY [25]: Detection of read pairs and split reads supporting the underlying rearrangement. Works only with paired tumor-normal samples. Can detect gene fusions including deletions, tandem duplications, inversions, and translocations. Sensitivity depends on the coverage and read-length.

BreakDancer [61]: Paired-end method that detects structural variants by identifying pairs of regions connected by discordant read pairs and assigns to each breakpoint a score based on a Poisson model.

BreaKmer [27]: Uses a split-read, assembly, and realignment approach for calling structural variants at gene level. "kmer" subtraction from reference for misaligned reads, and assembled contigs are aligned to the reference genome. Detects insertions, deletions, inversions, tandem duplications, and translocations at base-pair resolution.

Pindel [33]: Pattern growth split-read approach, to detect breakpoints of large deletions and medium-sized insertions from paired-end short reads.

LUMPY [62]: Probabilistic framework with distinct modules to integrate any number of input alignment signals such as read-pair, split-read, and read depth, along with prior evidence such as CNVs, used to detect deletions, tandem duplications, inversions, and translocations.

CREST [63]: Uses soft-clipped reads for assembly and remapping to determine the exact breakpoint of the variant.

MICROSATELLITE INSTABILITY

The FDA recently approved antiprogrammed death-1 (anti-PD-1) therapy for patients that are classified as MSI-high (MSI-H) [66]. At the DNA level, PCR assays have been used as the gold standard to calculate the MSI status of tumors, but many groups have established methods using existing NGS tests for cost-efficiency and leveraging an assay that is already run. These assays can capture a large number of relevant loci, found commonly near exon-intron boundaries, increasing the power of detection without any design changes. The MSI detection module has mainly been based on selecting loci with mononucleotide repeats covered by the target regions and using the distributions of reads across different repeat lengths. Table 3 lists some software approaches for MSI status detection. It is important to note that for each assay, when setting up an MSI method, it is important to set stringent criteria to select the assay-specific loci, including coverage and stability in normal controls. Each method uses different criteria to select the loci, including setting thresholds and creating baselines using normal samples, with MSI-Sensor being the only method using paired tumor-normal data [71–75].

TUMOR MUTATIONAL BURDEN

TMB is defined as the number of somatic mutations detected by NGS methods per megabase of coding genome examined. Most early research studies used tumor-normal WES for TMB calculations to demonstrate that a higher somatic TMB is predictive of durable clinical response in advanced melanoma [68] and non–small cell lung cancer (NSCLC) [69]. Subsequent studies showed that targeted hybrid-capture clinical panels could be used to estimate TMB with similar

TABLE 3
Microsatellite Instability Detection Software and Approaches

	MSIsensor [71]	**mSINGS [72]**	**Chalmers et al [73]**	**MANTIS [74]**	**MSI-ColonCare [75]**
	Tumor-Normal	**Tumor Only**	**Tumor Only**	**Tumor-Normal**	**Tumor Only**
Comparison metric	Read count distribution of diff repeat lengths	Read counts of diff repeat lengths	Mean and variances of repeat lengths	Stepwise difference between locus length distributions	Coverage ratio of repeat lengths
Criteria for instable locus	*p-val* < threshold	No. of types of repeat lengths > reference mean + 3 SD	Principal component analysis to generate "MSI score"	Average of difference scores	Coverage ratio < [mean − 3 SD] of reference set
Scoring approach	Positive markers	% of instable loci	% of instable loci	Aggregate instability score	% of instable loci
Thresholds					
MSI-H	Five & 7 markers are positive	>20%	Determined by manual unsupervised clustering	0.4	>40%
MSS		<20%			<15%
MSI-L					15%–40%

accuracy to that using WES [70], and higher TMB predicts favorable outcome across tumors beyond NSCLC and melanoma [76]. Targeted panel-derived TMB metrics are only useful for large panels with greater than 300 genes as the predictive accuracy is reduced for panels with less than 150 genes [77,78]. There is enough evidence to include TMB as a biomarker in clinical trials for anti-PD-1/PD-L1 therapies [73]; however, a major issue in this area is that there is no universal cutoff for TMB as each study has a custom method to calculate the metric based on panel size, content and presence of a matched normal, and also tumor type. Recent studies have suggested that 20 mutations per megabase is classified as high TMB using FoundationOne [76] and MSK-IMPACT [79] assays; however, there have not been any studies focused on how or whether the mutation load results differ by assay or whether the threshold should vary by any other factors. The 2 main ways for TMB calculation in literature is based on the presence or absence of a matched-normal, and Fig. 3 shows a representation of how the somatic mutational load has been estimated in both these scenarios across multiple studies [73,78,79].

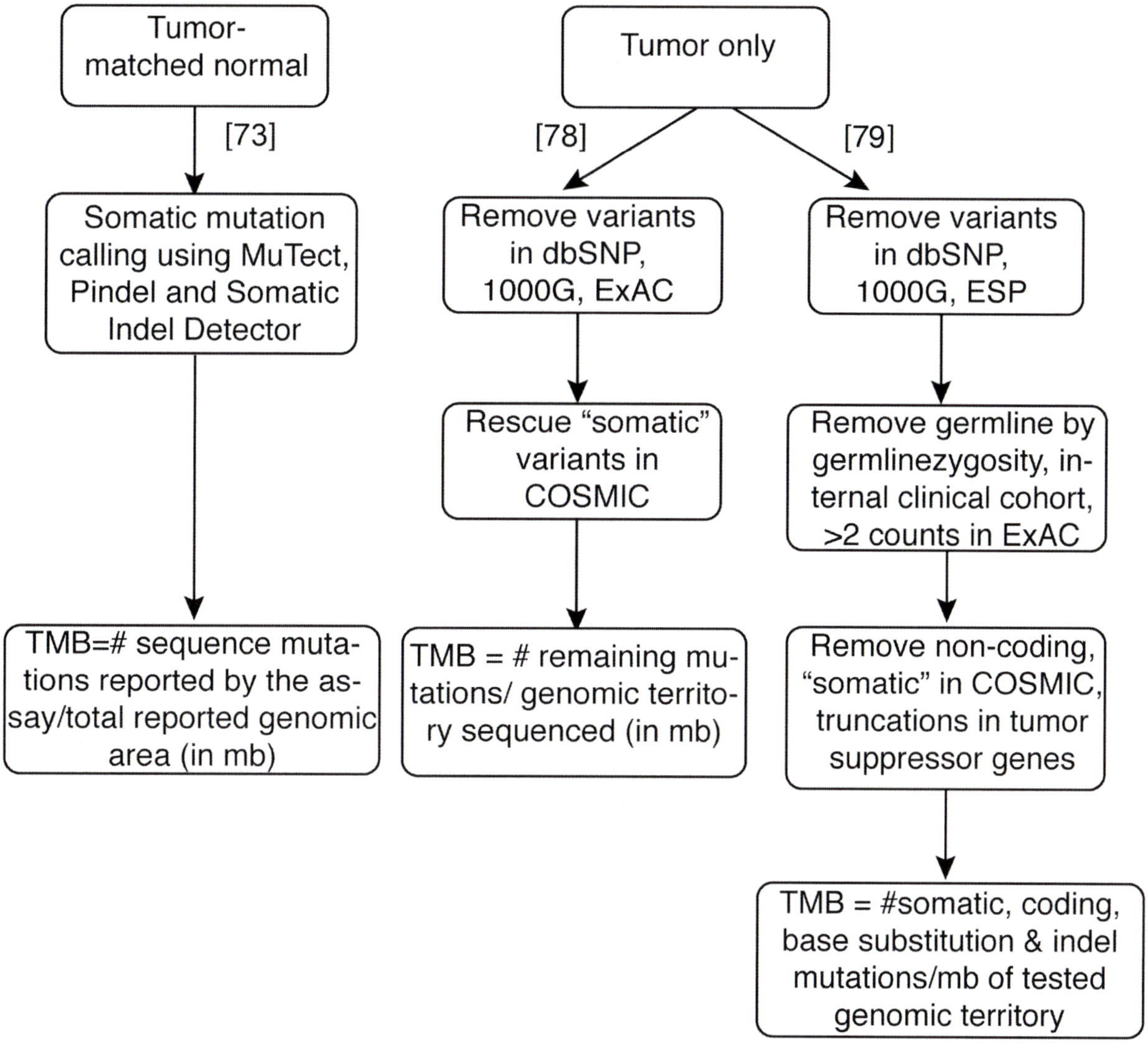

FIG. 3 Published approaches for TMB calculations with and without a matched normal. The tumor-only methods differ in the types of mutations that are used to calculate TMB.

Other Immunotherapy Biomarkers

Few studies have shown other biomarkers, fraction of copy number-altered genome (FGA) [70], aneuploidy [80] and gene expression [81], to be predictive of response to ICIs. However, much work needs to be done to perform a systematic investigation of the association of these with markers like TMB and their clinical use.

$$\text{FGA} = \frac{\text{Area with copy number gain or loss}}{\text{Size of genome profiled}}$$

$$\text{Aneuploidy} = \text{Abnormal number of chromosomes}$$

HOMOLOGOUS RECOMBINATION DEFICIENCY SIGNATURES

Recent studies have established the importance of homologous recombination deficiency (HRD) scores in predicting response to platinum-based therapy and PARP (poly (ADP ribose) polymerase) inhibitors [82,83]. Baits targeting SNPs could be added to an existing clinical gene panel, as described above, with slightly more sequencing, and HRD scores can be calculated in parallel in a more cost-effective way. First, allele specific copy number at each SNP is calculated, using methods such as Sequenza [84] or Abkevich and colleagues [85]. HRD score is computed as a combination of 3 scores, either as a non-weighted sum or as a mean (HRD-Mean) [83]:

i. HRD-loss of heterozygosity score =#LOH regions greater than 15 Mb (shorter than chromosome),
ii HRD-telomeric allelic imbalance score =#regions with allelic imbalance extending to one of the sub-telomeres but not crossing the centromere, and
iii. HRD-large-scale state transition score =#break points between regions greater than 10 Mb after filtering regions <3 Mb.

DNA NEXT-GENERATION SEQUENCING TECHNOLOGIES FOR LOW-LEVEL MUTATION DETECTION (LIQUID BIOPSY)

Cancer profiling by NGS approaches are no longer limited to the above-mentioned gene panels. The next wave of diagnostics is now focused on early (although cautious) detection of cancer and MRD using noninvasive "liquid biopsy." "Liquid biopsy" includes somatic testing of blood-based biomarkers in ctDNA, circulating free tumor DNA (cfDNA), or other tumor cell derivatives such as miRNAs and may offer an invaluable tool for future cancer therapy [86]. Companion diagnostics platforms for *EGFR* mutation detection in cfDNA are already available [87].

ctDNA fragments are released by tumor cells into blood and can be used to detect SNVs, rearrangements, and copy number abnormalities for

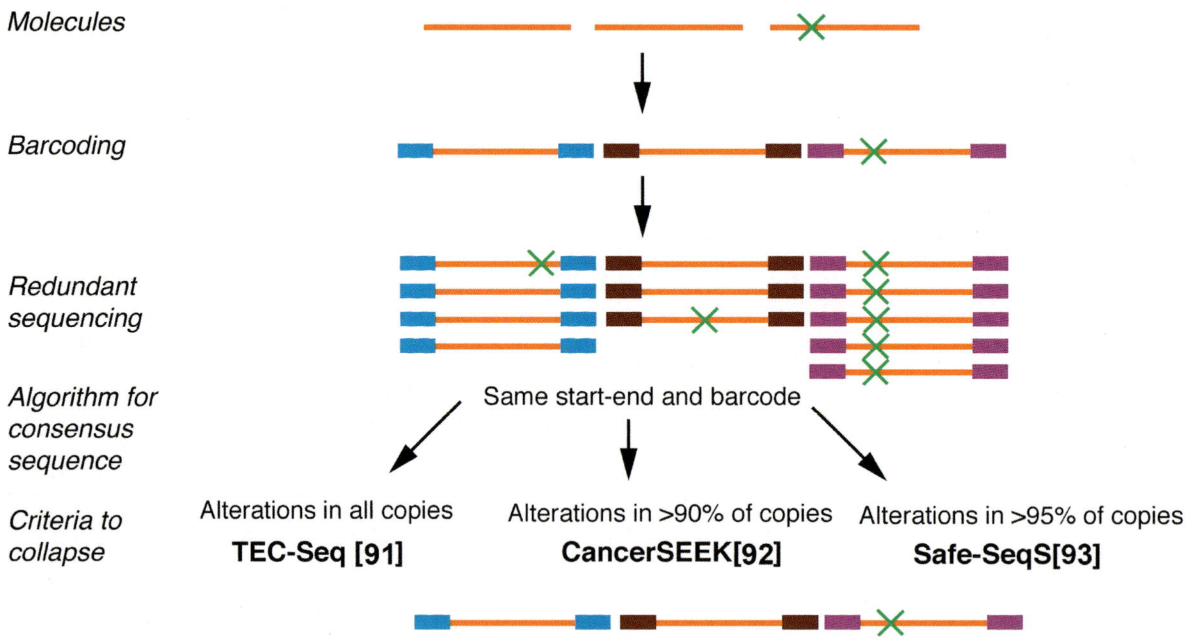

FIG. 4 Barcode collapsing for consensus read sequence in ctDNA methods. Methods use custom scripts and mainly differ in the basic criteria to collapse the redundant reads into a consensus sequence.

early detection of cancer or prediction of MRD or the presence of therapy resistance mutations, which may be associated with metastasis or relapse risk [88–90]. To remove the noise from inherent sequencing error rate and increase the sensitivity as well as specificity of detection, assays use interesting NGS strategies such as unique identifier sequences (UIDs)/molecular barcodes, careful targeted territory design and deep sequencing, as well as advanced computational methods. The bioinformatics challenge is to group reads from a common template to find a consensus sequence for the molecule, using a combination of mapping positions and barcodes, and has been tackled by various groups using custom software. Fig.4 demonstrates some published approaches [91–93] to identify the unique molecules.

Adequate tumor tissue may not always be available for larger molecular assays to calculate TMB, and thus, blood-based assays may be considered (bTMB). Initial studies have shown reliable bTMB calculation (high-confidence SNVs over 394 genes from cfDNA) and correlation with anti-PD-L1 activity [94]. However, there is need for further systematic studies and clinical trials to demonstrate the utility and feasibility of liquid biopsies for routine use. Numerous undertakings such as the European consortium CANCER-ID (13 countries) has been created for the clinical validation of blood-based biomarkers and to establish the clinical utility of these biomarkers.

Multiagent testing: There is some evidence that point to increased sensitivity of detection using a combination of genetics with other biomarkers like proteins, RNAs, metabolites. As an example, Cohen and colleagues [92] describe a new blood test called CancerSEEK combining genetic and protein biomarkers across 2001 genomic positions across 61 DNA amplicons and 8 protein levels to detect early cancers and localize the organ of origin [92]. The analysis of this novel test is a custom approach consisting of the following:

i. Calculation of MAFs by using UIDs (see Fig. 4),
ii. Normalization of MAFs across the wells using a normal control set,
iii. Computation of a P value for MAF against reference distributions of normal and cancer plasmas.

Finally, logistic regression using the log ratio of the P values and the protein concentrations that were calculated using vendor-supplied controls and software, Bioplex Manager (Biorad, Hercules CA), is used to calculate CancerSEEK scores.

RNA AND EPIGENETICS-BASED ASSAYS

(RNA) Fusion Detection

The role of RNA in clinical practice has gradually been increasing recently. RNA-based assays are a better alternative to DNA in gene fusion detection, because they do not require large intronic regions to be captured by the assay; however, there are technical limitations related to the quality of RNA. This concern is being addressed by multiplex PCR or probes to capture genes of interest in the RNA. With tests such as Archer RNA multiplex anchored multiplex PCR (AMP™) technology (ArcherDX, Boulder, CO, USA), for fusion detection from RNA, laboratories are getting increasingly interested in RNA-based assays for applications of RNA in the clinic. Data from Archer systems are typically processed using proprietary workflows (http://archerdx.com/software/analysis). RNA-based capture panels can also be used for fusion detection using various software such as STAR-fusion [95].

Gene Expression

Another major focus of cancer research studies has been transcriptomics using RNASeq, but until recently, gene expression signatures were not considered for their clinical applications. As mentioned above, gene expression has also been shown to be predictive of response to immunotherapy [81]. Other applications of RNA-based assays are studying splicing, exon skipping, and allele-specific expression.

microRNAs

Few studies have demonstrated the stability of miRNAs and creation of miRNA panels to potentially detect relapse in breast cancer; however, there has not been much progress to use miRNAs in the clinic as replacement markers for relapse [90].

5-Hydroxymethylcytosine

Recent studies have also identified 5-hydroxymethylcytosine, a chemically stable DNA mark, signatures in plasma cfDNA samples as superior biomarkers for detection of colorectal and gastric cancers from healthy individuals [96]. These signatures are usually calculated similarly to RNASeq signatures using featureCounts [97] for quantification and DESeq2 [98] for comparison between groups, correcting for batch effects and technician bias, after typical read processing of read trimming, quality filters, and alignments [96].

FUTURE CHALLENGES

There has been massive growth in NGS assay development for precision medicine in recent years. However, there are many bioinformatics challenges for clinical laboratories developing these complex tests. There is a lack of standardization with respect to workflows, methods, and even thresholds. Some of these have been discussed in previous sections.

One of the technical challenges is keeping up with the latest updates in the reference genome, which is designed to improve the quality of the results generated. The reference genome is the foundation of all NGS processing, determining the quality of the data and the final results. Currently, most assays and databases used for variant interpretation are based on using the GRCh37 (hg19) version of the human genome. Version GRCh38 (hg38) from December 2013 is an improved assembly with base corrections, introduction of centromere sequences, and better representation of diverse haplotypes. Databases have started to add entries for the new version, through either lift-over or remapping of data [99,100], and it is only a matter of time before bioinformatics pipelines will have adopted the new version of the genome. This update to the new genome version poses a major challenge in updating the knowledgebase, statistics, and mining operations.

As cloud computing and storage costs reduce and cloud-base services become HIPAA compliant, laboratories might be able to run analysis on NGS data without requiring on-site computing resources. Resources such as Basespace (https://basespace.illumina.com) are also available for pipeline development and execution.

Rapid sequencing and large-scale studies are identifying many potential biomarkers in oncology across transcriptomics, proteomics, and more, which might lead to more future integrative testing and novel mechanistic insights in oncology. Many strides have been made to develop new potential tools for early prognosis of cancer or monitoring patients for potential relapse using circulating DNA, including DNA methylation, histone modifications, miRNAs, and proteomics. However, it is critical to note that any such tests must be thoroughly tested prospectively across a large cohort, and bioinformatics methods must be trained for high specificity to avoid any errors in classification or risk stratification.

DISCUSSION

Clinical NGS bioinformatics has truly come into its own as an important component of the diagnosis and routine management of patients with cancer. Although hybrid-capture NGS technology has largely remained unchanged over the past 5 years, it is advancements in bioinformatics that have truly moved forward the testing capabilities in personalized oncology diagnostics. Computational methods have made this possible by driving the discovery of novel genetic markers and providing ways to perform simultaneous assessment of many complex biomarkers of various scales and sizes in a single assay. Today, NGS oncology tests are being used to make many standard treatment decisions for patients as well as match them to desirable clinical trials. Increasingly, these tests are also needed for rendering the correct primary diagnosis, as multiple disease entities are now classified based in part on molecular features according to the World Health Organization system. In this review, the author summarized the bioinformatics methods used by commonly reported somatic clinical assays, along with considerations for building a state-of-the-art modular pipeline designed to simultaneously detect alterations of different scales, including complex genomic signature biomarkers, such as MSI, TMB, and HRD.

There is an undeniable trend in the field toward biomarkers of increasing complexity, which presents an array of exciting challenges. Emerging biomarkers, such as ctDNA and other MRD assays, as well as a wealth of potential signals present within epigenetic and transcriptomic data are certain to ensure many years of continual growth in applications and capabilities. However, because of the increasing complexity of desired bioinformatics analyses and the growing importance of clinical NGS results to patient care, it is more important than ever that laboratories strive to develop pipelines with the highest possible performance standards and validate them as stringently as possible. Pathologists, clinicians, and patients need to be able to trust the assays they depend on to reliably detect this expanding range of genetic anomalies, and with applications expanding, it is only through intensive refinement and validation that this trust can be achieved. Likewise, it would be desirable for more laboratories to openly share with each other their pipelines and test datasets in the interest of developing best practices and minimizing errors. In this way, advancements in both capabilities and quality may be efficiently achieved across many institutions, such that the greatest number of patients can benefit from the continued advancement of this field.

REFERENCES

[1] Aziz N, Zhao Q, Bry L, et al. College of American Pathologists' laboratory standards for next-generation

sequencing clinical tests. Arch Pathol Lab Med 2015; 139(4):481–93.

[2] Roy S, Coldren C, Karunamurthy A, et al. Standards and guidelines for validating next-generation sequencing bioinformatics pipelines: a joint recommendation of the Association for Molecular Pathology and the College of American Pathologists. J Mol Diagn 2018; 20(1):4–27.

[3] Vogelstein B, Papadopoulos N, Velculescu VE, et al. Cancer genome landscapes. Science 2013;339(6127): 1546–58.

[4] Beadling C, Neff TL, Heinrich MC, et al. Combining highly multiplexed PCR with semiconductor-based sequencing for rapid cancer genotyping. J Mol Diagn 2013;15(2):171–6.

[5] Tsongalis GJ, Peterson JD, De A, et al. Routine use of the Ion Torrent AmpliSeq™ Cancer Hotspot Panel for identification of clinically actionable somatic mutations. Clin Chem Lab Med 2014;52(5):707–14.

[6] Singh RR, Patel KP, Routbort MJ, et al. Clinical validation of a next-generation sequencing screen for mutational hotspots in 46 cancer-related genes. J Mol Diagn 2013;15(5):607–22.

[7] Kadri S, Zhen CJ, Wurst MN, et al. Amplicon indel hunter is a novel bioinformatics tool to detect large somatic insertion/deletion mutations in amplicon-based next-generation sequencing data. J Mol Diagn 2015; 17(6):635–43.

[8] Hovelson DH, McDaniel AS, Cani AK, et al. Development and validation of a scalable next-generation sequencing system for assessing relevant somatic variants in solid tumors. Neoplasia 2015;17(4): 385–99.

[9] Davies KD, Farooqi MS, Gruidl M, et al. Multi-institutional FASTQ file exchange as a means of proficiency testing for next-generation sequencing bioinformatics and variant interpretation. J Mol Diagn 2016;18(4): 572–9.

[10] Au CH, Leung AYH, Kwong A, et al. INDELseek: detection of complex insertions and deletions from next-generation sequencing data. BMC Genomics 2017; 18(1):16.

[11] Yang R, Nelson AC, Henzler C, et al. ScanIndel: a hybrid framework for indel detection via gapped alignment, split reads and de novo assembly. Genome Med 2015;7:127.

[12] Au CH, Wa A, Ho DN, et al. Clinical evaluation of panel testing by next-generation sequencing (NGS) for gene mutations in myeloid neoplasms. Diagn Pathol 2016; 11:11.

[13] Daber R, Sukhadia S, Morrissette JJ. Understanding the limitations of next generation sequencing informatics, an approach to clinical pipeline validation using artificial data sets. Cancer Genet 2013;206(12):441–8.

[14] Albers CA, Lunter G, MacArthur DG, et al. Dindel: accurate indel calls from short-read data. Genome Res 2011; 21(6):961–73.

[15] Indelocator | www.broadinstitute.org/cancer/CGA. Available at: http://archive.broadinstitute.org/cancer/cga/indelocator. Accessed April 2, 2018.

[16] Cheng DT, Mitchell TN, Zehir A, et al. Memorial sloan kettering-integrated mutation profiling of actionable cancer targets (MSK-IMPACT): a hybridization capture-based next-generation sequencing clinical assay for solid tumor molecular oncology. J Mol Diagn 2015; 17(3):251–64.

[17] Garcia EP, Minkovsky A, Jia Y, et al. Validation of OncoPanel: a targeted next-generation sequencing assay for the detection of somatic variants in cancer. Arch Pathol Lab Med 2017;141(6):751–8.

[18] Frampton GM, Fichtenholtz A, Otto GA, et al. Development and validation of a clinical cancer genomic profiling test based on massively parallel DNA sequencing. Nat Biotechnol 2013;31(11):1023–31.

[19] Kadri S, Long BC, Mujacic I, et al. Clinical validation of a next-generation sequencing genomic oncology panel via cross-platform benchmarking against established amplicon sequencing assays. J Mol Diagn 2017;19(1):43–56.

[20] Martin M. Cutadapt removes adapter sequences from high-throughput sequencing reads. EMBnet.journal 2011;17(1):10–2.

[21] Li H. Aligning sequence reads, clone sequences and assembly contigs with BWA-MEM. ArXiv Prepr ArXiv13033997; 2013. p. 589–95.

[22] McKenna A, Hanna M, Banks E, et al. The genome analysis toolkit: a MapReduce framework for analyzing next-generation DNA sequencing data. Genome Res 2010;20(9):1297–303.

[23] Cibulskis K, Lawrence MS, Carter SL, et al. Sensitive detection of somatic point mutations in impure and heterogeneous cancer samples. Nat Biotechnol 2013; 31(3):213–9.

[24] Wang K, Li M, Hakonarson H. ANNOVAR: functional annotation of genetic variants from high-throughput sequencing data. Nucleic Acids Res 2010;38(16):e164.

[25] Rausch T, Zichner T, Schlattl A, et al. DELLY: structural variant discovery by integrated paired-end and split-read analysis. Bioinformatics 2012;28(18):i333–9.

[26] Pugh TJ, Amr SS, Bowser MJ, et al. VisCap: inference and visualization of germ-line copy-number variants from targeted clinical sequencing data. Genet Med 2016;18(7):712–9.

[27] Abo RP, Ducar M, Garcia EP, et al. BreaKmer: detection of structural variation in targeted massively parallel sequencing data using kmers. Nucleic Acids Res 2015; 43(3):e19.

[28] Bolger AM, Lohse M, Usadel B. Trimmomatic: a flexible trimmer for Illumina sequence data. Bioinformatics 2014;30(15):2114–20.

[29] Pritchard CC, Salipante SJ, Koehler K, et al. Validation and implementation of targeted capture and sequencing for the detection of actionable mutation, copy number variation, and gene rearrangement in clinical cancer specimens. J Mol Diagn 2014;16(1):56–67.

[30] Koboldt DC, Zhang Q, Larson DE, et al. VarScan 2: somatic mutation and copy number alteration discovery in cancer by exome sequencing. Genome Res 2012; 22(3):568–76.

[31] Thankaswamy-Kosalai S, Sen P, Nookaew I. Evaluation and assessment of read-mapping by multiple next-generation sequencing aligners based on genome-wide characteristics. Genomics 2017;109(3–4):186–91.

[32] Mose LE, Wilkerson MD, Hayes DN, et al. ABRA: improved coding indel detection via assembly-based realignment. Bioinformatics 2014;30(19):2813–5.

[33] Ye K, Schulz MH, Long Q, et al. Pindel: a pattern growth approach to detect break points of large deletions and medium sized insertions from paired-end short reads. Bioinformatics 2009;25(21):2865–71.

[34] Smith CC, Wang Q, Chin C-S, et al. Validation of ITD mutations in FLT3 as a therapeutic target in human acute myeloid leukaemia. Nature 2012;485(7397): 260–3.

[35] Saunders CT, Wong WSW, Swamy S, et al. Strelka: accurate somatic small-variant calling from sequenced tumor-normal sample pairs. Bioinformatics 2012; 28(14):1811–7.

[36] Strelka2: Fast and accurate variant calling for clinical sequencing applications | bioRxiv. Available at: https://www.biorxiv.org/content/early/2017/09/25/192872. Accessed April 2, 2018.

[37] Larson DE, Harris CC, Chen K, et al. SomaticSniper: identification of somatic point mutations in whole genome sequencing data. Bioinformatics 2012;28(3): 311–7.

[38] Rimmer A, Phan H, Mathieson I, et al. Integrating mapping-, assembly- and haplotype-based approaches for calling variants in clinical sequencing applications. Nat Genet 2014;46(8):912–8.

[39] Garrison E, Marth G. Haplotype-based variant detection from short-read sequencing. ArXiv12073907 Q-Bio. 2012. Available at: http://arxiv.org/abs/1207.3907. Accessed April 2, 2018.

[40] Wilm A, Aw PPK, Bertrand D, et al. LoFreq: a sequence-quality aware, ultra-sensitive variant caller for uncovering cell-population heterogeneity from high-throughput sequencing datasets. Nucleic Acids Res 2012;40(22):11189–201.

[41] den Dunnen JT, Dalgleish R, Maglott DR, et al. HGVS recommendations for the description of sequence variants: 2016 update. Hum Mutat 2016; 37(6):564–9.

[42] Thorvaldsdóttir H, Robinson JT, Mesirov JP. Integrative Genomics Viewer (IGV): high-performance genomics data visualization and exploration. Brief Bioinform 2013;14(2):178–92.

[43] Li MM, Datto M, Duncavage EJ, et al. Standards and guidelines for the interpretation and reporting of sequence variants in cancer: a joint consensus recommendation of the association for molecular pathology, American Society of Clinical Oncology, and College of American Pathologists. J Mol Diagn 2017;19(1):4–23.

[44] Sharma MK, Phillips J, Agarwal S, et al. Clinical genomicist workstation. AMIA Jt Summits Transl Sci Proc 2013;2013:156–7.

[45] Roy S, Durso MB, Wald A, et al. SeqReporter: automating next-generation sequencing result interpretation and reporting workflow in a clinical laboratory. J Mol Diagn 2014;16(1):11–22.

[46] Kang W, Kadri S, Puranik R, et al. System for Informatics in the Molecular Pathology Laboratory (SIMPL): an open-source end-to-end solution for next-generation sequencing clinical data management. J Mol Diagn 2018. https://doi.org/10.1016/j.jmoldx.2018.03.008.

[47] 1000 Genomes Project Consortium, Auton A, Brooks LD, Durbin RM, et al. A global reference for human genetic variation. Nature 2015;526(7571):68–74.

[48] Sherry ST, Ward MH, Kholodov M, et al. dbSNP: the NCBI database of genetic variation. Nucleic Acids Res 2001;29(1):308–11.

[49] Forbes SA, Beare D, Gunasekaran P, et al. COSMIC: exploring the world's knowledge of somatic mutations in human cancer. Nucleic Acids Res 2015;43(Database issue):D805–11.

[50] Gao J, Aksoy BA, Dogrusoz U, et al. Integrative analysis of complex cancer genomics and clinical profiles using the cBioPortal. Sci Signal 2013;6(269):pl1.

[51] Landrum MJ, Lee JM, Riley GR, et al. ClinVar: public archive of relationships among sequence variation and human phenotype. Nucleic Acids Res 2014; 42(Database issue):D980–5.

[52] Stenson PD, Ball EV, Mort M, et al. The Human Gene Mutation Database (HGMD) and its exploitation in the fields of personalized genomics and molecular evolution. Curr Protoc Bioinformatics 2012;Chapter 1: Unit1.13.

[53] Beroukhim R, Mermel CH, Porter D, et al. The landscape of somatic copy-number alteration across human cancers. Nature 2010;463(7283):899–905.

[54] Zare F, Dow M, Monteleone N, et al. An evaluation of copy number variation detection tools for cancer using whole exome sequencing data. BMC Bioinformatics 2017;18(1):286.

[55] Shen W, Paxton CN, Szankasi P, et al. Detection of genome-wide copy number variants in myeloid malignancies using next-generation sequencing. J Clin Pathol 2018;71(4):372–8.

[56] Olshen AB, Venkatraman ES, Lucito R, et al. Circular binary segmentation for the analysis of array-based DNA copy number data. Biostatistics 2004;5(4): 557–72.

[57] Talevich E, Shain AH, Botton T, et al. CNVkit: genome-wide copy number detection and visualization from targeted DNA sequencing. PLoS Comput Biol 2016;12(4): e1004873.

[58] CONTRA: copy number analysis for targeted resequencing. Available at: https://www.ncbi.nlm.nih.

gov/pmc/articles/PMC3348560/. Accessed April 2, 2018.
[59] Sathirapongsasuti JF, Lee H, Horst BAJ, et al. Exome sequencing-based copy-number variation and loss of heterozygosity detection: ExomeCNV. Bioinformatics 2011;27(19):2648–54.
[60] Abel HJ, Al-Kateb H, Cottrell CE, et al. Detection of gene rearrangements in targeted clinical next-generation sequencing. J Mol Diagn 2014;16(4): 405–17.
[61] Chen K, Wallis JW, McLellan MD, et al. Break-Dancer: an algorithm for high-resolution mapping of genomic structural variation. Nat Methods 2009; 6(9):677–81.
[62] Layer RM, Chiang C, Quinlan AR, et al. LUMPY: a probabilistic framework for structural variant discovery. Genome Biol 2014;15(6):R84.
[63] Wang J, Mullighan CG, Easton J, et al. CREST maps somatic structural variation in cancer genomes with base-pair resolution. Nat Methods 2011;8(8):652–4.
[64] Rosenberg JE, Hoffman-Censits J, Powles T, et al. Atezolizumab in patients with locally advanced and metastatic urothelial carcinoma who have progressed following treatment with platinum-based chemotherapy: a single-arm, multicentre, phase 2 trial. Lancet 2016; 387(10031):1909–20.
[65] Carbone DP, Reck M, Paz-Ares L, et al. First-line nivolumab in stage iv or recurrent non-small-cell lung cancer. N Engl J Med 2017;376(25):2415–26.
[66] Le DT, Uram JN, Wang H, et al. PD-1 blockade in tumors with mismatch-repair deficiency. N Engl J Med 2015;372(26):2509–20.
[67] Le DT, Durham JN, Smith KN, et al. Mismatch repair deficiency predicts response of solid tumors to PD-1 blockade. Science 2017;357(6349):409–13.
[68] Snyder A, Makarov V, Merghoub T, et al. Genetic basis for clinical response to CTLA-4 blockade in melanoma. N Engl J Med 2014;371(23):2189–99.
[69] Rizvi NA, Hellmann MD, Snyder A, et al. Cancer immunology. Mutational landscape determines sensitivity to PD-1 blockade in non-small cell lung cancer. Science 2015;348(6230):124–8.
[70] Rizvi H, Sanchez-Vega F, La K, et al. Molecular determinants of response to anti-programmed cell death (PD)-1 and anti-programmed death-ligand 1 (PD-L1) blockade in patients with non-small-cell lung cancer profiled with targeted next-generation sequencing. J Clin Oncol 2018;36(7):633–41.
[71] Niu B, Ye K, Zhang Q, et al. MSIsensor: microsatellite instability detection using paired tumor-normal sequence data. Bioinformatics 2014;30(7):1015–6.
[72] Salipante SJ, Scroggins SM, Hampel HL, et al. Microsatellite instability detection by next generation sequencing. Clin Chem 2014;60(9):1192–9.
[73] Chalmers ZR, Huang FW, Gay LM, et al. Analysis of tumor mutation burden (TMB) in >51,000 clinical cancer patients to identify novel non-coding PMS2 promoter mutations associated with increased TMB. J Clin Oncol 2016;34(15_suppl):9572.
[74] Kautto EA, Bonneville R, Miya J, et al. Performance evaluation for rapid detection of pan-cancer microsatellite instability with MANTIS. Oncotarget 2016;8(5): 7452–63.
[75] Zhu L, Huang Y, Fang X, et al. A novel and reliable method to detect microsatellite instability in colorectal cancer by next-generation sequencing. J Mol Diagn 2018;20(2):225–31.
[76] Goodman AM, Kato S, Bazhenova L, et al. Tumor mutational burden as an independent predictor of response to immunotherapy in diverse cancers. Mol Cancer Ther 2017;16(11):2598–608.
[77] Campesato LF, Barroso-Sousa R, Jimenez L, et al. Comprehensive cancer-gene panels can be used to estimate mutational load and predict clinical benefit to PD-1 blockade in clinical practice. Oncotarget 2015; 6(33):34221–7.
[78] Garofalo A, Sholl L, Reardon B, et al. The impact of tumor profiling approaches and genomic data strategies for cancer precision medicine. Genome Med 2016; 8(1):79.
[79] Zehir A, Benayed R, Shah RH, et al. Mutational landscape of metastatic cancer revealed from prospective clinical sequencing of 10,000 patients. Nat Med 2017; 23(6):703–13.
[80] Davoli T, Uno H, Wooten EC, et al. Tumor aneuploidy correlates with markers of immune evasion and with reduced response to immunotherapy. Science 2017; 355(6322) [pii:eaaf8399].
[81] Jamieson NB, Maker AV. Gene-expression profiling to predict responsiveness to immunotherapy. Cancer Gene Ther 2017;24(3):134–40.
[82] Telli ML, Timms KM, Reid J, et al. Homologous Recombination Deficiency (HRD) score predicts response to platinum-containing neoadjuvant chemotherapy in patients with triple-negative breast cancer. Clin Cancer Res 2016;22(15):3764–73.
[83] Maxwell KN, Wubbenhorst B, Wenz BM, et al. BRCA locus-specific loss of heterozygosity in germline BRCA1 and BRCA2 carriers. Nat Commun 2017;8(1): 319.
[84] Favero F, Joshi T, Marquard AM, et al. Sequenza: allele-specific copy number and mutation profiles from tumor sequencing data. Ann Oncol 2015; 26(1):64–70.
[85] Abkevich V, Timms KM, Hennessy BT, et al. Patterns of genomic loss of heterozygosity predict homologous recombination repair defects in epithelial ovarian cancer. Br J Cancer 2012;107(10):1776–82.
[86] Bardelli A, Pantel K. Liquid biopsies, what we do not know (Yet). Cancer Cell 2017;31(2):172–9.
[87] Li X, Zhou C. Comparison of cross-platform technologies for EGFR T790M testing in patients with non-small cell lung cancer. Oncotarget 2017;8(59): 100801–18.

[88] Leary RJ, Sausen M, Kinde I, et al. Detection of chromosomal alterations in the circulation of cancer patients with whole-genome sequencing. Sci Transl Med 2012; 4(162):162ra154.

[89] Dawson S-J, Tsui DWY, Murtaza M, et al. Analysis of circulating tumor DNA to monitor metastatic breast cancer. N Engl J Med 2013;368(13):1199–209.

[90] Beddowes E, Sammut SJ, Gao M, et al. Predicting treatment resistance and relapse through circulating DNA. Breast 2017;34(Suppl 1):S31–5.

[91] Phallen J, Sausen M, Adleff V, et al. Direct detection of early-stage cancers using circulating tumor DNA. Sci Transl Med 2017;9(403) [pii:eaan2415].

[92] Cohen JD, Li L, Wang Y, et al. Detection and localization of surgically resectable cancers with a multi-analyte blood test. Science 2018;359(6378):926–30.

[93] Kinde I, Wu J, Papadopoulos N, et al. Detection and quantification of rare mutations with massively parallel sequencing. Proc Natl Acad Sci U S A 2011;108(23): 9530–5.

[94] Gandara DR, Kowanetz M, Mok TSK, et al. Blood-based biomarkers for cancer immunotherapy: Tumor mutational burden in blood (bTMB) is associated with improved atezolizumab (atezo) efficacy in 2L+ NSCLC (POPLAR and OAK). Ann Oncol 2017;28(suppl_5).

[95] STAR-fusion: fast and accurate fusion transcript detection from RNA-Seq | bioRxiv. Available at: https://www.biorxiv.org/content/early/2017/03/24/120295. Accessed April 1, 2018.

[96] Li W, Zhang X, Lu X, et al. 5-Hydroxymethylcytosine signatures in circulating cell-free DNA as diagnostic biomarkers for human cancers. Cell Res 2017;27(10): 1243–57.

[97] Liao Y, Smyth GK, Shi W. featureCounts: an efficient general purpose program for assigning sequence reads to genomic features. Bioinformatics 2014;30(7): 923–30.

[98] Love MI, Huber W, Anders S. Moderated estimation of fold change and dispersion for RNA-seq data with DESeq2. Genome Biol 2014;15(12):550.

[99] Zhang X, Minikel EV, O'Donnell-Luria AH, et al. ClinVar data parsing. Wellcome Open Res 2017;2:33.

[100] Zheng-Bradley X, Streeter I, Fairley S, et al. Alignment of 1000 genomes project reads to reference assembly GRCh38. Gigascience 2017;6(7):1–8.

Solid Tumors

Advances in Molecular Pathology 1 (2018) 167–182
ADVANCES IN MOLECULAR PATHOLOGY

Clinical Next-Generation Sequencing Assays for Solid Tumors

Current Practices, Technological Advances, and Challenges in Clinical Practice

Susan J. Hsiao, MD, PhD[a], Dara L. Aisner, MD, PhD[b], Mark D. Ewalt, MD[c,*]

[a]Department of Pathology and Cell Biology, Columbia University Medical Center, 630 West 168th Street, PS17-414, New York, NY 10032, USA; [b]Department of Pathology, Colorado Molecular Correlates Laboratory, 12705 East Montview Boulevard, Suite 400, Aurora, CO 80045, USA; [c]Department of Pathology, University of Colorado, 12705 East Montview Boulevard, Suite 400, Aurora, CO 80045, USA

KEYWORDS

• Oncology • Next-generation sequencing • Cancer • Biomarkers • Variant interpretation

KEY POINTS

- Next-generation sequencing technologies are varied and offer possibilities for detection across multiple classes of alterations in solid tumors.
- Preanalytic factors can greatly impact success rate of testing, particularly for formalin-fixed, paraffin-embedded tissue.
- Tumor enrichment is a critical component of preanalytical sample processing to ensure confidence in next-generation sequencing–based testing.
- Interpretation of next-generation sequencing data involves technical review as well as clinical analysis to appropriately classify variants and guide clinical decisions.

INTRODUCTION

As our understanding of the pathobiology of cancer has evolved over time, we have come to understand it as a disease of the genome. Different cancer types show specific patterns of genomic alterations and identification of these alterations can be used to assist in diagnosis, monitor disease progression, and offer therapies aimed at the individual targets, enabling a personalized genomic approach to cancer. Given the diversity of alterations within each cancer type, technologies have evolved to test multiple genetic targets simultaneously. Next-generation sequencing (NGS), which is the focus of this article, has emerged as one of the leading technologies to allow this broad testing in a streamlined approach.

NEXT-GENERATION SEQUENCING TECHNOLOGIES

The term NGS has been used to describe many different technologies that allow for simultaneously sequencing numerous targets, compared with Sanger sequencing,

Disclosure Statement: Dr S.J. Hsiao has the following disclosure: Honoraria from Roche, Ventana. Dr D.L. Aisner has the following disclosures: Honoraria from Bristol-Meyers Squibb, Genentech, and AbbVie, and research support from Genentech. Dr M.D. Ewalt has no disclosures.

*Corresponding author, *E-mail address:* mark.ewalt@ucdenver.edu

https://doi.org/10.1016/j.yamp.2018.07.008
2589-4080/18/

which evaluates a single region. Although the available technologies differ in specific chemistry, performance characteristics, and cost, they share the following steps to enable large-scale sequencing: (1) library preparation, (2) physical separation of fragments, (3) signal amplification, (4) massively parallel sequencing, and (5) bioinformatics processing to resolve data. The specifics of individual sequencing platforms are beyond the scope of this article and can be found in other sources [1–3].

Library preparation refers to enrichment of a sample for the regions of interest and is defined during assay design. It is typically accomplished either by polymerase chain reaction (PCR) amplification of the region of interest (amplicon-based preparation) or by fragmentation of the nucleic acid sample and capture using complimentary probes (capture-based preparation). For RNA-based assays, reverse-transcription is performed to generate complementary DNA for downstream library preparation. The prepared library is composed of a population of DNA molecules corresponding to the regions of interest in the initial sample to which platform-specific adapters are added to the ends of each molecule for subsequent sequencing reactions.

After library preparation, the DNA molecules are physically separated from one another by hybridizing each molecule to a support, typically either a solid support (Illumina sequencing) or a bead (IonTorrent sequencing) through the adapter sequences. These individual DNA molecules are locally amplified to generate a clonal DNA population and allow resolution of a sequencing-by-synthesis signal. The exact chemistry underlying sequencing-by-synthesis depends on the platform used and is comprehensively reviewed elsewhere [2]. At the conclusion of sequencing, extensive bioinformatics processing is performed to resolve the data into an interpretable format, which is discussed briefly in this article and more extensively in Sabah Kadri's article, "Advances in Next Generation Sequencing Bioinformatics for Clinical Diagnostics: Taking Precision Oncology to the Next Level," elsewhere in this issue.

Just as there are different core technologies underlying DNA sequencing in NGS, there are a myriad of options for assays in solid tumor oncology testing. A large number of vendors make kits including single tumor type panels, pan-cancer panels, and others. In addition, many laboratories design and develop their own custom assays based on the clinical needs at their institution. The principle consideration in assay selection or design is identification of the target alterations for the assay. Other considerations that are discussed elsewhere in this article include the type, quantity, and quality of nucleic acid available and assay performance characteristics.

The most important consideration in assay design is the target alterations which the assay must detect. For assays that are focused on the detection of single nucleotide variants and small insertions and deletions (indels), assays using genomic DNA as an input are excellent. For assays focused on the detection of abnormal RNA products such as abnormal splicing (ie, *MET* exon 14 skipping) or gene fusions (ie, *EML4-ALK* fusion), RNA-based assays may be preferred because they do not require sequencing across the large intronic regions, where most of the variants occur.

Compounding these considerations is the challenge of available nucleic acid in clinical samples. The majority of clinical NGS testing for solid tumors is now performed on nucleic acids extracted from formalin-fixed paraffin-embedded tissue (FFPET). As discussed in the Preanalytics section, this may pose a challenge with regard to quality and availability of nucleic acid from these samples.

The final components of assay specification relate to the specific assay performance characteristics, including sensitivity, specificity, accuracy, limit of detection, and throughput. Regardless of the platform, every NGS assay has an upper limit of total sequencing data per run. This set amount of sequencing data must be split among the number of clinical samples and controls in each run and further split among all of the genomic regions that are sequenced. By carefully considering the depth required to achieve the desired sensitivity of the assay, an ideal number of samples can be determined per sequencing run. The number of a times a specific base position is interrogated is called the depth at that position. Regions with high depth are able to detect variants at a lower limit of detection with confidence. In addition, the use of specialized techniques such as molecular barcodes and optimized bioinformatics can further improve limit of detection and sensitivity. Specificity is often limited by assay artifacts; however, many of these artifacts can be identified during a careful validation study.

Several pitfalls are unavoidable in NGS. These include overestimation due to PCR artifacts, deamination artifacts, high sequencing artifact rates (particularly in regions of repetitive sequence), and barcode misassignment. The majority of approaches to managing these pitfalls center on use of sophisticated bioinformatic analysis to include deduplication and error correction through unique molecular indices (molecular barcodes), evaluation of read strand bias, and tracking of sample barcodes relative to instrument use and findings [4–7]. Artifacts related to a repetitive sequence can be identified by visual examination of the sequence, combined with ongoing assay tracking to identify those that are recurrent.

Although current NGS technologies offer great diversity in testing options, newer technologies are always in development. Some intriguing emerging technologies include single molecule and long read sequencing approaches. Although these technologies have not made it into routine clinical use, both offer potential benefits in cancer testing, namely in evaluating subclonal compositions and improved ability to detect larger genomic events than can be resolved by existing approaches. Specifically, single molecule sequencing has demonstrated the ability to understand subclonal processes and evolution, and may be applicable to clinical care in predicting therapeutic responsiveness [8]. Long-read sequencing technologies may also find clinical application in the improved ability to identify structural alterations; however, the limitations of archival tissue (eg, highly fragmented nucleic acids) may preclude widespread adoption. NGS technology is also being rapidly applied to the emerging area of circulating cell-free nucleic acid evaluation (see Siddhartha Sen and colleagues' article, "Emerging Concepts in Liquid Biopsy," in this issue). Regardless of the technology used, all clinical testing relies on appropriate preanalytics lest the adage "garbage in, garbage out" become a challenge for patient testing.

PREANALYTICAL SPECIMEN HANDLING AND EVALUATION

Molecular testing of solid tumors is complicated by the nature of the tested sample, most commonly FFPET; routine tissue processing damages nucleic acids, creating challenges for molecular assays, and makes consideration of the preanalytical sample processing critical. Numerous preanalytic variables can potentially impact the quality of subsequent molecular testing; however, the degree of impact has been variably quantified. A selection of major preanalytic considerations and their impact are noted here and more comprehensively reviewed elsewhere [9,10].

Warm and Cold Ischemic Times

There is a growing recognition that intraoperative and postoperative ischemic times have the potential to impact the quality and quantity of nucleic acids. For DNA-based NGS assays, warm and cold ischemic time are likely less impactful than subsequent FFPET processing. However, for studies involving RNA, both warm and cold ischemic time may significantly impact RNA quality and quantity [11]. Although this phenomenon is well-recognized, there are no widespread guidelines for prescribing or monitoring warm and cold ischemic times, with some exceptions, particularly in breast carcinoma [12].

Fixative

Standard histopathology practice is fixation of tissues in 10% neutral buffered formalin, which introduces extensive cross-linkages within tissue. Procedures to eliminate these cross-linkages (most commonly heat and proteinase K) result in a high degree of susceptibility to nucleic acid fragmentation [13]. Of critical note, alternative fixatives, such as Zenker's, Bouin's, B-5, and others, are essentially incompatible with downstream nucleic acid based studies; thus, careful consideration should be given to tissue fixative selection [14].

Fixation and Processing Conditions

A chief consideration in fixing tissues with molecular testing in mind is the duration of fixation, because nucleic acid quality decreases with longer fixation. With the exception of recommendations for breast carcinoma, there are few widely accepted standards for this variable. Although general recommendations have suggested that DNA-based studies can be performed on specimens fixed for up to 72 hours in neutral buffered formalin [9], these authors find that, when possible, exposure to neutral buffered formalin for longer than 48 hours should be avoided and best results are seen when specimens are fixed for less than 24 hours, particularly small samples.

Decalcification

A common dilemma in the testing of solid tumor specimens is the impact of decalcification treatment on nucleic acid, because bony metastases are commonly sampled. Traditionally, decalcification has been achieved with harsh acid fixatives, which render samples unsuitable for subsequent molecular studies. Recent studies have demonstrated that decalcification using EDTA is a suitable alternative to acid decalcification and preserves the ability to perform molecular studies [9]. In addition, in many cases of bony metastases, decalcification solutions may be completely avoided [15].

Maximizing Tissue

Another major challenge in solid tumor testing is performing analysis on small samples obtained through minimally invasive approaches such as core needle biopsy and fine needle aspiration. Although challenging, there are numerous potential solutions to preserve tissue and the ability to perform comprehensive molecular testing. These approaches are often more time consuming than standard histopathology procedures, but are increasingly important when a patient undergoes a tissue acquisition procedure for the sole purpose of molecular testing, as well as maximizing the opportunity for molecular testing in initial diagnostic samples. Several techniques to decrease tissue depletion include separate embedding of separate fragments of tissue, superficial facing of blocks (Fig. 1), and avoidance of immunohistochemistry (which may require a disclaimer) [15]. Another key element of maximizing tissue for molecular testing is the clear need for systems-based solutions to properly identify the cases in which such specialized handling is necessary. This typically requires a multidisciplinary approach and efficient systems that minimize one-at-a-time communications are preferred.

Another approach to maximizing opportunities for molecular testing involves use of non-FFPET materials, such as cytopathology materials (reviewed elsewhere in this article) and circulating cell-free tumor DNA (see Siddhartha Sen and colleagues' article, "Emerging Concepts in Liquid Biopsy," elsewhere in this issue).

Non–formalin-Fixed Paraffin-Embedded Specimens

Given the likely long-term persistence of FFPET as a standard in pathology and the increasing use of molecular testing, there has been substantial effort to identify alternate approaches to specimen acquisition, fixation, and storage to preserve high-quality nucleic acid(s). A highly attractive approach is the use of cytopathology preparations (such as touch preps, smears, and liquid-based cytology specimens) with molecular testing. Cytopathology specimens are often processed with nonformalin fixatives and result in higher quality nucleic acids. Numerous approaches to the use of cytopathology specimens have been described, including scraping or microdissecting stained slides, or using a liquid-based preparation with visualization of a small proportion to ensure adequate tumor cellularity [16].

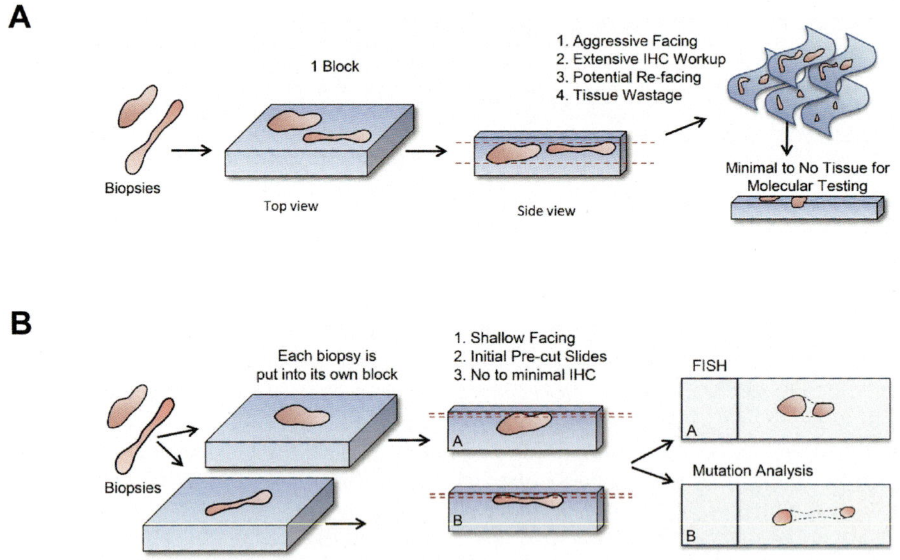

FIG. 1 Maximization approach for small biopsies. (**A**) Common pathology practice, in which multiple tissue fragments such as biopsies are embedded in a single paraffin block. When the tissue is faced to achieve a representative cross-section of all tissue, a significant amount of the specimen is discarded. (**B**) An approach that can be used to maximize tissue for molecular studies, in which each tissue fragment is separately embedded and sectioned only superficially. Such superficial facing may result in incomplete visualization of the tissue (*dotted line*); however, because the purpose in this context is to confirm the presence of tumor, this superficial facing is often sufficient and results in reduced tissue wastage. FISH, fluorescence in situ hybridization; IHC, immunohistochemistry. (*Courtesy of* Regents of the University of Colorado, Aurora, CO; with permission. Copyright 2016.)

These approaches have shown excellent success, particularly owing to generally excellent nucleic acid.

Specimen Assessment

A crucial component of testing in solid tumors is the assessment of tissue adequacy for the desired testing. This process entails a review to confirm that the tumor present in the specimen meets the analytical sensitivity requirements of the assay, potentially after tumor enrichment strategies are used. Pathologist assessment of tumor cellularity is known to be imprecise [17]; therefore, it is recommended that pathologists be conservative in their estimates to account for potentially inaccurate assessment. Additionally, specimens with low tumor cellularity may fail to detect certain clinically relevant alteration types, such as copy number alterations or subclonal mutations. There is ongoing debate as to whether primary lesions or metastases should be preferentially tested and some data suggest that this decision may be tumor-type specific, with additional information about prior lines of therapy needed to inform such decision making. For example, in colorectal carcinoma, primary and metastatic lesions are highly concordant with regard to driver alterations [18]; however, in non–small cell lung carcinoma, the use of a specimen after progression on targeted therapy may provide different results compared with a pretreatment specimen [8]. Tumor heterogeneity can potentially also impact findings; however, all current data suggest that primary driver mutations are truncal and should not be subject to significant variation based on regions of tumor selected for analysis [19].

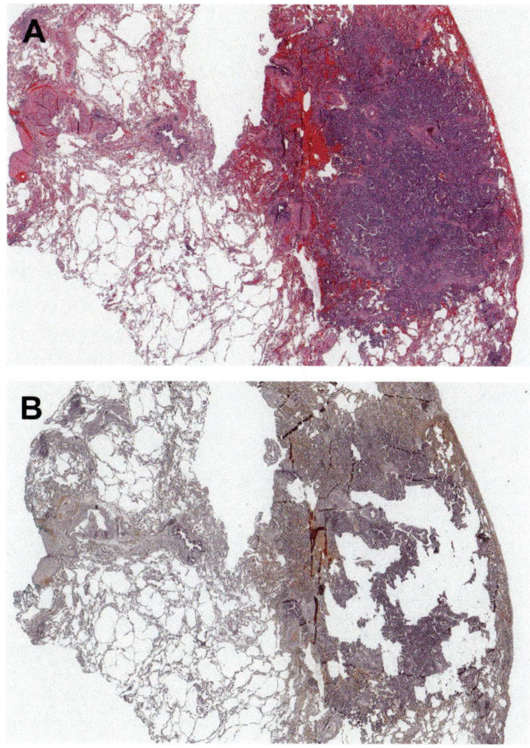

FIG. 2 Paired images demonstrating tumor enrichment when performed by microdissection. (**A**) Hematoxylin and eosin–stained slide with a region of pulmonary adenocarcinoma (original magnification x 2). (**B**) Slide stained with hematoxylin to facilitate microdissection, demonstrates selective removal of dense regions of tumor, minimizing the retrieval of surrounding nontumor tissue (original magnification x 2).

Tumor Enrichment

The majority of archival pathology specimens must undergo tumor enrichment to be suitable for molecular testing. Several common methods of tumor enrichment for FFPE materials include (1) boring, coring or gouging material directly from a paraffin block, (2) macrodissection of unstained slides using a razor or scalpel, and (3) microdissection, in which a microdissecting microscope is used in conjunction with fine tools, such as a needle or scalpel tip (Fig. 2, Table 1) [13]. These approaches involve the use of a hematoxylin and eosin–stained slide to direct efforts and may also involve a counterstain when performing dissection from slides to observe histologic features. Laser capture microdissection has been shown to be a technically acceptable approach [20]; however, the cost, timeframe of use, and labor-intensive features of laser capture microdissection have generally precluded widespread adoption. Newer technologies, some with automation, have been developed to decrease the manual burden of microdissection, including Roche Millisect and NeuroInDx Unipick+ [21,22].

Nucleic Acid Extraction and Evaluation

Numerous methodologies have been shown to be effective for the extraction of nucleic acids from FFPET specimens [23]. In general, the necessary steps include deparaffinization, cell lysis, protein digestion, reversal of FFPET induced cross-links, and isolation of nucleic acids from lysate. Although numerous automated solutions for extraction exist, scant samples may require manual processing, because automated instruments may have lower yields than manual methods. Some assays use RNA as input material for NGS testing and additional considerations, particularly care to prevent RNase contamination, are crucial. RNA quality and quantity decreases rapidly, even in FFPET format; therefore, the ability to use RNA-based assays may be more limited in older specimens. Once extracted, nucleic acids can be quantified through a variety of means with fluorometric measurement being recommended over spectrophotometric measurement because it is more accurate.

Owing to the complexity of library preparation, NGS may require a nuanced approach to determining assay input. In addition to a quantitative measurement, most NGS assays using FFPET are best performed if a qualitative measurement is included and used to modulate sample input [24]. For example, a sample with a very low qualitative measurement (indicating very highly fragmented nucleic acid) may require increased input, whereas a sample with excellent qualitative measurements may succeed with low levels of input material.

ALTERATION TYPES IN SOLID TUMORS AND THEIR CLINICAL RELEVANCE

A wide variety of somatic alteration types can be seen in cancer specimens and a careful understanding of the capabilities of each assay to detect the variety of alteration is of particular relevance.

Single nucleotide variants are colloquially referred to as point mutations and denote the alteration of a single nucleic acid base to a different base. In many cases, these variants contribute to disease pathogenesis through the activation of signal transduction pathways or inactivation of cellular checks and balances, such as DNA repair. A classic example of this phenomenon is the frequent mutation of *KRAS* in a variety of tumor types. The common mutations in *KRAS* result in constitutive activation of this G-protein by eliminating intrinsic GTPase activity, resulting in unregulated cellular proliferation.

Insertions/deletions (indels) collectively describe alterations in which nucleic acid sequence is either deleted or added. In many cases, indels cause a frameshift alteration, leading to premature protein truncation. In other situations, indels may occur in multiples of three, resulting in an in-frame change. Frameshift-causing indels are most commonly observed in tumor suppressor genes, resulting in a loss of function. A common example in this setting is frameshift alterations in *PTEN*, which result in loss of function of this negative regulator. In-frame indels are most commonly seen in oncogenes, where the alteration results in the impaired regulation of key signal transduction machinery. An example of an in-frame indel is the common deletion of a portion of the juxtamembrane region in *KIT*, resulting in unregulated kinase activity.

Structural Rearrangements

Chromosomal rearrangements have been long described in a variety of tumor types. The first discovery of a fusion event in tumorigenesis was the 1973 discovery of the canonical t(9;22) fusion in chronic myeloid leukemia, which eventually lead to the identification of the *BCR-ABL1* fusion transcript in 1985. These structural rearrangements are now part of the classification schema in the diagnosis of myeloid neoplasms, and evaluation of fusion events is often used for diagnostic clarification in sarcomas. Although a variety of recurrent rearrangements have been identified in other solid tumors (such as dermatofibrosarcoma protuberans), it is only with the more recent widespread use of nonbiased sequencing technologies that a far greater number of

TABLE 1
Comparison of Tumor Enrichment Methodologies

	Pros	Cons
Retrieving tissue directly from block (coring, gouging)	• Fastest • Dissecting microscope not needed	• May have reduced precision • May require extensive extraction time owing to increased paraffin and tissue burden
Macrodissection	• Fast • Dissecting microscope not needed	• Requires slide cutting • Intermediate precision • Paraffin profile may be challenging to align
Microdissection	• Most accurate • Concomitant histologic review accounts for changes within a block	• Most labor intensive • Dissecting microscope needed • Requires slide cutting • Requires extensive training

recurrent fusions across a spectrum of solid tumors has been realized [25]. Two major mechanisms underlie how structural rearrangements contribute to tumorigenesis. In one, the coding regions of the 2 fused genes remain intact and in-frame, and result in a functional chimeric protein, which leads to dysregulation of the signaling from one of the two partners. A common example of this type of fusion event is the *EML4-ALK* fusion identified in 3% to 5% of non–small cell lung cancer. The other mechanism is when an active region of a gene (most commonly full length) is placed behind an active promoter resulting in inappropriate expression of the protein. Most examples of this mechanism are seen in hematologic neoplasms.

Splice Site Alterations and Alternative Splicing

Splicing of pre-mRNA is a highly complex process that allows for increased diversity of expressed proteins encoded by a finite genome. Numerous examples of splicing defects as the molecular basis of disease have been documented, perhaps best documented in β-thalassemia. In solid tumors, oncogenic splice variants with potential clinical significance have only recently become evident. A notable example is the recently heterogeneous described group of alterations in *MET* that result in the skipping of the exon [14,26,27] that codes for a region containing a ubiquitination motif. Exon skipping alterations eliminate this motif and result in an accumulation of the protein product [28]. In cases of splicing alterations, the most common mechanism of oncogenesis is elimination of a regulatory region, leading to increased signaling.

Copy number variants

Copy number alterations have long been known to occur in multiple tumor types and, in many cases, the identification of these alterations can impact therapy choice. A canonical example is *ERBB2* (HER2) amplification in breast carcinoma. It is important to note that NGS technologies may not have the same resolution for copy number changes, particularly amplification, as older technologies, such as fluorescence in situ hybridization. Two of the most common bioinformatic approaches to CNV evaluation in NGS involve evaluation of deviations in coverage depth, and single nucleotide polymorphism plots (akin to microarray).

Microsatellite Instability

The role of microsatellite instability (MSI) testing in solid tumors is rapidly evolving. Recent studies have demonstrated that high-level MSI status is correlated with responsiveness to a class of immunotherapy agents (PD-1 and PD-L1 inhibitors), across all tested tumor types [29–31] and is further discussed elsewhere in this article. MSI is classically performed using a PCR-based fragment analysis; however, numerous approaches to incorporating MSI analysis into NGS testing exist and are increasingly used in lieu of separate MSI testing [32–34].

Nonsynonymous Mutation Burden

Mutational loads vary across tumor types, with some being much more prone to extensive mutagenesis. For example, melanoma and non–small cell lung carcinoma have some of the highest mutation burdens across tumor types [35]. However, numerous bioinformatic approaches for determining mutational load exist, and specific clinically relevant cutoffs have not yet been established. Some studies have demonstrated that mutation burden may be predictive of benefit from immunotherapy agents, however this biomarker remains poorly defined and lacks standardization [36].

BIOINFORMATICS

Bioinformatics processing plays a key role in the evaluation of NGS data with many key steps being shared across different NGS platforms and assays. Base calls from the sequencer are demultiplexed and converted to FASTQ files, which contain the sequence reads and the Phred-like quality score. These sequences are aligned to a reference genome and the alignment data is stored as a binary alignment (BAM) file. Next, variant calls are made by comparing the mapped reads with the reference and these calls are stored in a variant call format (VCF) file. Most bioinformatics pipelines will then take these variant calls and annotate, filter, and prioritize them before clinical interpretation/review.

Specific considerations for solid tumor NGS testing that may affect the bioinformatics processing needed include limited nucleic acid input (especially for small samples), which may lead to large numbers of PCR duplicates, particularly in amplicon based assays; the need for high sensitivity to detect low variant allelic fractions; and considerations of paired normal tissue, when evaluated. For detailed information on the bioinformatics of NGS testing please refer to Sabah Kadri's article, "Advances in Next Generation Sequencing Bioinformatics for Clinical Diagnostics: Taking Precision Oncology to the Next Level," elsewhere in this issue, for a detailed discussion.

TECHNICAL INTERPRETATION

Once the raw data from the sequencing run have been analyzed through the informatics pipeline, the data interpretation process begins. This process consists of technical and clinical analysis, the former assessing the accuracy and the latter assessing the clinical implications and reportability of variant calls. Technical interpretation begins by reviewing specific sequencing metrics from the instrument, such as total sequence generated and run quality metrics. Each laboratory should develop their own acceptance criteria based on their assay validation. The VCF and BAM files generated from the pipeline are then assessed.

At its most basic, a VCF lists all identified variants, including the chromosome number and position, reference sequence, sequence of the alteration, and depth of sequencing at that position. Informatics pipelines may add additional fields to the VCF such as gene name, amino acid changes encoded by the change, and presence of the variant in various databases. In addition to the VCF file, variants are reviewed in the BAM file using a browser such as the Integrated Genomics Viewer (IGV, http://software.broadinstitute.org/software/igv/home, accessed April 16, 2018). Once opened in a genome browser, the BAM file shows the individual sequencing reads as horizontal strings aligned to a reference genome, and highlights variants from this reference (Fig. 3).

By manually reviewing each variant in a VCF file within a genome browser, the reviewer is able to identify technical artifacts generated from sequencing. For example, deamination of cytosine residues to uracil or

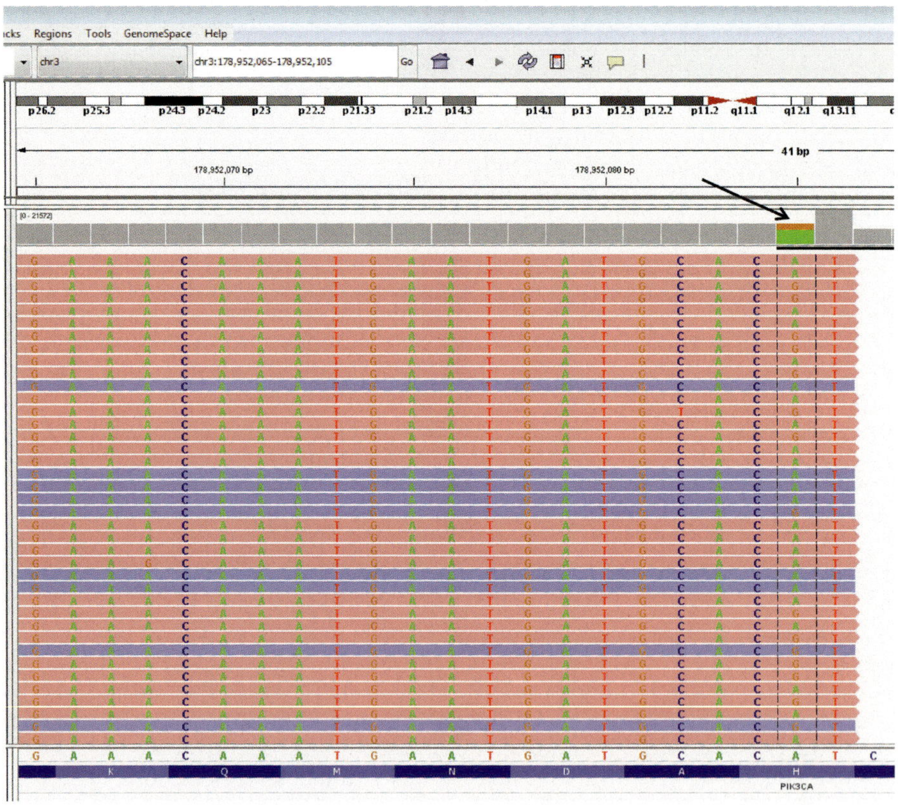

FIG. 3 A representative screenshot from IGV v2.3.97 (*Courtesy of* Broad Institute, Cambridge, MA. Available at http://software.broadinstitute.org/software/igv/.). The *red and blue lines* show the forward (sense strand, *red*) and reverse (antisense strand, *blue*) reads of a DNA sequence at each position. At the bottom of the panel is the genomic reference sequence at that position and the translation denoted by one letter amino acid code. The *red and green bars* denoted by the *arrow* reflects that there is a mixture of different calls between adenine (A; *green*) and guanine (G; *red*) at this position. The *gray bars* adjacent to this mixed color bar represent the depth of coverage at each adjacent position.

thymine can lead to the presence of artifactual C > T transitions [37]. When sequencing both strands of template DNA, this artifact will be present in the strand with a C at the position of interest, but will be absent in its complement. This results in strand bias or the presence of a variant preferentially in a single strand or direction of sequencing, which is often a sign of an artifact. Other types of artifacts that are easily identified are single base duplications and deletions at long homopolymer sites owing to enzymatic slippage, which is a particular problem with sequencing chemistries that do not use chain termination. In addition, the very ends of sequencing reads often show lower quality and this phenomenon can result in artifactual calls.

Other considerations when reviewing variant technical interpretation is the tumor content present in the sample and the variant allele fraction of the variant. It can be tempting to assume that all true variants in oncogenes will have a variant allele fraction of approximately one-half the tumor percentage of the sample being tested; however, this assumption fails to consider the overall genomic instability of cancer cells, including aneuploidy and focal events such as gene amplifications and deletions. In addition, many clinically important mutations arise as subclones and become increasingly dominant over time. Other challenging considerations in the technical interpretation of assays include the identification of reciprocal events in genomic fusions [38] and methodologies for copy number change detection (eg, single nucleotide polymorphism–based and coverage based algorithms may perform differently). At the conclusion of technical interpretation, the variants present in the VCF should be easily separable into true alterations and artifacts.

The Association for Molecular Pathology, the American Society of Clinical Oncology, and the College of American Pathologists recently released guidelines for the interpretation of somatic variants in cancer [39], which can aid in structuring clinical interpretation. The key steps in this process include review of population databases to identify polymorphisms; review of gene- and disease-specific databases to understand potential clinical impact of variants; review of clinical guidelines to understand how specific variants may relate to the use of a variant for diagnosis, prognosis, disease monitoring, and therapeutic selection; and review of the scientific literature to further investigate the significance of variants. In addition, atlases related to protein expression, functional domains, and computational predictions can aid in evaluation of novel variants. A list of useful data sources for variant interpretation is provided in Table 2. Using the information in these sources and the guidelines mentioned, laboratories can assess the clinical significance of sequencing variants along a spectrum. Following the schema proposed in the guideline, tier I variants are variants of strong clinical significance, tier II variants are variants of potential clinical significance, tier III variants are variants of unknown clinical significance, and tier IV variants are benign or likely benign variants (Fig. 4). The following section reviews specific tier I variants in several common solid tumors.

CLINICAL INTERPRETATION

Clinical molecular testing of solid tumors is most frequently performed for those biomarkers with strong evidence supporting clinical usefulness as a diagnostic, prognostic, or therapeutic biomarker. These biomarkers typically have extensive literature supporting their clinical use and are recommended by professional guidelines (selected examples are highlighted in Table 3). NGS-based testing, particularly targeted or hotspot panels, are increasingly being used for the routine evaluation of these biomarkers owing to the ability to detect multiple targets with high sensitivity and a fast turnaround time.

For lung cancer, updated guidelines from the College of American Pathologists/International Association for the Study of Lung Cancer/Association for Molecular Pathology were recently published [40]. In addition to *EGFR* testing of exons 18 to 21 and *ALK* fusion testing, testing for *ROS1* fusions has been recommended [40]. For laboratories that perform NGS testing, it is also recommended that *ERBB2*, *MET*, *BRAF*, *KRAS*, and *RET* be included in panels, based on the potential for enrollment in clinical trials of targeted agents. These oncogenic driver gene mutations generally are not co-occurring, and collectively account for the majority of driver mutations seen in lung adenocarcinoma.

In colorectal carcinoma, evidence-based guidelines from the American Society for Clinical Pathology/College of American Pathologists/Association for Molecular Pathology/American Society of Clinical Oncology were published in 2017 [41]. These guidelines recommend extended *RAS* testing (which should include *KRAS* and *NRAS* codons 12, 13, 59, 61, 117, and 146) in patients where anti-*EGFR* therapy (eg, cetuximab or panitumumab) is being considered. *BRAF* p.V600E mutation testing is also recommended as a prognostic marker. In addition, for those colorectal tumors that show evidence of defective mismatch repair, *BRAF* mutation testing shows additional usefulness, because the presence of the *BRAF* p.V600E mutation strongly favors

TABLE 2
Databases Relevant to Interpretation of Somatic Sequence Variants in Cancer

Usefulness/Function	Database	Location (Web Address)
Population databases to exclude polymorphisms	1000 Genomes Project	http://www.internationalgenome.org/
	Exome Variant Server	http://evs.gs.washington.edu/EVS
	dbSNP	http://www.ncbi.nlm.nih.gov/snp
	dbVar	http://www.ncbi.nlm.nih.gov/dbvar
	ExAC	http://exac.broadinstitute.org
	gnomAD	http://gnomad.broadinstitute.org/
Cancer-specific variant databases	Catalog of Somatic Mutations in Cancer	http://cancer.sanger.ac.uk/cosmic
	My Cancer Genome	http://www.mycancergenome.org
	Personalized cancer therapy, MD Anderson Cancer Center	https://pct.mdanderson.org
	cBioPortal, Memorial Sloan Kettering Cancer Center	http://www.cbioportal.org
	Intogen	https://www.intogen.org/search
	IARC (WHO) TP53 mutation database	http://p53.iarc.fr
	Pediatric Cancer Genome Project (St. Jude Children's Research Hospital - Washington University)	http://explorepcgp.org
	International Cancer Genome Consortium	https://dcc.icgc.org
	CIVic	https://civicdb.org/home
	Atlas of Genetics and Cytogenetics in Oncology and Hematology	http://atlasgeneticsoncology.org/
	DoCM	http://www.docm.info/
Sequence repositories and data hosts	NCBI Genome	http://www.ncbi.nlm.nih.gov/genome
	RefSeqGene	http://www.ncbi.nlm.nih.gov/refseq/rsg
	Locus Reference Genomic	http://www.lrg-sequence.org
	UCSC table browser	https://genome.ucsc.edu/cgi-bin/hgTables
	Ensemble BioMart	http://useast.ensembl.org/biomart/martview
Other disease/mutation databases useful in the context of variant interpretation for cancer genomics	ClinVar	http://www.ncbi.nlm.nih.gov/clinvar
	Human Gene Mutation Database	http://www.hgmd.org
	Leiden Open Variation Database	http://www.lovd.nl
	dbNSFP (compiled database of precomputed in silico prediction scores for nonsynonymous SNVs)	https://sites.google.com/site/jpopgen/dbNSFP
	Ensemble Variant Effect Predictor	https://www.ensembl.org/vep
	UniProt	http://www.uniprot.org/
	Mutalyzer	https://mutalyzer.nl/
	JAX-Clinical Knowledgebase	https://ckb.jax.org/
	The Human Protein Atlas	https://www.proteinatlas.org/

Abbreviations: SNV, single nucleotide variant; WHO, World Health Organization.

Modified from Li MM, Datto M, Duncavage EJ, et al. Standards and guidelines for the interpretation and reporting of sequence variants in cancer: a joint consensus recommendation of the Association for Molecular Pathology, American Society of Clinical Oncology, and College of American Pathologists. J Mol Diagn 2017;19(1):7; with permission.

the tumor being sporadic in origin (as opposed to arising in the context of Lynch syndrome). Currently, there is insufficient evidence for *PIK3CA* mutation testing in colorectal cancer for therapy selection outside of clinical trials. Of note, some studies have suggested *PIK3CA* mutational status to be associated with the improved survival resulting from postoperative aspirin use in patients with early stage colorectal carcinoma [42–44].

Molecular testing in melanoma has mainly focused on *BRAF* p.V600E mutation testing. *BRAF* mutations are frequently seen in melanoma, particularly in cutaneous melanomas [45]. The p.V600E mutation is the most common *BRAF* mutation identified, followed by p.V600K [46]. Other *BRAF* mutations affecting codon 600 or other codons are less common in melanoma. Patients with advanced or metastatic *BRAF* p.V600E (or p.V600 K) mutant melanomas may show response to BRAF inhibitors (which may be combined with MEK inhibitors) [47,48]. Newer studies suggest that BRAF inhibitors may be useful in the neoadjuvant setting in stage III disease [49,50].

Testing for *KIT* activating mutations (which are more common in acral or mucosal melanomas) in patients with metastatic melanoma may be helpful to inform treatment with imatinib [47,48]. Finally, testing for *NRAS, GNA11,* or *GNAQ* mutations may inform therapy in the context of clinical trials.

The majority of gastrointestinal stromal tumors harbor mutations in *KIT* or *PDGFRA*. *KIT* mutations typically involve exons 9, 11, or 13, and may confer sensitivity to imatinib or sunitinib [51]. *PDGFRA* mutations mostly involve exons 12, 14, or 18, and tumors harboring these mutations are typically sensitive to imatinib [52]. However, primary and secondary resistance mutations in *KIT* (such as p.D816V) or *PDGFRA* (such as p.D842V) may also occur [53,54]. Furthermore, not every mutation confers the same level of sensitivity to therapy. For example, those tumors harboring *KIT* exon 9 mutations may not respond to TKI therapy as well as those that harbor *KIT* exon 11 mutations and a higher starting dose of inhibitor may be required [55].

Several molecular markers have been described in glioma. Many of these markers have been included in the World Health Organization's classification of central nervous system tumors because they define subgroups with specific prognostic implications [56]. *IDH1* and *IDH2* mutational status is incorporated into the classification of diffuse gliomas: diffuse astrocytoma, anaplastic astrocytoma, and glioblastoma [56]. In oligodendrogliomas, both 1p/19q co-deletion along with *IDH1/2* mutation are seen. Diffuse midline gliomas are another group of tumors defined by molecular alterations; in this case with p.K27M mutations in the histones *H3F3A* or *HIST1H3B*. Other central nervous

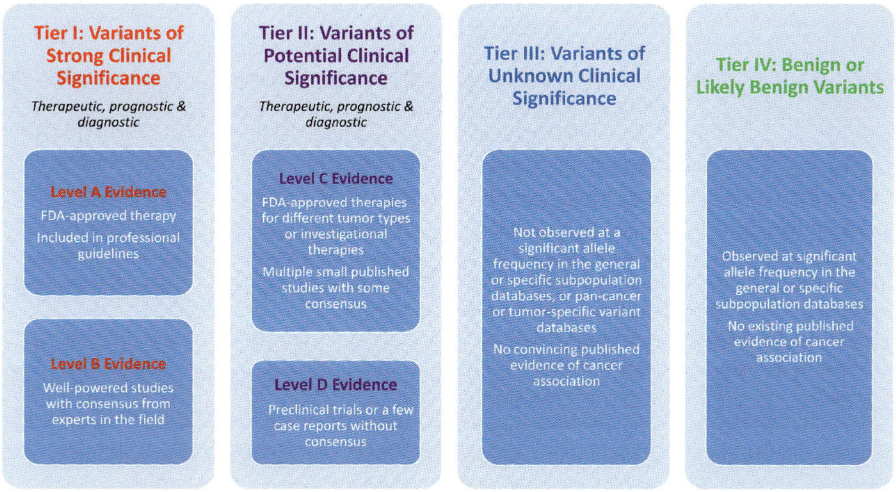

FIG. 4 Proposed categorization of somatic variants in cancer. FDA, US Food and Drug Administration. (*From* Li MM, Datto M, Duncavage EJ, et al. Standards and guidelines for the interpretation and reporting of sequence variants in cancer: a joint consensus recommendation of the Association for Molecular Pathology, American Society of Clinical Oncology, and College of American Pathologists. J Mol Diagn 2017;19(1):11; with permission.)

TABLE 3
Molecular Biomarkers in Cancer Commonly Assessed by NGS Technologies

Tumor	Gene	Clinical Usefulness	Interpretation
Lung	*ALK*	Therapeutic	Fusion predicts response to TKIs
	EGFR	Therapeutic	Activating mutations predict response to TKIs
	ROS1	Therapeutic	Fusion predicts response to TKIs
	KRAS	Other	*KRAS* mutation generally mutually exclusive with *EGFR* mutation or *ALK* or *ROS1* fusion. Presence of *KRAS* mutation may be used to exclude patients from expanded panel testing.
	BRAF	Therapeutic	Activating mutation predicts response to BRAF inhibitors
	ERBB2	Therapeutic	Activating mutations are a potential target in the context of clinical trials
	MET	Therapeutic	*MET* exon 14 skipping mutations are a potential target in the context of clinical trials
	RET	Therapeutic	Fusions are a potential target in the context of clinical trials
Colorectal	*KRAS*	Therapeutic	Activating mutations predict lack of response to anti-EGFR therapies
	NRAS	Therapeutic	Activating mutations predict lack of response to anti-EGFR therapies
	BRAF	Therapeutic	Activating mutation predicts lack of response to anti-EGFR therapies.
		Prognostic	Reduced PFS and OS in patients with *BRAF* mutation.
		Other	In a mismatch repair deficient tumor, presence of *BRAF* mutation favors a sporadic tumor.
	PIK3CA	Therapeutic	Activating mutations are a potential target in the context of clinical trials
Melanoma	*BRAF*	Therapeutic	Activating mutations predict response to BRAF inhibitors
	KIT	Therapeutic	Activating mutations predict response to TKIs
	NRAS	Therapeutic	Activating mutations are a potential target in the context of clinical trials
GIST	*KIT*	Therapeutic	Activating mutations predict response to TKIs
	PDGFRA	Therapeutic	Activating mutations predict response to TKIs
Glioma	*IDH1/IDH2*	Diagnostic Prognostic	Diffuse astrocytoma, *IDH*-mutant Anaplastic astrocytoma, *IDH*-mutant Glioblastoma, *IDH*-mutant Oligodendroglioma, *IDH*-mutant and 1p/19q-codeleted Anaplastic oligodendroglioma, *IDH*-mutant and 1p/19q-codeleted
	BRAF	Therapeutic	Activating mutations or fusions are a potential target in the context of clinical trials
	H3F3A	Diagnostic	Diffuse midline glioma, H3 family p.K27M-mutant
	HIST1H3B	Diagnostic	Diffuse midline glioma, H3 family p.K27M-mutant
Sarcoma	*PAX3-FOXO1* *PAX7-FOXO1*	Diagnostic	Alveolar rhabdomyosarcoma
	EWSR1-FLI1 *EWSR1-ERG*	Diagnostic	Ewing sarcoma
	SS18-SSX1 *SS18-SSX2*	Diagnostic	Synovial sarcoma
	ETV6-NTRK3	Diagnostic	Fibrosarcoma
	FUS-DDIT3	Diagnostic	Myxoid/round cell liposarcoma
	CIC-DUX4	Diagnostic	CIC-rearranged Ewing-like sarcoma
	BCOR-CCNB3	Diagnostic	BCOR-rearranged Ewing-like sarcoma

(*continued on next page*)

TABLE 3
(*continued*)

Tumor	Gene	Clinical Usefulness	Interpretation
Pan-tumor	Microsatellite instability	Therapeutic	Predicts response to PD-1/PD-L1 inhibitors
	Nonsynonymous mutation load	Therapeutic	May predict response to PD-1/PD-L1 inhibitors

Abbreviations: EGFR, epidermal growth factor receptor; GIST, gastrointestinal stromal tumor; NGS, next-generation sequencing; OS, overall survival; PFS, progression-free survival; TKI, tyrosine kinase inhibitors.

system tumors such as pilocytic astrocytoma, pleomorphic xanthastrocytoma, ganglioglioma, or epithelioid glioblastomas frequently have *BRAF* alteration (activating mutations or fusions), which may be targetable in the context of clinical trials.

Many sarcomas are driven by the presence of specific fusion proteins. Molecular testing to detect fusions plays an important role as ancillary testing to support histologic diagnoses of sarcoma. Several examples of these fusions are listed in Table 3. Although testing for fusions in sarcoma is primarily diagnostic, in some cases these fusions are targetable. For example, therapeutics targeting *NTRK1/2/3* fusions are currently being investigated in clinical trials [57,58].

In addition to tumor-specific biomarkers, the advent of immune checkpoint inhibitors such as PD-1/PD-L1 inhibitors, which are being used in multiple solid tumor malignancies, has led to the search for pan-tumor markers that best predict response. MSI has been proposed as one such marker and rapidly emerging data led to the first-of-its-kind FDA drug approval based on a molecular finding across all tumor types for pembrolizumab [59]. Tumors with MSI have high numbers of mutations, which is hypothesized to increase the production of tumor-specific neoantigens [30,60]. MSI, however, only accounts for a subset of cases that may respond to immunotherapy. Tumors harboring mutations in polymerases *POLE* or *POLD1* have impaired proofreading during DNA replication and often have very high mutation rates [61]. Additionally, some tumors without MSI or *POLE/POLD1* mutations may have high nonsynonymous mutation loads and it is postulated that a high level of nonsynonymous changes leads to increased neoantigen presentation. Studies suggest this may be a promising biomarker for predicting response to immunotherapy agents [31,36,62].

Additional tumor biomarkers continue to be rapidly identified and adopted into clinical use. Evidence supporting biomarkers may evolve rapidly, making clinical interpretation of these biomarkers challenging. Molecular tumor boards are increasingly being incorporated into clinical practice to review variants and develop treatment recommendations [63–66].

FUTURE DIRECTIONS AND APPLICATIONS

In a relatively short period of time, clinical NGS has become widely adopted in solid tumor oncology. Many new technologies including single molecule and long-read sequencing are being investigated for clinical use and the list of clinically relevant alterations continues to increase from simple single nucleotide variants to fusion events and genome-wide mutation assessment. With further advances in research and technology, this trend is expected to continue and grow in the coming years and NGS shows exceptional versatility in assessing many large genomic regions simultaneously.

REFERENCES

[1] Garrido-Cardenas JA, Garcia-Maroto F, Alvarez-Bermejo JA, et al. DNA sequencing sensors: an overview. Sensors (Basel) 2017;17(3) [pii:E588].

[2] Goodwin S, McPherson JD, McCombie WR. Coming of age: ten years of next-generation sequencing technologies. Nat Rev Genet 2016;17(6):333–51.

[3] Sheikine Y, Kuo FC, Lindeman NI. Clinical and technical aspects of genomic diagnostics for precision oncology. J Clin Oncol 2017;35(9):929–33.

[4] Smith T, Heger A, Sudbery I. UMI-tools: modeling sequencing errors in Unique Molecular Identifiers to improve quantification accuracy. Genome Res 2017;27(3):491–9.

[5] Kou R, Lam H, Duan H, et al. Benefits and challenges with applying unique molecular identifiers in next

generation sequencing to detect low frequency mutations. PLoS One 2016;11(1):e0146638.
[6] Kircher M, Sawyer S, Meyer M. Double indexing overcomes inaccuracies in multiplex sequencing on the Illumina platform. Nucleic Acids Res 2012;40(1):e3.
[7] MacConaill LE, Burns RT, Nag A, et al. Unique, dual-indexed sequencing adapters with UMIs effectively eliminate index cross-talk and significantly improve sensitivity of massively parallel sequencing. BMC Genomics 2018;19(1):30.
[8] Hsu PP, Shaw AT. Lung cancer: a wily genetic opponent. Cell 2017;169(5):777–9.
[9] Bass BP, Engel KB, Greytak SR, et al. A review of preanalytical factors affecting molecular, protein, and morphological analysis of formalin-fixed, paraffin-embedded (FFPE) tissue: how well do you know your FFPE specimen? Arch Pathol Lab Med 2014;138(11):1520–30.
[10] Srinivasan M, Sedmak D, Jewell S. Effect of fixatives and tissue processing on the content and integrity of nucleic acids. Am J Pathol 2002;161(6):1961–71.
[11] Guerrera F, Tabbo F, Bessone L, et al. The influence of tissue ischemia time on RNA integrity and Patient-Derived Xenografts (PDX) engraftment rate in a Non-Small Cell Lung Cancer (NSCLC) Biobank. PLoS One 2016;11(1): e0145100.
[12] Rakha EA, Starczynski J, Lee AH, et al. The updated ASCO/CAP guideline recommendations for HER2 testing in the management of invasive breast cancer: a critical review of their implications for routine practice. Histopathology 2014;64(5):609–15.
[13] Hunt JL. Molecular pathology in anatomic pathology practice: a review of basic principles. Arch Pathol Lab Med 2008;132(2):248–60.
[14] Greer CE, Peterson SL, Kiviat NB, et al. PCR amplification from paraffin-embedded tissues. Effects of fixative and fixation time. Am J Clin Pathol 1991;95(2):117–24.
[15] Aisner DL, Rumery MD, Merrick DT, et al. Do more with less: tips and techniques for maximizing small biopsy and cytology specimens for molecular and ancillary testing: the University of Colorado Experience. Arch Pathol Lab Med 2016. [Epub ahead of print].
[16] Roy-Chowdhuri S, Aisner DL, Allen TC, et al. Biomarker testing in lung carcinoma cytology specimens: a perspective from members of the pulmonary pathology society. Arch Pathol Lab Med 2016. [Epub ahead of print].
[17] Viray H, Li K, Long TA, et al. A prospective, multi-institutional diagnostic trial to determine pathologist accuracy in estimation of percentage of malignant cells. Arch Pathol Lab Med 2013;137(11):1545–9.
[18] Huhns M, Krohn S, Murua Escobar H, et al. Genomic heterogeneity in primary colorectal carcinomas and their metastases: born bad or brought up a villain? Hum Pathol 2018;74:54–63.
[19] Jamal-Hanjani M, Wilson GA, McGranahan N, et al. Tracking the evolution of non-small-cell lung cancer. N Engl J Med 2017;376(22):2109–21.
[20] Chowdhuri SR, Xi L, Pham TH, et al. EGFR and KRAS mutation analysis in cytologic samples of lung adenocarcinoma enabled by laser capture microdissection. Mod Pathol 2012;25(4):548–55.
[21] NeuroInDX. UNIPICK+. Available at: http://www.neuroindx.com/products-2/unipick/. Accessed July 9, 2018.
[22] Roche. AVENIO millisect system. Available at: https://sequencing.roche.com/en/products-solutions/by-category/sample-collection/avenio-millisect-system.html. Accessed July 9, 2018.
[23] Patel PG, Selvarajah S, Guerard KP, et al. Reliability and performance of commercial RNA and DNA extraction kits for FFPE tissue cores. PLoS One 2017;12(6):e0179732.
[24] Sah S, Chen L, Houghton J, et al. Functional DNA quantification guides accurate next-generation sequencing mutation detection in formalin-fixed, paraffin-embedded tumor biopsies. Genome Med 2013;5(8):77.
[25] Mertens F, Johansson B, Fioretos T, et al. The emerging complexity of gene fusions in cancer. Nat Rev Cancer 2015;15(6):371–81.
[26] Awad MM, Oxnard GR, Jackman DM, et al. MET Exon 14 mutations in non-small-cell lung cancer are associated with advanced age and stage-dependent MET genomic amplification and c-met overexpression. J Clin Oncol 2016;34(7):721–30.
[27] Frampton GM, Ali SM, Rosenzweig M, et al. Activation of MET via diverse exon 14 splicing alterations occurs in multiple tumor types and confers clinical sensitivity to MET inhibitors. Cancer Discov 2015;5(8):850–9.
[28] Drilon A. MET Exon 14 alterations in lung cancer: exon skipping extends half-life. Clin Cancer Res 2016; 22(12):2832–4.
[29] Le DT, Durham JN, Smith KN, et al. Mismatch repair deficiency predicts response of solid tumors to PD-1 blockade. Science 2017;357(6349):409–13.
[30] Le DT, Uram JN, Wang H, et al. PD-1 Blockade in tumors with mismatch-repair deficiency. N Engl J Med 2015; 372(26):2509–20.
[31] Rizvi NA, Hellmann MD, Snyder A, et al. Cancer immunology. Mutational landscape determines sensitivity to PD-1 blockade in non-small cell lung cancer. Science 2015;348(6230):124–8.
[32] Kautto EA, Bonneville R, Miya J, et al. Performance evaluation for rapid detection of pan-cancer microsatellite instability with MANTIS. Oncotarget 2017;8(5): 7452–63.
[33] Niu B, Ye K, Zhang Q, et al. MSIsensor: microsatellite instability detection using paired tumor-normal sequence data. Bioinformatics 2014;30(7):1015–6.
[34] Salipante SJ, Scroggins SM, Hampel HL, et al. Microsatellite instability detection by next generation sequencing. Clin Chem 2014;60(9):1192–9.
[35] Vogelstein B, Papadopoulos N, Velculescu VE, et al. Cancer genome landscapes. Science 2013;339(6127): 1546–58.
[36] Hellmann MD, Ciuleanu TE, Pluzanski A, et al. Nivolumab plus Ipilimumab in lung cancer with a high tumor

mutational burden. N Engl J Med 2018;378(22):2093–104.

[37] Do H, Dobrovic A. Sequence artifacts in DNA from formalin-fixed tissues: causes and strategies for minimization. Clin Chem 2015;61(1):64–71.

[38] Rosenbaum JN, Bloom R, Forys JT, et al. Genomic heterogeneity of ALK fusion breakpoints in non-small-cell lung cancer. Mod Pathol 2018;31(5):791–808.

[39] Li MM, Datto M, Duncavage EJ, et al. Standards and guidelines for the interpretation and reporting of sequence variants in cancer: a joint consensus recommendation of the Association for Molecular Pathology, American Society of Clinical Oncology, and College of American Pathologists. J Mol Diagn 2017;19(1):4–23.

[40] Lindeman NI, Cagle PT, Aisner DL, et al. Updated molecular testing guideline for the selection of lung cancer patients for treatment with targeted tyrosine kinase inhibitors: guideline from the College of American Pathologists, the International Association for the Study of Lung Cancer, and the Association for Molecular Pathology. J Mol Diagn 2018;20(2):129–59.

[41] Sepulveda AR, Hamilton SR, Allegra CJ, et al. Molecular biomarkers for the evaluation of colorectal cancer: guideline from the American Society for Clinical Pathology, College of American Pathologists, Association for Molecular Pathology, and American Society of Clinical Oncology. J Mol Diagn 2017;19(2):187–225.

[42] Domingo E, Church DN, Sieber O, et al. Evaluation of PIK3CA mutation as a predictor of benefit from nonsteroidal anti-inflammatory drug therapy in colorectal cancer. J Clin Oncol 2013;31(34):4297–305.

[43] Elwood PC, Morgan G, Pickering JE, et al. Aspirin in the treatment of cancer: reductions in metastatic spread and in mortality: a systematic review and meta-analyses of published studies. PLoS One 2016;11(4):e0152402.

[44] Liao X, Lochhead P, Nishihara R, et al. Aspirin use, tumor PIK3CA mutation, and colorectal-cancer survival. N Engl J Med 2012;367(17):1596–606.

[45] Maldonado JL, Fridlyand J, Patel H, et al. Determinants of BRAF mutations in primary melanomas. J Natl Cancer Inst 2003;95(24):1878–90.

[46] Lovly CM, Dahlman KB, Fohn LE, et al. Routine multiplex mutational profiling of melanomas enables enrollment in genotype-driven therapeutic trials. PLoS One 2012;7(4):e35309.

[47] National Comprehensive Cancer Network, Clinical practice guidelines in oncology, melanoma, Version 1.2018. 2018. Available at: https://www.nccn.org/professionals/physician_gls/default.aspx. Accessed January 18, 2018.

[48] Dummer R, Hauschild A, Lindenblatt N, et al. Cutaneous melanoma: ESMO clinical practice guidelines for diagnosis, treatment and follow-up. Ann Oncol 2015;26(Suppl 5):v126–32.

[49] Long GV, Hauschild A, Santinami M, et al. Adjuvant dabrafenib plus trametinib in stage III BRAF-mutated melanoma. N Engl J Med 2017;377(19):1813–23.

[50] Maio M, Lewis K, Demidov L, et al. Adjuvant vemurafenib in resected, BRAF(V600) mutation-positive melanoma (BRIM8): a randomised, double-blind, placebo-controlled, multicentre, phase 3 trial. Lancet Oncol 2018;19(4):510–20.

[51] Heinrich MC, Corless CL, Demetri GD, et al. Kinase mutations and imatinib response in patients with metastatic gastrointestinal stromal tumor. J Clin Oncol 2003;21(23):4342–9.

[52] Corless CL, Schroeder A, Griffith D, et al. PDGFRA mutations in gastrointestinal stromal tumors: frequency, spectrum and in vitro sensitivity to imatinib. J Clin Oncol 2005;23(23):5357–64.

[53] Cassier PA, Fumagalli E, Rutkowski P, et al. Outcome of patients with platelet-derived growth factor receptor alpha-mutated gastrointestinal stromal tumors in the tyrosine kinase inhibitor era. Clin Cancer Res 2012;18(16):4458–64.

[54] Heinrich MC, Maki RG, Corless CL, et al. Primary and secondary kinase genotypes correlate with the biological and clinical activity of sunitinib in imatinib-resistant gastrointestinal stromal tumor. J Clin Oncol 2008;26(33):5352–9.

[55] National Comprehensive Cancer Network, Clinical practice guidelines in oncology, soft tissue sarcoma, Version 1.2018. 2018. Available at: https://www.nccn.org/professionals/physician_gls/default.aspx. Accessed January 18, 2018.

[56] World Health Organization. WHO Classification of Tumours of the Central Nervous System. vol 1. 4th edition. Geneva (Switzerland): World Health Organization; 2016.

[57] Drilon A, Siena S, Ou SI, et al. Safety and antitumor activity of the multitargeted Pan-TRK, ROS1, and ALK inhibitor entrectinib: combined results from two phase I trials (ALKA-372-001 and STARTRK-1). Cancer Discov 2017;7(4):400–9.

[58] Laetsch TW, DuBois SG, Mascarenhas L, et al. Larotrectinib for paediatric solid tumours harbouring NTRK gene fusions: phase 1 results from a multicentre, open-label, phase 1/2 study. Lancet Oncol 2018;19(5):705–14.

[59] FDA approves first cancer treatment for any solid tumor with a specific genetic feature. 2017. Available at: https://www.fda.gov/newsevents/newsroom/pressannouncements/ucm560167.htm. Accessed April 18, 2018.

[60] Llosa NJ, Cruise M, Tam A, et al. The vigorous immune microenvironment of microsatellite instable colon cancer is balanced by multiple counter-inhibitory checkpoints. Cancer Discov 2015;5(1):43–51.

[61] Briggs S, Tomlinson I. Germline and somatic polymerase epsilon and delta mutations define a new class of hypermutated colorectal and endometrial cancers. J Pathol 2013;230(2):148–53.

[62] Rizvi H, Sanchez-Vega F, La K, et al. Molecular determinants of response to anti-programmed cell death (PD)-1 and anti-programmed death-ligand 1 (PD-L1) blockade in patients with non-small-cell lung cancer

profiled with targeted next-generation sequencing. J Clin Oncol 2018;36(7):633–41.

[63] Bryce AH, Egan JB, Borad MJ, et al. Experience with precision genomics and tumor board, indicates frequent target identification, but barriers to delivery. Oncotarget 2017;8(16):27145–54.

[64] Harada S, Arend R, Dai Q, et al. Implementation and utilization of the molecular tumor board to guide precision medicine. Oncotarget 2017;8(34):57845–54.

[65] Hyman DM, Solit DB, Arcila ME, et al. Precision medicine at Memorial Sloan Kettering Cancer Center: clinical next-generation sequencing enabling next-generation targeted therapy trials. Drug Discov Today 2015;20(12): 1422–8.

[66] Knepper TC, Bell GC, Hicks JK, et al. Key lessons learned from Moffit's molecular tumor board: the clinical genomics action committee experience. Oncologist 2017; 22(2):144–51.

Advances in Molecular Pathology 1 (2018) 183–191
ADVANCES IN MOLECULAR PATHOLOGY

Emerging Concepts in Liquid Biopsy

Siddhartha Sen, MD, PhD, Michael Datto, MD, PhD, Sarah Rapisardo, PhD*
Department of Pathology, Duke University Medical Center, Durham, NC 27710, USA

KEYWORDS
• Liquid biopsy • Next-generation sequencing (NGS) • Bioinformatics • Circulating tumor DNA (ctDNA)

KEY POINTS

- Liquid biopsy is a minimally invasive approach that relies on analyzing traces of tumor from body fluids like blood or urine.
- Circulating tumor DNA (ctDNA) testing may be used to monitor for recurrence and for the evolution of new resistance mutations, particularly when the risk of biopsy exceeds the benefit.
- Liquid biopsy has demonstrated utility in only limited indications to date, such as non–small cell lung cancer.
- The complex informatics processing required to meaningfully use the sequencing data remains one of the greatest challenges of next-generation sequencing for mutation detection in ctDNA.
- Tumor genotyping by ctDNA will require technological and bioinformatic advances in addition to proven clinical utility for future applications.

INTRODUCTION

Despite advances in targeted therapies in the management of cancer, its diagnosis, treatment, and posttherapy surveillance are still heavily reliant on tissue biopsies and imaging. Traditional methods like needle biopsies, although still considered "gold standard," are beset with limitations. In addition to being invasive, they provide limited information and may not account for heterogeneity that exists between different areas within the same tumor mass (spatial heterogeneity), or may incompletely demonstrate the evolution of the clonal changes over time, which can be evident when comparing the primary tumor to distant metastases (temporal heterogeneity) [1]. Optimum tumor sampling is often not possible due to inaccessible and remote tumor locations. Thus, a traditional needle biopsy may not provide accurate and adequate information, possibly compromising treatment decisions. Minimally invasive tests that can accurately reflect the molecular signature of tumors or biomarkers of disease can overcome some such limitations. The term "liquid biopsy" denotes an approach that relies primarily on analyzing traces of tumor in the form of circulating cancer cells or nucleic acid molecules from body fluids like blood or urine. Although the science of this approach is still evolving, liquid biopsy holds enormous potential, with emerging clinical utility that can complement, and perhaps eventually replace, tissue biopsies.

There are several sources of cellular and tumor-derived material that can be noninvasively assessed by a liquid biopsy. These sources include circulating tumor cells (CTCs) [2], exosomes [3,4], cell-free DNA (cfDNA), and tumor-educated platelets (TEPs) [5], to name a few. CTCs are viable tumor cells that are shed into the circulation from a primary tumor or metastases. They can be distinguished from normal cells in circulation based on expression of certain molecules. Exosomes are nanometer-sized membrane encapsulated vesicles that

Disclosure Statement: The authors have nothing to disclose.

*Corresponding author. 2351 Erwin Road, Room 0213A, Wadsworth Building, Durham, NC 27705. *E-mail address:* sarah.horn@duke.edu

https://doi.org/10.1016/j.yamp.2018.07.009
2589-4080/18/

are released from tumor cells via exocytosis. Once considered cellular artifact or debris, exosomes have attracted much attention of late. Several studies have demonstrated that these exosomes are enriched in certain micro-RNAs and proteins derived from their cell of origin [6,7] and can thus be important tumor cell surrogates in liquid biopsy. TEPs are part of the tumor microenvironment and contain tumor-derived RNA, which can aid in identifying the location of a tumor and determining treatment strategies [8]. Compared with CTCs, the level of circulating tumor DNA (ctDNA) has been shown to be higher than that of CTCs and can provide a more accessible source for tumor genotyping [9]. This review focuses primarily on the current applications of ctDNA, next-generation sequencing (NGS), and other technologies for mutation detection, and the unique challenges for this promising biomarker.

HISTORY AND BIOLOGY OF CELL-FREE DNA

The presence of cfDNA in blood was first described in 1948 [10], but its first link to any kind of disease was demonstrated almost 20 years later when high levels of cfDNA were seen in lupus patients [11]. In 1997, increased levels of cfDNA were first reported in the circulation of patients with cancer [12]. However, the potential of cfDNA as a clinical biomarker was realized much later, when Lo and colleagues [13] demonstrated that small amounts of DNA originating from the fetus could be reliably identified in maternal plasma. They further showed that significantly high concentrations of fetal DNA were present in the maternal plasma (mean ranging from 3.4% to 6.2% of the total plasma DNA), depending on the stage of pregnancy [14]. These findings were seminal findings that eventually culminated in the development of noninvasive prenatal screening (NIPS). NIPS is now in widely used to screen for common chromosomal and single-gene disorders.

cfDNA is double-stranded DNA approximately 167 bp in length, which matches that of DNA occupied by a nucleosome along with the associated linker DNA [15,16]. Apoptosis, necrosis, as well as active secretion [17], have been postulated as the primary mechanisms via which cfDNA is released into the circulation. cfDNA is cleared from the body by the liver and kidneys, with its half-life varying from 15 minutes to a few hours [18]. Tumor-specific cfDNA (ctDNA) consists of fragments of DNA originating from the tumor and is present in the circulation along with cfDNA. ctDNA has been seen in several cancers [19], but its amount in the circulation shows considerable variation. Importantly, ctDNA contains genetic alterations specific to the tumor; mutations in oncogenes, tumor suppressor genes, genetic alterations like microsatellite instability, loss of heterozygosity, as well as DNA hypermethylation can be detected in the ctDNA [20]. The presence of recurrent mutations can be helpful in discriminating ctDNA from normal cfDNA in an individual, although the presence of such mutations does not necessarily correlate with the presence of a tumor [21]. Although cfDNA can be detected in certain physiologic as well as various nonmalignant conditions, it has been shown that the amount of ctDNA is significantly higher in patients with malignancies in comparison to normal healthy subjects and other pathologic conditions like chronic inflammation [22].

ctDNA testing to detect mutations depends on the ability of cancer cells to actively shed tumor DNA into the circulation. Not all tumors, however, shed detectable amounts of ctDNA. Certain tumors like melanoma, and advanced pancreatic, ovarian, and colorectal cancers have been shown to have readily detectable amounts of ctDNA in the circulation [9]. Significantly high yields of ctDNA have also been reported in patients of multiple myeloma, likely due to increased shedding of tumor DNA into circulation by the malignant plasma cells [23]. On the other hand, renal cancers, and primary brain tumors like glioma and medulloblastoma, are examples of tumors with extremely low ctDNA shedding [9]. Therefore, the amount of tumor DNA shedding and clearance from the circulation may greatly influence the amount of detectable ctDNA, independent of tumor size, extent of necrosis, or presence of metastases [24].

APPLICATIONS AND APPROACHES TO CIRCULATING TUMOR DNA TESTING

In addition to prenatal screening with NIPS, current applications of cfDNA testing (specifically ctDNA) also include the diagnosis and management of cancer. At the time of a new cancer diagnosis, ctDNA testing can be performed to complement tumor testing, both to assess for driver mutations (also present in the tumor) and for additional mutations not evident in the tumor due to spatial heterogeneity. ctDNA testing may also be used to monitor for recurrence and for the evolution of new resistance mutations, particularly when the risk of biopsy exceeds the benefit.

Although the potential applications of ctDNA are numerous, liquid biopsy has demonstrated utility in only limited indications to date. The current National Comprehensive Cancer Network guidelines for non–small cell lung cancer (NSCLC) suggest that plasma genotyping may be considered instead of tissue biopsy for patients with metastatic disease (although tissue biopsy is recommended if feasible and if the plasma biopsy is negative) [25]. The recent US Food and Drug Administration (FDA) approval of a targeted polymerase chain reaction (PCR) assay for epidermal growth factor receptor (EGFR) mutation detection in peripheral blood, which can be run without bioinformatics expertise or anything other than standard laboratory equipment, is a testament to the fact that this technology has come of age. In June 2016, the FDA approved a real-time PCR test, the cobas EGFR Mutation Test v2 (Roche Molecular Systems, Inc) for detecting EGFR mutations in NSCLC patients [26]. The use of ctDNA in NSCLC is a success story, driven in part by the availability of targeted therapies and by the underlying biology: a limited number of recurrent hotspot mutations in oncogenes are interrogated. In contrast, tumors driven by large-scale structural variation or chromosomal alterations require a whole genome-wide scale of analysis, with a corresponding decrease in sensitivity. A genome-wide copy number analysis requires a relatively high allele frequency for ctDNA of at least 5% to 10% of cfDNA [27], whereas targeted sequencing of ctDNA (with error correction using molecular barcodes) can detect mutations present at less than 0.2% [28,29].

Mutation-specific, targeted approaches to the detection cell-free ctDNA fill a niche in the care of patients with cancer. They answer a single clinical question at the time when it is most relevant and actionable, for example, Does this new diagnosis of patients with lung cancer have an EGFR mutation, and thus are they a candidate for targeted therapy? Several technologies are now routinely used for targeted mutation detection in cfDNA. Each has its strengths. For example, Droplet Digital PCR (ddPCR) can detect specific mutations down to less than 0.01% mutant allele fraction, thus providing an ultrasensitive approach to mutation detection [30]. Targeted, real-time PCR assays, although not as sensitive, can be implemented in most clinical molecular diagnostics laboratories. Both of these PCR approaches have high specificity with few "false positives" [30,31].

Targeted approaches like the cobas EGFR Mutation Test have a significant limitation, however. They are targeted. Other targeted methods like ddPCR show very good quantification and high sensitivity, but are likewise limited in their multiplexing capacity and are restricted to interrogating hotspot mutations in coding regions [30,32,33]. In contrast to the demonstrated clinical validity for biomarkers such as mutated EGFR in NSCLC, establishing the validity with broad NGS-based approaches is more challenging, because of the multiple targets across multiple tumor types [34]. Nevertheless, NGS-based approaches have the benefit of being able to interrogate the sequence of one hundred, one thousand, or more targets in a single assay. They are, in turn, able to answer multiple clinical questions simultaneously about the possible efficacy of a variety of targeted therapies or the patient-specific prognosis based on diverse tumor markers. The value and applicability of NGS in ctDNA detection are evidenced by the use of this technology by several commercial vendors (Foundation Medicine, Guardant Health, PGDx, and others) that provide NGS-based ctDNA solutions in a clinical setting to patients with cancer (Table 1). The commercially available panels evaluate multiple mutation types (single nucleotide variants, small insertions and deletions [indels], copy number alterations, and rearrangements/gene fusions) across a large number of genes and tumor types by NGS.

The intended use of any ctDNA assay guides both the test design and the methodology. Although targeted assays like the cobas EGFR Mutation Test identify specific variants associated with drug responsiveness in a single tumor type, a broader NGS panel allows versatility for a wider spectrum of targets across different tumor types. For advanced stage patients, NGS of ctDNA with larger panels of 50+ genes have identified at least one mutation in more than three-quarters of patients [28,35]. Such NGS panels may be informative across multiple cancer types at the time of diagnosis, and the inclusion of multiple targets allows for sensitive tracking of an individual's tumor over time. For example, the probability of detecting a single mutant genotype at a ctDNA fraction of 0.01% is around 40%, compared with a theoretic probability of more than 80% when monitoring for multiple mutations as part of a particular clonal signature [29].

BIOINFORMATICS APPROACHES TO ACCURATE MUTATION DETECTION IN NEXT-GENERATION SEQUENCING–BASED CIRCULATING TUMOR DNA TESTING

Despite the widespread applicability of NGS in ctDNA detection, the complex informatics processing required to meaningfully use the sequencing data remains one of the greatest challenges of NGS. This limitation is even greater in the context of detecting rare events. Analysis pipelines that are tuned to the detection of inherited

TABLE 1
Commercial Vendors (Foundation Medicine, Guardant Health, PGDx, and Others) that Provide Next-Generation Sequencing–Based Circulating Tumor DNA Solutions in a Clinical Setting to Cancer Patients

	ctDNA Product	Technology	Gene Number/ Cancer Types	Stated Limit of Detection
Roche Molecular Diagnostics	Cobas EGFR Mutation test v2 Available in 2016 as FDA-approved companion diagnostic	Real-time PCR	1 gene (EGFR)/ NSCLC	25–100 copies/mL
Guardant Health	Guardant 360 Available in 2014 as LDT in a CLIA-certified laboratory	NGS	73 genes/multiple cancer types	0.1% mutant allele fraction
Foundation Medicine	Foundation ACT Available in 2016 as LDT in a CLIA-certified laboratory	NGS	62 genes/multiple cancer types	Single base substitutions/indels with a sensitivity of >99% at mutant allele fraction of $\geq$0.5%
Personal Genome Diagnostics (PGDx)	Plasma SELECT 64 + MSI Available since 2015 as LDT in a CLIA-certified laboratory	NGS	64 genes/multiple caner types	Single base substitutions/indels with a sensitivity of >99% at mutant allele fraction of $\geq$0.5%

Data from Refs. [21,35,64–68]

mutations have the benefit of only considering variants that are present at a high allele fraction. This high percentage makes them insensitive to noise and artifact. These pipelines fail when trying to detect variants that make up a minority of sequences in a sea of normal DNA. Even pipelines that are designed to detect acquired variants are largely limited to the detection of sequence changes with a mutant allele fraction of greater than 5%. Less than 5%, artifact and noise confound results. There have been several innovations to remove artifacts or "noise" from NGS data. However, an understanding of the nature of NGS noise is required to discuss these approaches.

There are 3 main sources of noise, (1) true chemical changes to the DNA template (cytosine deamination), (2) variants that are introduced through library preparation (PCR artifact), (3) errors in the final "on-instrument" sequencing step. Cytosine deamination is a hydrolytic process in which cytosines are converted into uracil. This deamination leads to C:G to T:A conversions. Deamination occurs in vivo, in living cells, and is a means of mutation and perhaps evolution. Deamination can also occur artifactually, in vitro, at high temperatures (eg, those associated with PCR). Deamination, even if it is a rare event, can be a significant contributor to noise when sequencing individual molecules with NGS [36]. The process of amplifying DNA to create a sequencing library is another large source of noise. PCR error rates range from approximately 1×10^{-6} to 5×10^{-5} errors/bp using high-fidelity modern DNA polymerases [37]. Both amplicon-based and capture-based target enrichment strategies use PCR to amplify individual low-abundance DNA targets. Although there are typically higher cycle number PCR steps in amplicon-based approaches, no library preparations are immune to this artifact. Finally, it is well known that the quality of NGS sequence data decreases as read lengths increase. Bases near the end of a single molecule read have lower quality score and are less reliable than bases at the beginning. The nature of this noise is well demonstrated by a consistent lack of perfect overlap between "paired" reads (forward and reverse reads) on the Illumina platforms [38,39]. When taken together, these various sources of error combine to give mean error rates between 0.01% and 0.1% with loci-specific mutation rates as high as 1% or greater [28,40–42]. Without further noise reduction, such a high error rate would preclude meaningful use in ctDNA mutation detection.

The main approach to noise reduction in NGS data is elegant in its simplicity. The approach has been given a variety of names by a variety of laboratories (TEC-seq [28], Safe-seq [40], CAPP-Seq [29,43], and others [44–50]). It relies on the use of unique molecular identifiers (UMIs) and was first described in 2011 [40,51]. UMIs are short sequences, 4 to 12 bp, that uniquely identify each individual starting DNA molecule. When using capture-based library preparations, UMIs may be incorporated through ligation of random short DNA oligonucleotide sequences. UMIs may also simply be the sequence at the end of the random fragments of captured DNA. When using amplicon-based approaches, UMIs may be incorporated through the inclusion of a random string of Ns in the primers used for the first cycle DNA extension step. When sequencing is complete, these UMIs can be used to group reads into UMI "families." Each family consists of DNA derived from the same starting individual DNA fragment and all share the same UMI. All members of a given family should be identical. However, this is rarely the case. Differences found among individual family members represent PCR artifacts that were introduced during library preparation or errors in the "on-instrument" sequencing. This noise can be significantly reduced by developing a consensus sequence among the members of a UMI family. There is a balance between coverage depth (sensitivity) and specificity when writing the rules for developing a consensus sequence. At one extreme, one could use only large families with complete consensus among its members. Developing a consensus sequence from these families is easy; it is the sequence of its member, all of which are the same. Using only these families would lead to the exclusion of a large number of UMI families, poor coverage depth, but the near complete elimination of error. In the other extreme, one could force consensus among family members even with families with great diversity among individual reads, or use families with only a single read. This forced consensus would undoubtedly lead to the inclusion of noise/artifact. When striking the right balance, true read depths in the 1000s can be achieved for targeted gene panels with error rates of less than 1 error in 3 billion bases [28]. In addition, instrument-specific noise can be understood and perhaps corrected for short DNA fragments (of the type found in cfDNA) by pairing or stitching together paired end reads. Like members of a UMI family, the paired end reads from a single Illumina flow cell cluster should be identical. A variety of algorithms have be developed that can force this identity, each leading to a reduction in noise [39]. No approach could correct for artifacts that were introduced before library creation (eg, deamination). To account for this, groups are developing specific error cutoffs for individual genetic loci by sequencing cfDNA from large numbers of normal, otherwise healthy individuals. If each single nucleotide at each position of each gene is considered as a different "analyte" (to borrow a term from clinical chemists), this is just a return to the fundaments of developing cutoff values for a "negative" result. Using this approach, a mutation would only be detected if it was present at a level above that seen in the otherwise healthy, normal population.

VALIDATION OF CIRCULATING TUMOR DNA–next-GENERATION SEQUENCING ASSAYS

Although the clinical utility for testing ctDNA by NGS has yet to be proven for most indications, the increasing availability of packaged kits and bioinformatics solutions make ctDNA testing an appealing addition to laboratory testing menus. Upfront evaluation of the intended use of the panel to guide selection of the appropriate testing platform and to guide the validation study is essential, followed by analytical validation and clinical validation. The recently published Association for Molecular Pathology and College of American Pathologists (CAP) guidelines for validation of NGS-based oncology panels [52] and the joint review from the American Society for Clinical Oncology and CAP [34] are valuable resources for the design and validation of ctDNA testing within the laboratory.

The first phase of the validation establishes the performance characteristics of the assay, including analytical specificity and sensitivity. In the published Guardant laboratory developed test (LDT) validation, sensitivity was assessed by performing serial dilution studies with genomic DNA from healthy individuals (and reported at 2%–10% for single nucleotide variants) [35], whereas others have performed dilution series using genomes from combinations of annotated tumor cell lines [32]. Such methods are limited in their ability to replicate the unique biological characteristics of ctDNA. Newly available ctDNA reference materials (such as those available from SeraCare, Horizon Discovery, and others) contain synthetic variants at defined allelic frequencies and are engineered to approximate the biological features of ctDNA; such reference materials offer a convenient means of evaluating the analytical sensitivity across mutation types. In addition, standardized reference materials facilitate precision studies and allow for cross-platform comparisons that were previously challenging or unfeasible. This phase of validation also addresses the optimization of laboratory workflow, including plasma collection requirements, and DNA isolation to enrich for the maximum level of ctDNA within the cfDNA fraction.

Factors such as tumor type, size, disease stage, and the rate of DNA shedding into the circulation can limit the detection of ctDNA within the cfDNA fraction. Because analytical performance does not account for the biological variability of a disease, determining the clinical validity of a cfDNA assay is an essential next step [52]. A well-defined patient cohort, with samples representing the range of tumor types and intended uses, is required and can be accomplished using matched tumor and cfDNA samples. The presence of a mutation observed in the diagnostic tissue biopsy in ctDNA from a relapse sample can provide an internal positive control for the presence of ctDNA within the cfDNA [53].

Concordance rates between tissue and ctDNA NGS are reported in the range of 70% to 95% [29,54], but such concordance studies can be complicated by tumor heterogeneity and the presence of genomic variants from metastases within the ctDNA fraction that may not be present in the original tumor biopsy. Concordance rates for ctDNA NGS between laboratories, however, are not well characterized. In a recent report, Torga and Pienta compared ctDNA results from 40 patients with metastatic prostate cancer, collected during a single blood draw and shipped to 2 different Clinical Laboratory Improvement Amendments (CLIA)-certified laboratories [55]. Genetic alterations in the 42 genes covered by both platforms were compared, with very low overall congruence (3/40 samples or 7.5% with complete congruence with one or more reported alterations; 9/40 or 22.5% with complete congruence for no reported alterations; and 16/40 or 40% with no congruence). The disturbingly low congruence for commercially available testing (marketed to show high accuracy, specificity, and sensitivity) underscores the need for additional standardization and proficiency testing in this new arena of testing.

Additional considerations for validation include reporting of the quantity of ctDNA, in addition to mutations identified. Two metrics, mutant allele concentration (copies per volume) and mutant allele fraction (mutant as percent of total cfDNA), are used to quantify ctDNA, and when both are reported, these metrics can provide complementary information [21]. However, if serial assessment of mutation status over the course of disease is to be performed, a quantitative assessment of ctDNA (as a mutant allele concentration) instead of a relative metric (percent reactions that are mutant) is likely to be more precise, particularly at low concentrations [30].

In addition to the "technical noise" that can be reduced by bioinformatically, the presence of "biological noise" in the form of mutations associated with clonal hematopoiesis, observed in 5% to 10% of individuals over the age of 65, is another consideration for both assay design and interpretation for NGS testing of ctDNA [21,56].

FUTURE APPLICATIONS OF CIRCULATING TUMOR DNA

Circulating Tumor DNA as an Indicator of Treatment Response and Therapy Optimization

The amount of ctDNA in the serum or plasma is directly proportional to the size and stage of a tumor [9,57] and has been shown to also decrease in response to therapy [58,59]. Owing to its short half-life and rapid turnover, ctDNA may provide a more accurate snapshot of cancer cell dynamics in real time. A recent study in patients with metastatic colorectal cancers showed that early changes in ctDNA during chemotherapy strongly correlated with and could predict the later radiologic response. ctDNA fold-reduction was also a predictor for progression-free survival [60]. Similar studies in patients receiving treatment for metastatic melanoma have shown that resistance conferring mutations can be detected much earlier in the ctDNA of patients, before the evidence seen on imaging [61]. Thus, serial measurements of ctDNA can be extremely useful in monitoring clonal evolution and in identifying genomic changes that may predict development of resistance, at an earlier time point than radiographic detection and likely at a lower cost than medical imaging [30,62]. Limited studies report the detection of tumor response or resistance by ctDNA well before radiographic evidence of progression.

Circulating Tumor DNA in Cancer Screening

In the setting of a known cancer diagnosis, mutation detection from ctDNA has many advantages to tissue biopsy. However, the clinical utility of ctDNA testing in the asymptomatic patient is still unproven and quite challenging. A recent joint review emphasized prospective clinical trials as the most reliable demonstration of clinical utility, defined by the authors as high levels of evidence demonstrating that use of a test improves patient outcomes [34]. In 2016, both Guardant Health and Illumina announced initiatives (LUNAR and GRAIL, respectively) for the detection of early stage cancers, heralding a shift toward applying ctDNA analysis to early cancer detection in an asymptomatic patient with early-stage cancer. With this fundamental shift in application comes a need for increased sensitivity. In the context of a known cancer diagnosis, with the internal control of a known mutation or mutations from a diagnostic tissue biopsy, test specificity can be high; indeed, some groups have even focused assay development on maximizing specificity over sensitivity for the highest positive predictive value in this context [30]. However, the development of a ctDNA-based approach for cancer screening requires high sensitivity in addition to high specificity, as well as a large scale of clinical evidence and a sequencing approach that is both "broad and deep" [63,64].

Despite the enthusiasm, the use of ctDNA for screening will require technological and bioinformatic advances in addition to large prospective studies. A recently published study by Bettegowda and colleagues [9] evaluated the ability of ctDNA to detect the presence of tumor in a large cohort of patients; 640 patients with different tumor types were tested. They found that ctDNA was detectable in more than 75% of patients with advanced cancer, but only in about 47% of patients with stage I cancers. Another recent study on NSCLCs showed that ctDNA could be detected in 100% of the patients with stage II–IV disease, but dropped to only 50% in those with stage I disease [62]. Encouraging as they may be, unfortunately, these numbers are insufficient for cancer screening purposes and underscore the need for additional research and innovation for this application.

ctDNA is showing great promise as a biomarker, both in its presence as a proxy for tumor responsiveness or resistance and in its relative accessibility. Nevertheless, detecting the mutations harbored by ctDNA presents unique technical and bioinformatic challenges. Although the clinical utility for many ctDNA-based applications has yet to be established, tumor genotyping by ctDNA will play an integral role in the future diagnosis and care of patients with cancer.

REFERENCES

[1] McGranahan N, Swanton C. Clonal heterogeneity and tumor evolution: past, present, and the future. Cell 2017;168(4):613–28.

[2] Pantel K, Speicher MR. The biology of circulating tumor cells. Oncogene 2016;35(10):1216–24.

[3] Kai K, Dittmar RL, Sen S. Secretory microRNAs as biomarkers of cancer. Semin Cell Dev Biol 2018;78:22–36.

[4] Li A, Zhang T, Zheng M, et al. Exosomal proteins as potential markers of tumor diagnosis. J Hematol Oncol 2017;10(1):175.

[5] Joosse SA, Pantel K. Tumor-educated platelets as liquid biopsy in cancer patients. Cancer Cell 2015;28(5):552–4.

[6] Rabinowits G, Gercel-Taylor C, Day JM, et al. Exosomal microRNA: a diagnostic marker for lung cancer. Clin Lung Cancer 2009;10(1):42–6.

[7] Thakur BK, Zhang H, Becker A, et al. Double-stranded DNA in exosomes: a novel biomarker in cancer detection. Cell Res 2014;24(6):766–9.

[8] Best MG, Sol N, Kooi I, et al. RNA-Seq of tumor-educated platelets enables blood-based pan-cancer, multiclass, and molecular pathway cancer diagnostics. Cancer Cell 2015;28(5):666–76.

[9] Bettegowda C, Sausen M, Leary RJ, et al. Detection of circulating tumor DNA in early- and late-stage human malignancies. Sci Transl Med 2014;6(224):224ra224.

[10] Mandel P, Metais P. Les acides nucléiques du plasma sanguin chez l'homme. C R Seances Soc Biol Fil 1948; 142(3–4):241–3 [in Undetermined Language].

[11] Tan EM, Schur PH, Carr RI, et al. Deoxybonucleic acid (DNA) and antibodies to DNA in the serum of patients with systemic lupus erythematosus. J Clin Invest 1966; 45(11):1732–40.

[12] Leon SA, Shapiro B, Sklaroff DM, et al. Free DNA in the serum of cancer patients and the effect of therapy. Cancer Res 1977;37(3):646–50.

[13] Lo YM, Corbetta N, Chamberlain PF, et al. Presence of fetal DNA in maternal plasma and serum. Lancet 1997; 350(9076):485–7.

[14] Lo YM, Tein MS, Lau TK, et al. Quantitative analysis of fetal DNA in maternal plasma and serum: implications for noninvasive prenatal diagnosis. Am J Hum Genet 1998;62(4):768–75.

[15] Lo YM, Chan KC, Sun H, et al. Maternal plasma DNA sequencing reveals the genome-wide genetic and mutational profile of the fetus. Sci Transl Med 2010;2(61): 61ra91.

[16] Snyder MW, Kircher M, Hill AJ, et al. Cell-free DNA comprises an in vivo nucleosome footprint that informs its tissues-of-origin. Cell 2016;164(1–2):57–68.

[17] Wang W, Kong P, Ma G, et al. Characterization of the release and biological significance of cell-free DNA from breast cancer cell lines. Oncotarget 2017;8(26): 43180–91.

[18] Diehl F, Schmidt K, Choti MA, et al. Circulating mutant DNA to assess tumor dynamics. Nat Med 2008;14(9): 985–90.

[19] Alix-Panabieres C, Schwarzenbach H, Pantel K. Circulating tumor cells and circulating tumor DNA. Annu Rev Med 2012;63:199–215.

[20] Lecomte T, Ceze N, Dorval E, et al. Circulating free tumor DNA and colorectal cancer. Gastroenterol Clin Biol 2010;34(12):662–81.

[21] Wan JCM, Massie C, Garcia-Corbacho J, et al. Liquid biopsies come of age: towards implementation of circulating tumour DNA. Nat Rev Cancer 2017;17(4):223–38.

[22] Szpechcinski A, Chorostowska-Wynimko J, Struniawski R, et al. Cell-free DNA levels in plasma of patients with non-small-cell lung cancer and inflammatory lung disease. Br J Cancer 2015;113(3):476–83.

[23] Kis O, Kaedbey R, Chow S, et al. Circulating tumour DNA sequence analysis as an alternative to multiple myeloma bone marrow aspirates. Nat Commun 2017; 8:15086.

[24] Corro C, Hejhal T, Poyet C, et al. Detecting circulating tumor DNA in renal cancer: An open challenge. Exp Mol Pathol 2017;102(2):255–61.

[25] NCCN (National Comprehensive Cancer Network) Clinical Practice Guidelines. Non-small cell lung cancer (Version 3.2018). 2018.

[26] Kwapisz D. The first liquid biopsy test approved. Is it a new era of mutation testing for non-small cell lung cancer? Ann Transl Med 2017;5(3):46.

[27] Heitzer E, Ulz P, Geigl JB, et al. Non-invasive detection of genome-wide somatic copy number alterations by liquid biopsies. Mol Oncol 2016;10(3):494–502.

[28] Phallen J, Sausen M, Adleff V, et al. Direct detection of early-stage cancers using circulating tumor DNA. Sci Transl Med 2017;9(403) [pii:eaan2415].

[29] Newman AM, Lovejoy AF, Klass DM, et al. Integrated digital error suppression for improved detection of circulating tumor DNA. Nat Biotechnol 2016;34(5): 547–55.

[30] Oxnard GR, Paweletz CP, Kuang Y, et al. Noninvasive detection of response and resistance in EGFR-mutant lung cancer using quantitative next-generation genotyping of cell-free plasma DNA. Clin Cancer Res 2014; 20(6):1698–705.

[31] Thress KS, Brant R, Carr TH, et al. EGFR mutation detection in ctDNA from NSCLC patient plasma: a cross-platform comparison of leading technologies to support the clinical development of AZD9291. Lung Cancer 2015;90(3):509–15.

[32] Paweletz CP, Sacher AG, Raymond CK, et al. Bias-corrected targeted next-generation sequencing for rapid, multiplexed detection of actionable alterations in cell-free DNA from advanced lung cancer patients. Clin Cancer Res 2016;22(4):915–22.

[33] Luke JJ, Oxnard GR, Paweletz CP, et al. Realizing the potential of plasma genotyping in an age of genotype-directed therapies. J Natl Cancer Inst 2014;106(8) [pii: dju214].

[34] Merker JD, Oxnard GR, Compton C, et al. Circulating tumor DNA analysis in patients with cancer: american society of clinical oncology and college of American pathologists joint review. J Clin Oncol 2018;36(16): 1631–41.

[35] Lanman RB, Mortimer SA, Zill OA, et al. Analytical and clinical validation of a digital sequencing panel for quantitative, highly accurate evaluation of cell-free circulating tumor DNA. PLoS One 2015;10(10):e0140712.

[36] Chen G, Mosier S, Gocke CD, et al. Cytosine deamination is a major cause of baseline noise in next-generation sequencing. Mol Diagn Ther 2014;18(5):587–93.

[37] Cline J, Braman JC, Hogrefe HH. PCR fidelity of pfu DNA polymerase and other thermostable DNA polymerases. Nucleic Acids Res 1996;24(18):3546–51.

[38] Kwon S, Lee B, Yoon S. CASPER: context-aware scheme for paired-end reads from high-throughput amplicon sequencing. BMC Bioinformatics 2014;15(Suppl 9):S10.

[39] Zhang J, Kobert K, Flouri T, et al. PEAR: a fast and accurate Illumina Paired-End reAd mergeR. Bioinformatics 2014;30(5):614–20.

[40] Kinde I, Wu J, Papadopoulos N, et al. Detection and quantification of rare mutations with massively parallel sequencing. Proc Natl Acad Sci U S A 2011;108(23): 9530–5.

[41] Nothnagel M, Herrmann A, Wolf A, et al. Technology-specific error signatures in the 1000 Genomes Project data. Hum Genet 2011;130(4):505–16.

[42] Quail MA, Kozarewa I, Smith F, et al. A large genome center's improvements to the Illumina sequencing system. Nat Methods 2008;5(12):1005–10.

[43] Newman AM, Bratman SV, To J, et al. An ultrasensitive method for quantitating circulating tumor DNA with broad patient coverage. Nat Med 2014;20(5):548–54.

[44] Stahlberg A, Krzyzanowski PM, Jackson JB, et al. Simple, multiplexed, PCR-based barcoding of DNA enables sensitive mutation detection in liquid biopsies using sequencing. Nucleic Acids Res 2016;44(11):e105.

[45] Kou R, Lam H, Duan H, et al. Benefits and challenges with applying unique molecular identifiers in next generation sequencing to detect low frequency mutations. PLoS One 2016;11(1):e0146638.

[46] Eijkelenboom A, Kamping EJ, Kastner-van Raaij AW, et al. Reliable next-generation sequencing of formalin-fixed, paraffin-embedded tissue using single molecule tags. J Mol Diagn 2016;18(6):851–63.

[47] Schmitt MW, Fox EJ, Prindle MJ, et al. Sequencing small genomic targets with high efficiency and extreme accuracy. Nat Methods 2015;12(5):423–5.

[48] Kukita Y, Matoba R, Uchida J, et al. High-fidelity target sequencing of individual molecules identified using barcode sequences: de novo detection and absolute quantitation of mutations in plasma cell-free DNA from cancer patients. DNA Res 2015;22(4):269–77.

[49] Schmitt MW, Kennedy SR, Salk JJ, et al. Detection of ultra-rare mutations by next-generation sequencing. Proc Natl Acad Sci U S A 2012;109(36):14508–13.

[50] Kivioja T, Vaharautio A, Karlsson K, et al. Counting absolute numbers of molecules using unique molecular identifiers. Nat Methods 2011;9(1):72–4.

[51] Jabara CB, Jones CD, Roach J, et al. Accurate sampling and deep sequencing of the HIV-1 protease gene using a Primer ID. Proc Natl Acad Sci U S A 2011;108(50): 20166–71.

[52] Jennings LJ, Arcila ME, Corless C, et al. Guidelines for validation of next-generation sequencing-based oncology panels: a joint consensus recommendation of the association for molecular pathology and College of American Pathologists. J Mol Diagn 2017;19(3): 341–65.

[53] Sholl LM, Aisner DL, Allen TC, et al. Liquid biopsy in lung cancer: a perspective from members of the

pulmonary pathology society. Arch Pathol Lab Med 2016;140(8):825–9.
[54] Schwaederle M, Husain H, Fanta PT, et al. Use of Liquid biopsies in clinical oncology: pilot experience in 168 patients. Clin Cancer Res 2016;22(22):5497–505.
[55] Torga G, Pienta KJ. Patient-paired sample congruence between 2 commercial liquid biopsy tests. JAMA Oncol 2018;4(6):868–70.
[56] Jaiswal S, Fontanillas P, Flannick J, et al. Age-related clonal hematopoiesis associated with adverse outcomes. N Engl J Med 2014;371(26):2488–98.
[57] Thierry AR, Mouliere F, Gongora C, et al. Origin and quantification of circulating DNA in mice with human colorectal cancer xenografts. Nucleic Acids Res 2010; 38(18):6159–75.
[58] Shinozaki M, O'Day SJ, Kitago M, et al. Utility of circulating B-RAF DNA mutation in serum for monitoring melanoma patients receiving biochemotherapy. Clin Cancer Res 2007;13(7):2068–74.
[59] Calapre L, Warburton L, Millward M, et al. Circulating tumour DNA (ctDNA) as a liquid biopsy for melanoma. Cancer Lett 2017;404:62–9.
[60] Tie J, Kinde I, Wang Y, et al. Circulating tumor DNA as an early marker of therapeutic response in patients with metastatic colorectal cancer. Ann Oncol 2015;26(8): 1715–22.
[61] Gray ES, Rizos H, Reid AL, et al. Circulating tumor DNA to monitor treatment response and detect acquired resistance in patients with metastatic melanoma. Oncotarget 2015;6(39):42008–18.
[62] Bratman SV, Newman AM, Alizadeh AA, et al. Potential clinical utility of ultrasensitive circulating tumor DNA detection with CAPP-Seq. Expert Rev Mol Diagn 2015; 15(6):715–9.
[63] Aravanis AM, Lee M, Klausner RD. Next-generation sequencing of circulating tumor DNA for early cancer detection. Cell 2017;168(4):571–4.
[64] Webb S. The cancer bloodhounds. Nat Biotechnol 2016; 34(11):1090–4.
[65] Guardant Health. Guardant 360. Available at: http://www.guardanthealth.com/guardant360/. Accessed August 24, 2018.
[66] Personal genome diagnostics. PlasmaSELECT™ 64 + MSI. Available at: http://www.personalgenome.com/wp-content/uploads/2017/04/PS-64_MSI-_TESTBUL_CS-002-002.pdf. Accessed August 24, 2018.
[67] Foundation ACT. Analytical validation of the FoundationACT™ ctDNA assay. Available at: http://info.foundationmedicine.com/hubfs/New%20Corporate%20Site%20Documents/FoundationACT_AVWhitePaper.pdf. Accessed August 24, 2018.
[68] US Food & Drug Administration. Premarket approval P150044: Cobas EGFR MUTATION TEST V2. Available at: https://www.accessdata.fda.gov/scripts/cdrh/cfdocs/cfpma/pma.cfm?id=P150044. Accessed August 24, 2018.

Advances in Molecular Pathology 1 (2018) 193–208
ADVANCES IN MOLECULAR PATHOLOGY

Therapy Implications of DNA Mismatch Repair Deficiency, Microsatellite Instability, and Tumor Mutation Burden

Maryam Shirazi, MD, Antonia R. Sepulveda, MD, PhD*
Department of Pathology and Cell Biology, Columbia University Medical Center, 630 West 168th Street, VC14-212, New York, NY 10032, USA

KEYWORDS

• Microsatellite instability • DNA mismatch repair • Tumor mutation burden • Solid tumors • Cancer treatment • Cancer immunotherapy

KEY POINTS

- Microsatellite instability testing in cancers is conventionally used for Lynch syndrome screening and prognosis stratification.
- Recently, microsatellite instability has been introduced as a biomarker of tumor response to immunotherapy regardless of tumor site.
- All tumors with microsatellite instability have high tumor mutation burden, which may be used as a genomic biomarker of response to immunotherapy in some settings.
- Microsatellite instability is detected across a wide range of epithelial and nonepithelial tumors, highlighting the need of extending microsatellite instability testing to different cancer types.
- Immunohistochemistry and polymerase chain reaction assays are able to adequately detect tumors with microsatellite instability; however, newer testing approaches like next-generation sequencing platforms are emerging.

CANCER PRECISION THERAPY: PAST, PRESENT, AND FUTURE

Cancer therapy has evolved extensively over the past few years with the recognition of different cancer subtypes with distinct molecular signatures for which novel targeted and precision therapies can be used. One of these distinct molecular phenotypes is microsatellite instability (MSI), which has been reported in a diverse group of cancers, including colorectal, endometrial, gastric, prostate, ovarian cancer, and glioblastomas [1,2]. MSI status, in particular high levels of MSI (MSI-H), is known to be a prognostic biomarker across different cancer types, especially colorectal cancer (CRC) [3]. However, the recent introduction of MSI status as a predictive biomarker of cancer response to immune checkpoint blockade regardless of tumor site [4] and the subsequent approval of pembrolizumab as a programmed cell death-1 (PD-1) inhibitor by the US Food and Drug Administration (FDA) in 2017 for the treatment of all unresponsive or metastatic MSI-H cancers irrespective

Disclosure Statement: The authors have nothing to disclose.

*Corresponding author, *E-mail address:* as4400@cumc.columbia.edu

https://doi.org/10.1016/j.yamp.2018.07.010
2589-4080/18/

of tissue origin, warrants a more in-depth understanding of MSI frequency across a wider range of cancers as well as diagnostic tools available for the detection of MSI status and the potential pitfalls and limitations associated with each one of them, prognostic and predictive value of MSI status in the treatment of different cancers, and a review of the current available data on treating MSI-H cancers with immune checkpoint inhibitors across different tumor types. The relevance of MSI as a biomarker to identify tumors that are candidates for immune checkpoint blockade therapy continues to increase as more drugs become available and receive approval by FDA and the regulatory agencies in other countries.

MOLECULAR BASIS OF MICROSATELLITE INSTABILITY

Microsatellites are tandem repeats of short nucleotide sequences across the genome that are more prone to errors during DNA replication than other genomic segments, resulting in length alterations of these repeats within coding and noncoding regions of genes [5]. The DNA mismatch repair (MMR) system is responsible for the correction of these errors and preserving genetic fidelity through its active proteins, MLH1, PMS2, MSH2, and MSH6 [6]. Deficiency of the MMR system (dMMR) occurs through a number of different mechanisms including germline mutations in MMR genes that usually underlie hereditary nonpolyposis colorectal cancer (Lynch syndrome), whereas somatic mutations and inherited epigenetic modifications such as germline 3′-end deletions in *EPCAM* gene and subsequent methylation and silencing of the downstream *MSH2* gene rarely occur in patients with the Lynch syndrome [7]. The most frequent alterations in sporadic cancers are epigenetic alterations in MMR genes, especially hypermethylation of the *MLH1* gene promotor resulting in *MLH1* gene silencing [8]. Other alterations that occur in sporadic dMMR cancers include decreased histone acetylation [9] and microRNA-induced downregulation of MMR proteins expression, particularly through pathways related to miR-155 and miR-21 [10,11]. Impairment of the MMR system results in a mutator phenotype [12] and subsequent hypermutability state called "microsatellite instability" (MSI). MSI tumors accumulate numerous frameshift mutations and to a lesser extent single nucleotide alterations and small insertions and deletions (indels) within microsatellites in coding and noncoding regions of the genome, resulting in the production of truncated and nonfunctional proteins that are necessary for DNA repair, cell signaling, and apoptosis [13,14], leading to the eventual development of cancer.

DNA POLYMERASE EPSILON AND DNA POLYMERASE DELTA 1 EXONUCLEASE DOMAIN MUTATIONS IN ULTRAMUTATED CANCERS

The proofreading activity of exonuclease domains of DNA polymerases Pol δ-1 and Pol ε is another essential mechanism for the correction of mispaired bases during DNA replication and tumors with germline or somatic mutations in exonuclease domains of *POLE* and *POLD1* genes, which encode the catalytic subunits of Pol δ-1 and Pol ε, display an ultramutated phenotype with a high rate of single nucleotide mutations (>100 mutations/megabase (Mb) of genome) [15]. Somatic mutations in *POLE* have been described in 1% to 3% of CRCs [16] and about 7% of endometrial cancers (EC) [17], whereas very few cases of somatic mutations in *POLD1* have been described. Overall, it has been shown that CRCs and ECs with *POLE* somatic mutations have a favorable prognosis, which is thought to be due to high antigenicity that provokes a strong antitumor immune response. Interestingly, these tumors are usually microsatellite stable (MSS), with just a few *POLE* mutated tumors reported to be MSI due to somatic mutations in MMR genes. Germline mutations in the exonuclease domains of *POLE* and *POLD1* genes have been recently reported to be associated with "polymerase proofreading-associated polyposis", a condition that is characterized by multiple colon adenomas and familial CRCs [18]. *POLD1* germline mutations are associated with familial CRCs and these patients are also more predisposed to other cancers, such as ECs and breast cancers [19]. *POLE* germline mutations have also been associated with familial cases of CRC in addition to EC [20]. Patients with germline mutations in *POLE* and *POLD1* genes, carry a spectrum of phenotypes ranging from several adenomas with slow progression to cancer, to large adenomas, or early onset cancer [21]. Further insight into the mechanisms behind DNA polymerase proofreading domain mutations will help with implication of these genetic variants as cancer biomarkers and potential therapeutic targets.

DETECTION OF MISMATCH REPAIR DEFICIENCY BY IMMUNOHISTOCHEMICAL STAINS AND MICROSATELLITE STATUS BY POLYMERASE CHAIN REACTION

Immunohistochemical stains (IHC) to evaluate the expression of the main 4 MMR proteins and polymerase chain reaction (PCR) to determine MSI status using stablished panels of microsatellites or short tandem repeats are the main approaches used in the clinical setting for the detection of MMR deficiency in tumors. IHC to evaluate the expression of the 4 main DNA MMR proteins (MLH1, PMS2, MSH2, and MSH6) is performed on formalin-fixed paraffin-embedded sections of tumors. MLH1 dimerizes with PMS2 or MLH3, whereas MSH2 dimerizes with MSH6 or MSH3 to form heterodimers, resulting in stable protein complexes. However, PMS2 and MSH6 only form heterodimers with MLH1 and MSH2, respectively; hence, PMS2 and MSH6 are unstable in the absence of their obligatory partners, resulting in concurrent loss of MLH1/PMS2 or MSH2/MSH6 in *MLH1* or *MSH2* gene mutations, respectively; whereas, mutations in *PMS2* or *MSH6* genes result in isolated loss of PMS2 or MSH6 proteins [22,23]. The advantages of IHC include wide availability, reliable detection of deficiency in MMR protein expression, and the identification of which MMR protein(s) are lost in the tumor. However, IHC may not detect some qualitative protein changes, such as some missense mutations where the protein is dysfunctional yet antigenically active [22,23]. Furthermore, IHC is prone to technical errors, occasional false-deficient MMR reported results owing to heterogeneous staining patterns in MSS tumors [24], false-proficient MMR results presumably due to defects in other proteins involved in the MMR pathway (which are not examined by IHC), and interobserver variability, especially in aberrant or indeterminate expression patterns [25].

MSI PCR testing is an effective method to detect MMR-deficient tumors by comparing the alterations in the length of microsatellite short tandem repeats in the tumor with nonneoplastic tissue and it is widely considered as the gold standard diagnostic tool. This assay is highly reproducible between different centers owing to the availability of proficiency testing programs for the assay; furthermore, it allows for the detection of MSI that results from nontruncating missense mutations in MMR proteins, which may not be detected by IHC, as well as the MMR deficiency caused by genes other than those tested by IHC [26]. The National Cancer Institute (NCI) consensus meeting in 1997 recommended a reference panel (NCI-MSI panel) of 5 microsatellite markers to be tested in CRC, including 2 mononucleotide (BAT25 and BAT26) and 3 dinucleotide markers (D2S123, D5S346, and D17S250). Using this panel, a tumor is classified into 3 possible categories: MSI-H if 2 or more of the 5 markers or more than 30% of markers show instability, MSI-low if 1 of the 5 markers or fewer than 30% of markers shows instability, and MSS if no markers show instability [27]. Although this panel is currently widely used, the results should be interpreted with caution due to some limitations. Dinucleotide repeats are less sensitive than mononucleotide repeats for the detection of MSI-H tumors. Dinucleotide repeats in the NCI-MSI panel show instability in only 60% to 80% of MSI-H tumors [28], leading to an underestimation of MSI-H tumors in cases with instability at a large number of dinucleotide repeats and an overestimation of MSI-low tumors due to a smaller number of mononucleotide repeats tested in the panel. When only dinucleotide repeats are mutated in the NCI-MSI panel, a secondary panel of markers with mononucleotide repeats is recommended to exclude an MSI-low tumor [29]. To overcome part of these limitations, updated NCI guidelines in 2004 suggested that a pentaplex panel of 5 quasimonomorphic mononucleotide repeats might be more sensitive and specific to detect MSI-H colorectal and gastric tumors than other microsatellite markers [29,30]. Furthermore, because there is great diversity in the microsatellite loci which are altered in different MSI-H tumor types, additional markers may be needed to be added to the current panel to make it applicable to a wider range of tumors [31]. More recently, multiple next-generation sequencing platforms have been described for MSI detection in tumors with reportedly comparable sensitivity and specificity to MMR IHC and MSI PCR [32–34]. In summary, both IHC and MSI PCR testing are highly accurate diagnostic tools with more than 95% concordance in the clinical setting; however, owing to the limitations with each of these methods, they remain complementary to one another, with PCR detecting the functional defects of MMR pathway proteins and MMR IHC highlighting the specific protein(s) that are deficient [14].

TUMOR MUTATION BURDEN AS A PREDICTIVE GENOMIC BIOMARKER OF RESPONSE TO IMMUNE CHECKPOINT BLOCKADE THERAPY

Tumor mutation burden (TMB) refers to the total number of mutations per coding region of a tumor genome and has recently emerged as a potential predictive biomarker of response to immunotherapy. Initially, it was noted that tumors such as melanomas and non–small cell lung cancers, which carry a high number of somatic mutations and resultant neoantigens due to exposure to mutagenic factors such as ultraviolent light or smoking, show a striking response to immunotherapy [35,36], highlighting that the cancer genomic landscape may predict the response to immune checkpoint blockade. Further research revealed that TMB could help to predict response to immunotherapy across a wider range of tumors. In a study conducted by FoundationMedicine, more than 100,000 human cancer genomes across hundreds of tumor types were analyzed and it was concluded that a subset of patients across almost all cancer types, including very rare tumors, show high TMB levels and could potentially benefit from immunotherapy [37].

In a study of 2013 patients with CRC in which TMB levels were compared with the results of MSI status, 100% of MSI-H tumors were also TMB-high, but also almost 22% of MSS tumors were identified as TMB-high with mutations in *POLE* and *POLD1*, indicating that using TMB levels as a biomarker of response to immunotherapy may help with including a larger number of patients who could benefit from these therapies [38].

ASSESSMENT OF TUMOR MUTATION BURDEN USING NEXT-GENERATION SEQUENCING PLATFORMS

Measuring the total mutational load in tumors could be done through whole exome sequencing, but this method is expensive and labor intensive. More recently, tumor DNA sequencing with a hybrid capture-based next-generation sequencing diagnostic platform was introduced by FoundationOne, enabling the profiling of a smaller fraction of the genome (approximately 1.2 Mb, accounting for about 3% of the genome), which could act as a substitute to calculate the mutation burden in tumors. To determine TMB, the number of detected somatic mutations in this by next-generation sequencing in this fraction of genome id quantified and this value is extrapolated to the whole exome using a validated algorithm in which all short variant alterations, base substitutions, indels, and coding variants (including the silent alterations) are counted; whereas, noncoding variants, alterations with known or likely pathogenic (known somatic alterations in the COSMIC database and truncations in tumor suppressor genes, respectively), and predicted germline mutations are excluded. TMB is measured as the number of eligible alterations per Mb of genome and is divided into 3 groups: low (1–5 mutations/Mb), intermediate (6–19 mutations/Mb), and high ($\geq$ 20 mutations/Mb) [39,40].

IDENTIFICATION OF NEOANTIGEN-SPECIFIC LYMPHOCYTES IN THE PERIPHERAL BLOOD

Functional analysis in patients with MSI-H tumors responding to immunotherapy shows an expansion in cancer-resident monoclonal cytotoxic T lymphocytes, which are specific and reactive to mutant neoantigens in tumor [4]. These neoantigen-specific lymphocytes have been detected at low levels in the serum of patients with melanomas and they seem to be similar to tissue-resident lymphocytes and able to recognize autologous tumors [41]. Although these approaches are in early stages, they provide noninvasive strategies to detect biomarkers for targeted therapies and precision medicine.

FREQUENCY OF MICROSATELLITE INSTABILITY ACROSS HUMAN CANCERS

MSI has been studied extensively in specific cancers, such as colorectal, endometrial, and gastric adenocarcinomas [3,42–44]. DNA MMR deficiency and the MSI phenotype have been shown to have 3 main clinical implications, including screening for Lynch syndrome, prognosis stratification (these tumors generally have a more favorable prognosis), and prediction of response to chemotherapeutic agents in early stage CRC, although the latter is controversial [2,3]. With the introduction of MSI as an actionable biomarker for immune checkpoint blockade therapy, an increasing number of studies have been carried out to determine the dMMR and MSI status across a wider range of cancers to recognize tumors that may show response to immunotherapy [1,45,46] (Fig. 1, Table 1). Cortes-Ciriano and colleagues [46] analyzed the frequency of MSI events in 7919 tumors across 23 cancer types and showed that there was a significant variation in MSI events within and between tumors, ranging from 0.2% in lung adenocarcinomas to 28.3% in endometrial adenocarcinomas, concluding that the frequency of MSI was approximately 10 times higher in 5 MSI-prone tumors (uterine corpus endometrial carcinoma, stomach, colon, rectal, and esophageal adenocarcinomas) compared with other tumors. Bonneville and colleagues [45] identified MSI in 3.8% of cases across 27 different cancer types with a widely variable prevalence of MSI from 31.4% in endometrial adenocarcinoma to 0.25% in glioblastoma multiforme (see Fig. 1, Table 1). Interestingly, these studies detected MSI in tumors in which this phenotype had not been well-described previously, notably adrenocortical tumor (~5%), cervical squamous cell carcinoma (~2.5%), and mesothelioma (2.4%) [1,46], highlighting the value of extending MSI testing to a wider range of tumors to identify potential candidates for immunotherapy. Overall, current frequency data demonstrate significant interstudy variability with regard to MSI status in different tumor types partially due to lack of standardized testing. In addition, these

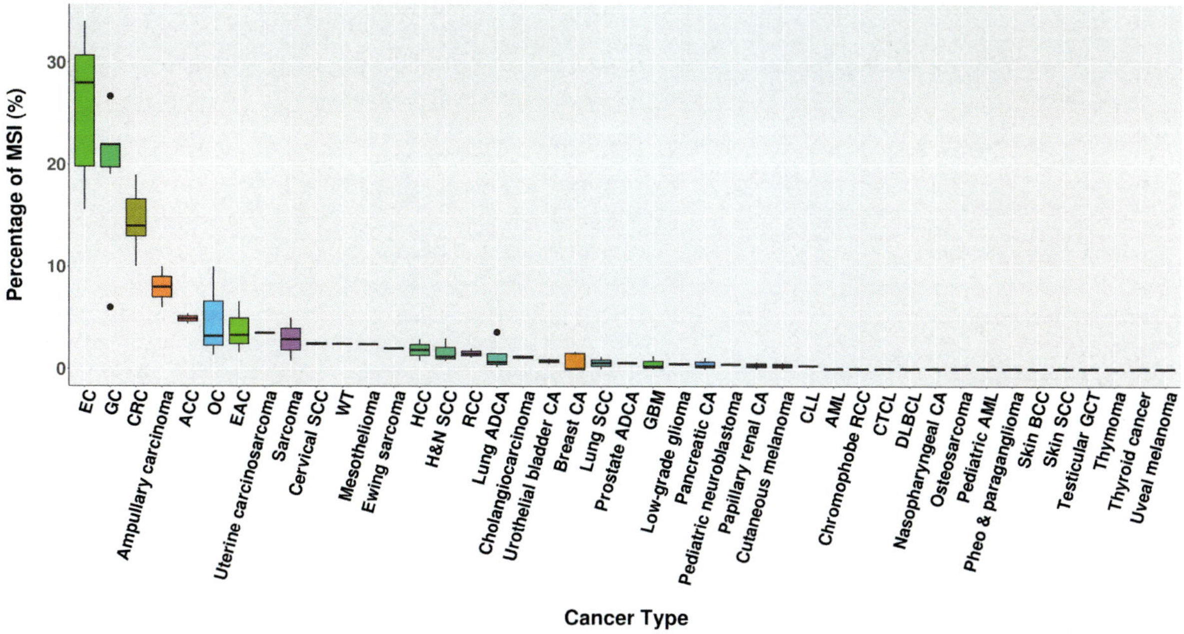

FIG. 1 Boxplot of microsatellite instability (MSI) frequencies by cancer type reported in the literature. Each bar represents 25th to 75th quartile ranges of MSI percent for cancer type. Whiskers extend to $\pm$1.5 of the interquartile range (IQR). ACC, adrenocortical carcinoma; AML, acute myeloid leukemia; breast CA, breast carcinoma; cervical SCC, cervical squamous cell carcinoma; chromophobe RCC, chromophobe renal cell carcinoma; CLL, chronic lymphocytic leukemia; CRC, colorectal cancer; CTCL, cutaneous T-cell lymphoma; DLBCL, diffuse large B-cell lymphoma; EAC, esophageal adenocarcinoma; EC, endometrial cancer; GBM, glioblastoma multiforme; GC, gastric cancer; H&N SCC, head and neck squamous cell carcinoma; HCC, hepatocellular carcinoma; lung ADCA, lung adenocarcinoma; lung SCC, lung squamous cell carcinoma; nasopharyngeal CA, nasopharyngeal carcinoma; OC, ovarian cancer; pancreatic CA, pancreatic carcinoma; papillary renal CA, papillary renal cell carcinoma; pediatric AML, pediatric acute myeloid leukemia; prostate ADCA, prostate adenocarcinoma; RCC, renal cell carcinoma; skin BCC, skin basal cell carcinoma; skin SCC, skin squamous cell carcinoma; testicular GCT, testicular germ cell tumor; urothelial bladder CA, urothelial bladder carcinoma; WT, Wilms tumor.

data underline the necessity of expanding MSI testing to a larger group of patients with different cancers who are not routinely examined.

PROGNOSTIC AND PREDICTIVE IMPLICATIONS OF MICROSATELLITE INSTABILITY TESTING

Prognostic and Predictive Role of Microsatellite Instability in Colorectal Cancer

MSI is detected in approximately 15% of all CRCs, including sporadic cases (12%) and hereditary nonpolyposis CRC–Lynch syndrome (3%) [47]. MSI CRCs have a distinctive phenotypic and clinical picture consisting of poor differentiation, mucin production, increased tumor infiltrating lymphocytes, right-side predominance, Crohn's-like lymphoid reaction, diagnosis at earlier stages, and less metastasis [48]. Several systematic reviews have shown that MSI CRCs are associated with a more favorable prognosis [49–51] and a significantly lower recurrence rate [52,53]. The colorectal molecular testing guidelines released by the American Society for Clinical Pathology, College of American Pathologists, Association for Molecular Pathology, and American Society of Clinical Oncology recommend that clinicians should order MMR status testing in patients with CRCs for the identification of patients at high risk for Lynch syndrome and/or prognostic stratification [3].

The better prognosis of MSI-H CRCs is believed to be associated with an accelerated antitumor immune response with an increase in tumor infiltrating T cells in response to specific tumor antigens, at least in part owing to the production of truncated peptides (neoantigens) as the result of numerous frameshift mutations.

TABLE 1
The Frequency of Microsatellite Instability Across Different Cancer Types Reported in the Literature

Cancer Type	MSI Frequency % (Method of Detection)	References
Endometrial cancer	31.37 (NGS), 28.3 (NGS), 34 (MSI, IHC), 20 (MSI), 32 (MSI, IHC), 22 (MSI), 17 (MSI, IHC), 15.6 (MSI), 19.6 (MSI, IHC), 28 (MSI, IHC)	[45,46,66,68–73,75]
Stomach adenocarcinoma	26.7 (MSI), 19 (NGS), 21.9 (NGS), 22 (NGS), 22 (MSI, IHC), 6 (NGS)	[43,45,79,109,110]
Colorectal adenocarcinoma	(19/5)[a] (NGS),16.6 (NGS),14 (NGS), 10 (MSI, methylation assay)	[45,46,110,111]
Ampullary carcinoma	10 (MSI, IHC), 6 (IHC)	[112,113]
Adrenocortical carcinoma	5.4 (NGS), 4.4 (NGS)	[45,46]
Ovarian cancer	1.37 (NGS), 3.2 (NGS),10[b] (MSI,IHC)	[45,46,114]
Esophageal adenocarcinoma	1.6 (NGS), 3.3 (NGS), 6.6 (MSI, IHC)	[45,46,115]
Uterine carcinosarcoma	3.51 (NGS)	[45]
Sarcoma	0.78 (NSG), 5 (MSI, IHC)	[45,116]
Cervical squamous cell carcinoma	2.62 (NGS), 2.3 (NGS)	[45,46]
Wilms tumor	2.44 (NGS)	[45]
Mesothelioma	2.41 (NGS)	[45]
Ewing sarcoma	2 (MSI, IHC)	[117]
Hepatocellular carcinoma	0.8 (NGS), 2.9 (NGS), 16[c] (MSI, IHC)	[45,46,136]
Head and neck squamous cell carcinoma	0.78 (NGS),1.2 (NGS), 3 (MSI)	[45,46,118]
Renal cell carcinoma	1.47 (NGS),1.1 (NGS), 2 (MSI, IHC)	[45,46,119]
Lung adenocarcinoma	0.53 (NGS), 0.2 (NGS), 3.6 (MSI), 0.8 (IHC)	[45,46,120,121]
Cholangiocarcinoma	1.35 (NGS), 0.98 (MSI, IHC)	[45,122]
Urothelial bladder cancer	0.49 (NGS), 0.8 (NGS), 1[d] (MSI, IHC)	[45,46,123]
Breast cancer	1.53 (NGS), 1.7 (NGS), 0 (MSI), 0 (MSI), 0 (MSI, IHC)	[45,46,124–126]
Lung squamous cell carcinoma	0.6 (NGS), 1.2 (NGS), 0 (MSI)	[45,46,120]
Prostate adenocarcinoma	0.6 (NGS), 0.6 (NGS)	[45,46]
Glioblastoma multiforme	0.25 (NGS),1.3 (NGS), 0 (MSI, IHC)	[45,46,127]
Low-grade glioma	0.39 (NGS), 0.6 (NGS)	[45,46]
Pancreatic cancer	0 (NGS), 1.1 (NGS), 0.3 (MSI, IHC)	[45,46,128]
Skin sebaceous neoplasm	25.7 (MSI,IHC), 60 (MSI)	[134,135]
Pediatric neuroblastoma	0.45 (NGS)	[45]
Papillary renal cell carcinoma	0 (NGS), 0.7 (NGS)	[45,46]
Cutaneous melanoma	0.64 (NGS), 0 (NGS), 11 (MSI)	[45,46,129]
Chronic lymphocytic leukemia	0.3 (NGS)	[45]
Acute myeloid leukemia	0 (NGS)	[45]
Chromophobe renal cell carcinoma	0 (NGS)	[45]

(continued on next page)

TABLE 1
(continued)

Cancer Type	MSI Frequency % (Method of Detection)	References
Cutaneous T-cell lymphoma	0 (NGS)	[45]
Diffuse large B-cell lymphoma	0 (NGS)	[45]
Nasopharyngeal carcinoma	0 (NGS)	[45]
Osteosarcoma	0 (MSI)	[130]
Pediatric acute myeloid leukemia	0 (NGS)	[45]
Pheochromocytoma and paraganglioma	0 (NGS), 0 (NGS)	[45,46]
Skin basal cell carcinoma	0 (MSI)	[131]
Skin squamous cell carcinoma	0 (MSI)	[131]
Testicular germ cell tumor	0 (NGS), 0 (MSI, IHC)	[45,132]
Thymoma	0 (NGS)	[45]
Thyroid cancer	0 (NGS), 0 (NGS), 50[c] (MSI)	[45,46,133]
Uveal melanoma	0 (NGS)	[45]

Abbreviations: IHC, immunohistochemical stain; MSI, microsatellite instability analysis by polymerase chain reaction for microsatellite marker; NGS, next-generation sequencing.

[a] In this study, MSI frequency was determined separately in colon cancer (~19%) and rectal cancer (~5%).

[b] Meta-analysis of 1234 patients in 22 studies.

[c] Studies with <50 cases enrolled.

[d] MSI detection rate of 1% by polymerase chain reaction, whereas IHC showed a decreased expression of mismatch repair proteins in 26 of 111 cases (23%).

These neoantigens are presented to cytotoxic T cells to mount an antitumor immune response and upregulation of immunomodulatory genes such as antigen chaperone molecules, proinflammatory cytokines, and cytotoxic mediators [54–56].

Additionally, MSI in CRCs is reported to be predictive of nonresponse to 5-fluorouracil–based adjuvant chemotherapy in early stage disease (stages II and III) [57], but this finding remains controversial [50,58].

In recent years, MMR deficiency has been established as a predictive biomarker of response to immune checkpoint blockade therapy, which is described in further detail elsewhere in this article [4].

Prognostic Role of Microsatellite Instability in Endometrial Cancer

ECs are histologically and clinically divided into 2 types [59]: type 1 (endometrioid) accounting for 70% to 80% of ECs and type 2 (nonendometrioid; including serous and clear cell carcinomas) accounting for the remaining cases. Type 1 ECs are hormone dependent, more differentiated, less aggressive, and generally associated with younger age and a more favorable prognosis. By contrast, type 2 ECs are less differentiated, more aggressive, less hormone dependent, associated with older age, and harbor a less favorable prognosis [60–62]. In addition, ECs have been further classified according to integrated genomic, transcriptomic, and proteomic data into 4 categories: POLE ultramutated (7%), MSI hypermutated (28%), copy number low (39%), and copy number high (36%) [63]. Looking closer at the MSI-H tumors in this study, the majority of these tumors harbored *MLH1* promotor hypermethylation and were frequently associated with alterations in the *KRAS*, *ARID5B*, and *PIK3CA* genes, lower *PTEN* expression, and rare *TP53* mutations. In addition, *POLE* mutations were seen in 5% of these MSI-H tumors and were mutually exclusive of *MLH1* hypermethylation.

The frequency of MSI in ECs ranges from 9% to 45% in different studies [64–76]. Approximately one-third of MSI cases are found in type 1 ECs with this phenotype being rare in type 2 cancers [67,68,73]. Considering the relatively high frequency of MSI in ECs, the prognostic role of MSI in these cancers has been investigated in multiple studies with conflicting and controversial results. In a systematic review and metaanalysis of MMR status and clinical outcome in ECs, Diaz-Padilla and colleagues [77] analyzed 23 related studies and found a significant association between MSI status and outcome in 32% of the studies with marked inter-study heterogeneity for estimated overall survival (OS) and disease-free survival, and it was concluded that there was no definitive evidence of significant association between MSI status and survival in ECs. Although the majority of studies show no significant difference in OS between MSI and MSS ECs [64,65,66,72,74,76], with 1 study associating MSI with adverse outcomes [67], there are a few studies with contradicting results. In a retrospective cohort of 473 patients with ECs, MSI status was associated with advanced stage cancer (92% vs 81%; $P = .01$) as well as myometrial invasion (92% vs 78%; $P = .01$), with significantly improved disease-free survival (hazard ratio, 0.3; 95% confidence interval, 0.2–0.7) and disease specific survival (hazard ratio, 0.3; 95% confidence interval, 0.1–0.8) on multivariate analysis [68]. Maxwell and colleagues [70] showed better survival in univariate and multivariate analyses of MSI tumors in 131 patients with EC in addition to an increased rate of molecular alterations associated with a better prognosis, such as *PTEN* mutations and less *p53* overexpression. Pijnenborg and colleagues [78] investigated 44 patients with recurrent stage I EC and compared them with the same number of patients who were free of disease for a minimum period of 3 years. These investigators concluded that MSI status does not predict recurrence in these tumors. Eventually, some studies have shown that MSI status is associated with advanced cancer stage and higher tumor grade, but none of these studies highlighted any definitive prognostic role for MSI in these tumors [66,69,71].

Prognostic Role of Microsatellite Instability in Gastric Cancer

The Cancer Genome Atlas proposed a molecular classification for gastric cancers and divided these tumors into 4 subtypes: tumors positive for Epstein-Barr virus (9%), microsatellite unstable tumors (22%), genomically stable tumors (20%), and tumors with chromosomal instability (50%). Each gastric cancer molecular subtype shows distinct molecular features that may provide a base for guidance of targeted therapies in clinical trials in these tumors [79]. Patients with MSI gastric cancer tend to be predominantly female and diagnosed at relatively older ages; these tumors have a better overall prognosis. Although MSI gastric cancers lack targetable amplifications, mutations in the *PIK3CA*, *ERBB3*, *ERBB2*, and *EGFR* genes are seen in these tumors, with many other mutations at hotspot sites seen in other cancer types. Of note, these tumors do not show *BRAF* V600E mutation, which is commonly seen in MSI CRCs [79]. Additionally, the mechanism of MMR deficiency and MSI in gastric cancer seems to be associated with chronic gastritis, in particular *Helicobacter pylori* infections, and MSI can be detected in the atrophic stomach with intestinal metaplasia [42,43].

MSI occurs in 15% to 30% of gastric cancers, with most of them arising in a sporadic fashion without a known genetically inherited MMR gene defect (Lynch syndrome) [80]; however, there is a known frequency difference across diverse populations. Data generally show that MSI status is associated with a better outcome in these patients [56]. In a meta-analysis of 24 studies with 5438 participants including 712 cases of MSI gastric cancers, Choi and colleagues [81] estimated that the hazard ratio for OS of MSI versus non-MSI gastric cancer was 0.72 (95% confidence interval, 0.59–0.88; $P = .001$); however, most recent studies have pointed toward heterogeneity in this group of cancers [81]. In another systematic review and meta-analysis of 8 studies including 1976 patients with gastric cancer, Zhu and colleagues [82] showed that MSI frequency was in a range of 11.68% to 33.82%. Patients with MSI gastric cancer were found to have less lymph node metastasis, superficial tumor invasion, and overall had an improved prognosis with a lower mortality rate.

Predictive Role of Microsatellite Instability in Gastric Cancer

The predictive role of MSI-H status in response to chemotherapy in gastric cancer is controversial; some studies show similar survival benefits as MSI-H CRCs. In a large cohort performed on 1276 patients with stages II and III gastric cancers who underwent surgical resection, MSI-H tumors were associated with a good prognosis in stage II and III gastric cancers when patients were treated by surgery alone, and the benefits of MSI-H status were attenuated by chemotherapy [83].

PRINCIPLES OF CANCER IMMUNOTHERAPY AND BIOMARKERS

Cancer immunotherapy or immunooncology is defined as therapeutic approaches that involve an interaction with the immune system aiming to treat and potentially cure cancer [84]. These interventions stimulate the immune system to initiate a new antitumor response and enhance the response of cancer cells to therapy [85]. Over the past years, immunooncology and cancer immunotherapy have evolved into one of the most promising alternative treatment options for patients with cancer. Cancer immunotherapy approaches could be classified as passive or active. Passive approaches exert their effect through the enhancement of the existing antitumor responses by providing the immune system with synthetic agents such as tumor-specific monoclonal antibodies and cytokines. Active immunotherapies aim at activating the host's own immune system to attack cancer cells, such as different vaccine therapy strategies [85,86]. These therapies depend on molecules expressed on the surface of cancer cells owing to their genetic instability, known as tumor-specific antigens or neoantigens, presenting new epitopes to be recognized by the immune system [87] to initiate an antitumor immune response to eliminate cancer cells and prevent disease spread. These advances have led to a number of immunotherapeutic agents being approved by the FDA for use in cancer therapy in recent years such as sipuleucel-T (an immunotherapy vaccine), ipilimumab (an inhibitor of cytotoxic T-lymphocyte–associated protein 4), and pembrolizumab (a PD-1 inhibitor). It should be noted that, although the immune system is capable of recognizing tumor cells and eliminating them, tumor cells have their own mechanisms to interfere with immune response and evade it [88], such as downmodulation of tumor antigen presentation, immunologic barriers within the tumor microenvironment, and through various components of innate and adaptive immune systems [89].

CANCER IMMUNOTHERAPY USING IMMUNE CHECKPOINT BLOCKADE

Immune checkpoints are immune system regulatory molecules that are involved in pathways essential for self-tolerance and prevention of autoimmunity. PD-1 is an inhibitory checkpoint protein that is expressed by activated T lymphocytes. The interaction between PD-1 on activated T cells and its ligands, PD-L1 and PD-L2, which are expressed by a wide variety of hematopoietic and nonhematopoietic tissues, plays an important role in downregulating the immune response by suppressing T-cell inflammatory activity [84]. This mechanism leads to the prevention of autoimmunity under physiologic conditions; however, this pathway can also be used by neoplastic cells, due to overexpression of PD-L1 and to lesser extent PD-L2 on these cells, to evade immune system control [90–92]. It has been shown that overexpression of PD-L1 is associated with a poor prognosis in cancers such as renal cell carcinoma, hepatocellular carcinoma, esophageal cancer, gastric cancer, pancreatic cancer, ovarian cancer, and bladder cancer. An abundance of PD-L1 on tumor cells correlates with a better prognosis in some other malignancies like breast cancer, whereas the outcomes of PD-L1 overexpression is not clearly defined in colorectal carcinoma, lung cancer, and melanomas [93]. Considering the significant role of the PD-1/PD-L1 pathway in tumor growth and disease outcome, there has been great emphasis on cancer therapy with immune checkpoint inhibitors over the past few years and it has become potentially one of the most promising approaches in the treatment of advanced malignancies. Recent observations have confirmed that cancer treatment with anti–PD-1/PD-L1 agents results in significant antitumor response through the restoration of the host immune response [91,94–96]. These observations resulted in FDA approval of several monoclonal antibodies such as nivolumab (anti–PD-1), pembrolizumab (anti–PD-1), and atezolizumab (anti–PD-L1) for the treatment of a range of cancers such as melanomas, non–small cell lung cancers, renal cell carcinomas, urothelial carcinomas, and head and neck squamous cell carcinomas due to their high efficacy and relatively low toxicity [95]. Despite significant recent advances in the field of cancer immunotherapy and a growing number of agents that are currently used in the clinical setting to treat a range of different cancer types, it has been shown that only a small subset of patients benefits from these treatment strategies [91,96,97] and the identification of these patients at early stages of disease remains a challenge. Furthermore, even though there is evidence of a correlation between the PD-L1 expression level and response to treatment, PD-L1 expression has limited value as the sole predictor of response to treatment, because a response can still be seen in some tumors without detectable PD-L1 expression [98]. This limitation is due to several factors, such as the detection of PD-L1 through different IHC platforms that use different monoclonal antibodies, heterogeneous expression of these molecules in the tumor tissue, and challenges with setting a significant expression level cutoff associated with response to therapy across different tumor types. These issues highlight the need to establish more reliable biomarkers of response to immunotherapy to identify the subset of patients who would benefit from these treatments at earlier stages of disease. Tumor MSI status is one of the biomarkers that has been shown to be a promising predictor of response to immunotherapy regardless of PD-1/PD-L1 expression levels or tumor site across a wide range of cancers [4].

MICROSATELLITE INSTABILITY AND IMMUNE CHECKPOINT BLOCKADE THERAPY

Microsatellite Instability and Immunogenicity

It has been known that tumors with high tumor-infiltrating lymphocytes (TILs) have a better prognosis with less growth and metastasis [99]. In addition, there is a correlation between high TILs in the tumor microenvironment and MMR deficiency/MSI in a subset of CRCs [100–102]. The mechanism responsible for the stronger immunogenic response of MSI-H tumors is believed to be due to a dysfunctional MMR system and the subsequently higher mutational load in these tumors, which results in the production and expression of a large number of proteins known as mutation-associated neoantigens on the surface of neoplastic cells. These neoantigens are subsequently presented to cytotoxic T cells to elicit an endogenous antitumor immune response [103,104]. These responses are counterbalanced by high expression of multiple immune checkpoint proteins including PD-1, PD-L1, and cytotoxic T-lymphocyte–associated protein-4 on either neoplastic cells or tumor microenvironment in MSI-H tumors, leading to the downregulation of the antitumor immune response and tumor survival [102]. Of note, expression levels of PD-1 and PD-L1 are significantly higher on TILs and tumor cells in MSI-H tumors compared with MSS tumors (PD-1 expression on TILs in 77% of MSI-H tumors vs in 39% of MSS tumors and PD-L1 expression in 32% of MSI-H tumors vs in 13% of MSS tumors) [14]. Overall, immunotherapy strategies through the blockade of the PD-1/PD-L1 pathway in dMMR/MSI-H tumors lead to a robust continuous immune response against neoplastic cells and subsequent tumor elimination owing to the high mutational burden and strong antigenicity of these tumors as well as high expression of immune checkpoint molecules in their microenvironment. Additionally, as discussed elsewhere in this article, given the high mutational burden of *POLE* and *POLD1* ultramutated tumors, these tumors also represent targets for immunotherapy, based on the same mechanisms that apply to MSI-H cancers.

Microsatellite Instability as a Novel Predictor of Response to Immunotherapy

In the early studies evaluating the response of human tumors to PD-1 blockade, it was noticed that just 1 of 33 patients with CRC had a response in contrast with a significantly greater proportion of patients with other tumor types, such as renal cell carcinoma, non–small cell lung carcinomas, and melanomas [91,96]. Subsequently, it was confirmed that this CRC was MMR deficient and this observation led to the hypothesis that MSI status could potentially be used as a biomarker of response to immunotherapy. This hypothesis was confirmed in a phase II study of 41 patients with stage IV colorectal and noncolorectal carcinomas with and without MMR deficiency (11 patients with MMR-deficient CRC, 21 patients with MMR-proficient CRC, and 9 patients with MMR-deficient non-CRC tumors including 4 ampullary or cholangiocarcinoma, 2 EC, 2 small bowel carcinomas, and 1 gastric cancer) who had failed other prior treatment regimens. Upon treatment with pembrolizumab, the immune-related objective response rate was 40% for MMR-deficient CRCs, 71% for MMR-deficient non-CRCs, and 0% in MMR-proficient CRCs; the immune-related progression-free survival rate was 78% in MMR-deficient CRCs, 67% in MMR-deficient non-CRCs, and 11% for MMR-proficient tumors, indicating that tumor MSI status is a significant predictor of response to immunotherapy [105]. Interestingly, all of the patients with MMR deficiency had an immediate clinical and biomarker response to treatment. This study was followed by a larger cohort to investigate the effect of treatment with pembrolizumab on 86 patients across 12 different MMR-deficient cancer types who had received at least 1 treatment before permbrolizumab therapy, which demonstrated objective radiographic responses in 53% of the patients as well as complete response in 21% of the study population. Although neither median progression-free survival nor median OS has yet been achieved for this study, the 1- and 2-year progression-free survival estimates were 64% and 53%, respectively, and the estimates of OS at 1 and 2 years were 76% and 64%, respectively, with no significant difference seen between patients with or without the Lynch syndrome. No evidence of cancer recurrence was seen in 11 patients who achieved a complete response and were taken off the therapy over a period of 8.3 months [14]. Functional analysis of responsive tumors showed a neoantigen-specific expansion of T cells to mutation-associated neoantigens in MMR-deficient tumor cells, leading to response to immune checkpoint blockade, regardless of tumor site.

In light of the reported data, the FDA granted accelerated approval to pembrolizumab for adult and pediatric patients with unresectable or metastatic, MSI-H or MMR-deficient solid tumors that have progressed after prior treatment and who have no satisfactory alternative treatment options, or MSI-H or MMR-deficient CRC that has progressed after treatment with a fluoropyrimidine, oxaliplatin, and irinotecan. The approval was based on data from 149 patients with MSI-H/MMR-deficient cancers enrolled across 5 uncontrolled, multicohort, multicenter, single-arm clinical trials. Ninety patients had CRC and 59 patients were diagnosed with 1 of 14 other cancer types. Patients were treated with pembrolizumab for a maximum of 24 months. The objective response rate was 36% in CRC and 46% in patients with other tumor types, with a pooled response rate of 36.9% including complete and partial responses in 11 patients with CRC and 48 patients with other tumor types. Of the patients who responded to pembrolizumab, 78% had a durable response that lasted 6 months or more [106].

Shortly after, nivolumab (an anti–PD-1 monoclonal antibody) was granted an accelerated approval by FDA for the treatment of patients with MMR-deficient and MSI-H metastatic CRC that has progressed after treatment with a fluoropyrimidine, oxaliplatin, and irinotecan. The approval was based on pooled data from 53 patients in a multicenter, open-label, single-arm study. The objective response rate was 28% and responses lasted for 6 months or more in 67% of the patients, with a complete response seen in 1 patient and partial responses in 14 patients [107].

Limitations of Microsatellite Instability as a Biomarker for Immunotherapy

Resistance to immune checkpoint blockade is seen in a subset of MSI-H tumors. *JAK 1/2;*–inactivating mutations are involved in primary resistance to anti–PD-1 therapy in MMR-deficient tumors with a high mutational burden, most likely owing to the lack of reactive PD-L1 expression and response to interferon-gamma [108]. Furthermore, acquired resistance after an initial objective response has been seen in a subset of patients, with the progressive disease observed in occult sites including brain and bone [4]. Eventually, despite impressive results, the majority of the studies that have been carried out on the response of MSI-H tumors to immune checkpoint blockades are short term and these studies need to be validated in larger cohorts.

SUMMARY

We are in a very exciting era of cancer therapy in which an increasing number of biomarkers of response to more targeted and individualized therapies are emerging that can enable us to identify patients who will benefit the best from these therapeutic approaches. MSI testing has long been used to screen patients for hereditary cancers as well as for prognostic purposes, predominantly in patients with colorectal and endometrial cancers (ECs), with limited application in choosing treatment strategies. However, the recent advancements in the molecular characterization of different cancers, better understanding of cancer immunology, and significant response of MSI-H tumors to immunotherapy across different cancer types has opened a new era in applying MSI testing to treatment of patients across a wide range of tumors, regardless of site. Several recent studies have shown MSI phenotype across a wide range of cancers beyond the limited number of cancer types, which have been traditionally tested. In an evaluation of 12,019 cancers representing 32 distinct cancer types for MMR deficiency, it was shown that more than 5% of adenocarcinomas of endometrium, stomach, small intestine, colon and rectum, cervix, prostate, bile duct and liver, neuroendocrine tumors, nonepithelial ovarian cancers, and uterine sarcomas were MMR deficient. Taking into account the stage of these cancers, this represents approximately 40,000 annual stage I to III and 20,000 stage IV diagnoses in the United States alone [4]. These data emphasize extending MSI testing to a larger spectrum of solid tumors to recognize a larger pool of patients who could potentially benefit from more individualized therapies. This finding also highlights the importance of optimizing the current methods of detecting MSI status, because these methods are mainly optimized for CRCs; however, MSI loci that are currently used according to the Bethesda Consensus are not applicable to all cancer types. Further attention should be given to *POLE* and *POLD1* ultramutated cancers, which could potentially benefit from immunotherapy through the same mechanisms that apply to MSI-H tumors.

REFERENCES

[1] Hause RJ, Pritchard CC, Shendure J, et al. Corrigendum: classification and characterization of microsatellite instability across 18 cancer types. Nat Med 2017; 23(10):1241.

[2] Vilar E, Gruber SB. Microsatellite instability in colorectal cancer-the stable evidence. Nat Rev Clin Oncol 2010;7(3):153–62.

[3] Sepulveda AR, Hamilton SR, Allegra CJ, et al. Molecular biomarkers for the evaluation of colorectal cancer: guideline from the American Society for Clinical Pathology, College of American Pathologists, Association for Molecular Pathology, and the American Society of Clinical Oncology. J Clin Oncol 2017;35(13):1453–86.

[4] Le DT, Durham JN, Smith KN, et al. Mismatch repair deficiency predicts response of solid tumors to PD-1 blockade. Science 2017;357(6349):409–13.

[5] Ogino S, Goel A. Molecular classification and correlates in colorectal cancer. J Mol Diagn 2008;10(1):13–27.

[6] Kunkel TA, Erie DA. Eukaryotic mismatch repair in relation to DNA replication. Annu Rev Genet 2015;49:291–313.

[7] Ligtenberg MJ, Kuiper RP, Chan TL, et al. Heritable somatic methylation and inactivation of MSH2 in families with Lynch syndrome due to deletion of the 39 exons of TACSTD1. Nat Genet 2009;41:112–7.

[8] Kane MF, Loda M, Gaida GM, et al. Methylation of the hMLH1 promoter correlates with lack of expression of hMLH1 in sporadic colon tumors and mismatch repair-defective human tumor cell lines. Cancer Res 1997;57(5):808–11.

[9] Edwards RA, Witherspoon M, Wang K, et al. Epigenetic repression of DNA mismatch repair by inflammation and hypoxia in inflammatory bowel disease-associated colorectal cancer. Cancer Res 2009;69(16):6423–9.

[10] Valeri N, Gasparini P, Braconi C, et al. MicroRNA-21 induces resistance to 5-fluorouracil by down-regulating human DNA MutS homolog 2 (hMSH2). Proc Natl Acad Sci U S A 2010;107(49):21098–103.

[11] Valeri N, Braconi C, Gasparini P, et al. MicroRNA-135b promotes cancer progression by acting as a downstream effector of oncogenic pathways in colon cancer. Cancer Cell 2014;25(4):469–83.

[12] Grilley M, Holmes J, Yashar B, et al. Mechanisms of DNA-mismatch correction. Mutat Res 1990;236(2–3):253–67.

[13] Boland CR, Goel A. Microsatellite instability in colorectal cancer. Gastroenterology 2010;138(6):2073–87.

[14] Lee V, Murphy A, Le DT, et al. Mismatch repair deficiency and response to immune checkpoint blockade. Oncologist 2016;21:1200–11.

[15] Nebot-Bral L, Brandao D, Verlingue L, et al. Hypermutated tumours in the era of immunotherapy: the paradigm of personalised medicine. Eur J Cancer 2017;84:290–303.

[16] Cancer Genome Atlas Network. Comprehensive molecular characterization of human colon and rectal cancer. Nature 2012;487(7407):330–7.

[17] Church DN, Briggs SEW, Palles C, et al. DNA polymerase 1 and d exonuclease domain mutations in endometrial cancer. Hum Mol Genet 2013;22(14):2820–8.

[18] Palles C, Cazier JB, Howarth KM, et al. Germline mutations affecting the proofreading domains of POLE and POLD1 predispose to colorectal adenomas and carcinomas. Nat Genet 2013;45(2):136–44.

[19] Bellido F, Pineda M, Aiza G, et al. POLE and POLD1 mutations in 529 kindred with familial colorectal cancer and/or polyposis: review of reported cases and recommendations for genetic testing and surveillance. Genet Med 2016;18(4):325–32.

[20] Rayner E, Van Gool IC, Palles C, et al. A panoply of errors: polymerase proofreading domain mutations in cancer. Nat Rev Cancer 2016;16(2):71–81.

[21] Heitzer E, Tomlinson I. Replicative DNA polymerase mutations in cancer. Curr Opin Genet Dev 2014;24:107–13.

[22] Harada S, Sepulveda AR. Molecular mechanisms and pathology of gastric carcinogenesis: sporadic cancers. In: Sepulveda AR, Lynch JP, editors. Molecular pathology of neoplastic gastrointestinal diseases. New York: Springer, LLC; 2013. p. 67–81.

[23] Shia J. Immunohistochemistry versus microsatellite instability testing for screening colorectal cancer patients at risk for hereditary nonpolyposis colorectal cancer syndrome. Part I. The utility of immunohistochemistry. J Mol Diagn 2008;10(4):293–300.

[24] Watson N, Grieu F, Morris M, et al. Heterogeneous staining for mismatch repair proteins during population-based prescreening for hereditary nonpolyposis colorectal cancer. J Mol Diagn 2007;9(4):472–8.

[25] Overbeek LI, Ligtenberg MJ, Willems RW, et al. Interpretation of immunohistochemistry for mismatch repair proteins is only reliable in a specialized setting. Am J Surg Pathol 2008;32(8):1246–51.

[26] Zhang L. Immunohistochemistry versus microsatellite instability testing for screening colorectal cancer patients at risk for hereditary nonpolyposis colorectal cancer syndrome. Part II. The utility of microsatellite instability testing. J Mol Diagn 2008;10(4):301–7.

[27] Boland CR, Thibodeau SN, Hamilton SR, et al. A National Cancer Institute workshop on microsatellite instability for cancer detection and familial predisposition: development of international criteria for the determination of microsatellite instability in colorectal cancer. Cancer Res 1998;58(22):5248–57.

[28] Sutter C, Gebert J, Bischoff P, et al. Molecular screening of potential HNPCC patients using a multiplex microsatellite PCR system. Mol Cell Probes 1999;13(2):157–65.

[29] Umar A, Boland CR, Terdiman JP, et al. Revised Bethesda Guidelines for hereditary nonpolyposis colorectal cancer (Lynch syndrome) and microsatellite instability. J Natl Cancer Inst 2004;96(4):261–8.

[30] Suraweera N, Duval A, Reperant M, et al. Evaluation of tumor microsatellite instability using five quasimonomorphic mononucleotide repeats and pentaplex PCR. Gastroenterology 2002;123(6):1804–11.

[31] Sood Ak, Holmes R, Hendrix MJ, et al. Application of the National Cancer Institute international criteria for determination of microsatellite instability in ovarian cancer. Cancer Res 2001;61(11):4371–4.

[32] Hempelmann JA, Scroggins SM, Pritchard CC, et al. MSIplus for Integrated colorectal cancer molecular testing by next-generation sequencing. J Mol Diagn 2015;17(6):705–14.

[33] Nowak JA, Yurgelun MB, Bruce JL, et al. Detection of mismatch repair deficiency and microsatellite instability in colorectal adenocarcinoma by targeted next-generation sequencing. J Mol Diagn 2017;19(1):84–91.

[34] Stadler ZK, Battaglin F, Middha S, et al. Reliable detection of mismatch repair deficiency in colorectal cancers using mutational load in next-generation sequencing panels. J Clin Oncol 2016;34(18):2141–7.

[35] Snyder A, Makarov V, Merghoub T, et al. Genetic basis for clinical response to CTLA-4 blockade in melanoma. N Engl J Med 2014;371(23):2189–99.
[36] Rizvi NA, Hellmann MD, Snyder A, et al. Mutational landscape determines sensitivity to PD-1 blockade in non-small cell lung cancer. Science 2015;348(6230):124–8.
[37] Chalmers ZR, Connelly CF, Fabrizio D, et al. Analysis of 100,000 human cancer genomes reveals the landscape of tumor mutational burden. Genome Med 2017;9:34.
[38] George TJ, Frampton GM, Sun J, et al. Tumor mutational burden as a potential biomarker for PD1/PD-L1 therapy in colorectal cancer. J Clin Oncol 2016; 34(15_suppl):3587.
[39] Johnson DB, Frampton GM, Rioth MJ, et al. Targeted Next Generation Sequencing Identifies Markers of Response to PD-1 Blockade. Cancer Immunol Res 2016;4(11):959–67.
[40] Goodman AM, Kato S, Bazhenova L, et al. Tumor Mutational Burden as an Independent Predictor of Response to Immunotherapy in Diverse Cancers. Mol Cancer Ther 2017;16(11):2598–608.
[41] Gros A, Parkhurst MR, Tran E, et al. Prospective identification of neoantigen-specific lymphocytes in the peripheral blood of melanoma patients. Nat Med 2016; 22(4):433–8.
[42] Sepulveda JL, Gutierrez-Pajares JL, Luna A, et al. High-definition CpG methylation of novel genes in gastric carcinogenesis identified by next-generation sequencing. Mod Pathol 2016;29(2):182–93.
[43] Leung WK, Kim JJ, Kim JG, et al. Microsatellite instability in gastric intestinal metaplasia in patients with and without gastric cancer. Am J Pathol 2000;156(2):537–43.
[44] Kim TM, Laird PW, Park PJ. The landscape of microsatellite instability in colorectal and endometrial cancer genomes. Cell 2013;155(4):858–68.
[45] Bonneville R, Krook MA, Kautto EA, et al. Landscape of microsatellite instability across 39 cancer types. JCO Precis Oncol 2017. https://doi.org/10.1200/PO.17.00073.
[46] Cortes-Ciriano I, Lee S, Park WY, et al. A molecular portrait of microsatellite instability across multiple cancers. Nat Commun 2017;8:15180.
[47] Jass JR. Molecular heterogeneity of colorectal cancer: implications for cancer control. Surg Oncol 2007; 16(Suppl 1):S7–9.
[48] Colle R, Cohen R, Cochereau D, et al. Immunotherapy and patients treated for cancer with microsatellite instability. Bull Cancer 2017;104(1):42–51.
[49] Popat S, Hubner R, Houlston RS. Systematic review of microsatellite instability and colorectal cancer prognosis. J Clin Oncol 2005;23(3):609–18.
[50] Guastadisegni C, Colafranceschi M, Ottini L, et al. Microsatellite instability as a marker of prognosis and response to therapy: a meta-analysis of colorectal cancer survival data. Eur J Cancer 2010;46(15):2788–98.
[51] Gelsomino F, Barbolini M, Spallanzani A, et al. The evolving role of microsatellite instability in colorectal cancer: a review. Cancer Treat Rev 2016;51:19–26.
[52] Sinicrope FA, Yang ZJ. Prognostic and predictive impact of DNA mismatch repair in the management of colorectal cancer. Future Oncol 2011;7(3):467–74.
[53] Hutchins G, Southward K, Handley K, et al. Value of mismatch repair, KRAS, and BRAF mutations in predicting recurrence and benefits from chemotherapy in colorectal cancer. J Clin Oncol 2011;29(10):1261–70.
[54] Phillips SM, Banerjea A, Feakins R, et al. Tumour-infiltrating lymphocytes in colorectal cancer with microsatellite instability are activated and cytotoxic. Br J Surg 2004;91(4):469–75.
[55] Banerjea A, Ahmed S, Hands RE, et al. Colorectal cancers with microsatellite instability display mRNA expression signatures characteristic of increased immunogenicity. Mol Cancer 2004;3:21.
[56] Yamamoto H, Imai K. Microsatellite instability: an update. Arch Toxicol 2015;89(6):899–921.
[57] Des Guetz G, Schischmanoff O, Nicolas P, et al. Does microsatellite instability predict the efficacy of adjuvant chemotherapy in colorectal cancer? A systematic review with meta-analysis. Eur J Cancer 2009;45(10):1890–6.
[58] Kawakami H, Zaanan A, Sinicrope FA. Microsatellite instability testing and its role in the management of colorectal cancer. Curr Treat Options Oncol 2015; 16(7):30.
[59] Lax SF, Kurman RJ. A dualistic model for endometrial carcinogenesis based on immunohistochemical and molecular genetic analyses. Verh Dtsch Ges Pathol 1997;81:228–32.
[60] Amant F, Moerman P, Neven P, et al. Endometrial cancer. Lancet 2005;366(9484):491–505.
[61] Lax SF. Molecular genetic pathways in various types of endometrial carcinoma: from a phenotypical to a molecular-based classification. Virchows Arch 2004; 444(3):213–23.
[62] Prat J, Gallardo A, Cuatrecasas M, et al. Endometrial carcinoma: pathology and genetics. Pathology 2007;39(1): 72–87.
[63] Kandoth C, Schultz N, Cherniack AD, et al. Integrated genomic characterization of endometrial carcinoma. Nature 2013;497(7447):67–73.
[64] Zighelboim I, Goodfellow PJ, Gao F, et al. Microsatellite instability and epigenetic inactivation of MLH1 and outcome of patients with endometrial carcinomas of the endometrioid type. J Clin Oncol 2007;25(15): 2042–8.
[65] Basil JB, Goodfellow PJ, Rader JS, et al. Clinical significance of microsatellite instability in endometrial carcinoma. Cancer 2000;89(8):1758–64.
[66] Baldinu P, Cossu A, Manca A, et al. Microsatellite instability and mutation analysis of candidate genes in unselected Sardinian patients with endometrial carcinoma. Cancer 2002;94(12):3157–68.
[67] Caduff RF, Johnston CM, Svoboda-Newman SM, et al. Clinical and pathological significance of microsatellite instability in sporadic endometrial carcinoma. Am J Pathol 1996;148(5):1671–8.

[68] Black D, Soslow RA, Levine DA, et al. Clinicopathologic significance of defective DNA mismatch repair in endometrial carcinoma. J Clin Oncol 2006;24(11):1745–53.
[69] Muresu R, Sini MC, Cossu A, et al. Chromosomal abnormalities and microsatellite instability in sporadic endometrial cancer. Eur J Cancer 2002;38(13):1802–9.
[70] Maxwell GL, Risinger JI, Alvarez AA, et al. Favorable survival associated with microsatellite instability in endometrioid endometrial cancers. Obstet Gynecol 2001; 97(3):417–22.
[71] Fiumicino S, Ercoli A, Ferrandina G, et al. Microsatellite instability is an independent indicator of recurrence in sporadic stage I-II endometrial adenocarcinoma. J Clin Oncol 2001;19(4):1008–14.
[72] Kanopiene D, Vidugiriene J, Valuckas KP, et al. Endometrial cancer and microsatellite instability status. Open Med (Wars) 2015;10(1):70–6.
[73] Tibiletti MG, Furlan D, Taborelli M, et al. Microsatellite instability in endometrial cancer: relation to histological subtypes. Gynecol Oncol 1999;73(2):247–52.
[74] Wong YF, Ip TY, Chung TKH, et al. Clinical and pathologic significance of microsatellite instability in endometrial cancer. Int J Gynecol Cancer 1999;9(5):406–10.
[75] Catasus L, Machin P, Matias-Guiu X, et al. Microsatellite instability in endometrial carcinomas: clinicopathologic correlations in a series of 42 cases. Hum Pathol 1998;29(10):1160–4.
[76] MacDonald ND, Salvesen HB, Ryan A, et al. Frequency and prognostic impact of microsatellite instability in a large population-based study of endometrial carcinomas. Cancer Res 2000;60(6):1750–2.
[77] Diaz-Padilla I, Romero N, Amir E, et al. Mismatch repair status and clinical outcome in endometrial cancer: a systematic review and meta-analysis. Crit Rev Oncol Hematol 2013;88(1):154–67.
[78] Pijnenborg JM, Dam-de Veen GC, de Haan J, et al. Defective mismatch repair and the development of recurrent endometrial carcinoma. Gynecol Oncol 2004;94(2):550–9.
[79] Cancer Genome Atlas Research Network. Comprehensive molecular characterization of gastric adenocarcinoma. Nature 2014;513(7517):202–9.
[80] Velho S, Fernandes MS, Leite M, et al. Causes and consequences of microsatellite instability in gastric carcinogenesis. World J Gastroenterol 2014;20(44):16433–42.
[81] Choi YY, Bae JM, An JY, et al. Is microsatellite instability a prognostic marker in gastric cancer? a systematic review with meta-analysis. J Surg Oncol 2014;110(2): 129–35.
[82] Zhu L, Li Z, Wang Y, et al. Microsatellite instability and survival in gastric cancer: a systematic review and meta-analysis. Mol Clin Oncol 2015;3(3):699–705.
[83] Kim SY, Choi YY, An JY, et al. The benefit of microsatellite instability is attenuated by chemotherapy in stage II and stage III gastric cancer: results from a large cohort with subgroup analyses. Int J Cancer 2015;137(4): 819–25.
[84] Konsoulova A. Principles of cancer immunobiology and immunotherapy of solid tumors. In: Metodiev K, editor. Immunopathology and immunomodulation. Rijeka (Croatia): InTech; 2015. p. 77–99, Ch. 05.
[85] Galluzzi L, Vacchelli E, Bravo-San Pedro JM, et al. Classification of current anticancer immunotherapies. Oncotarget 2014;5(24):12472–508.
[86] Mellman I, Coukos G, Dranoff G. Cancer immunotherapy comes of age. Nature 2011;480(7378):480–9.
[87] Mitra AK, Agrahari V, Mandal A, et al. Novel delivery approaches for cancer therapeutics. J Control Release 2015;219:248–68.
[88] Blattman JN, Greenberg PD. Cancer immunotherapy: a treatment for the masses. Science 2004;305(5681): 200–5.
[89] Drake CG, Jaffee E, Pardoll DM. Mechanisms of immune evasion by tumors. Adv Immunol 2006;90: 51–81.
[90] Dong H, Strome SE, Salomao DR, et al. Tumor-associated B7-H1 promotes T-cell apoptosis: a potential mechanism of immune evasion. Nat Med 2002;8(8): 793–800.
[91] Topalian SL, Drake CG, Pardoll DM. Targeting the PD-1/B7-H1(PD-L1) pathway to activate anti-tumor immunity. Curr Opin Immunol 2012;24(2):207–12.
[92] Boussiotis VA. Molecular and Biochemical Aspects of the PD-1 Checkpoint Pathway. N Engl J Med 2016; 375(18):1767–78.
[93] Wang X, Teng F, Kong L, et al. PD-L1 expression in human cancers and its association with clinical outcomes. Onco Targets Ther 2016;9:5023–39.
[94] Philips GK, Atkins M. Therapeutic uses of anti-PD-1 and anti-PD-L1 antibodies. Int Immunol 2015;27(1):39–46.
[95] Hashem O, Alsaab SS, Alzhrani R, et al. PD-1 and PD-L1 checkpoint signaling inhibition for cancer immunotherapy: mechanism, combinations, and clinical outcome. Front Pharmacol 2017;8:561.
[96] Brahmer JR, Drake CG, Wollner I, et al. Phase I study of single-agent anti-programmed death-1 (MDX-1106) in refractory solid tumors: safety, clinical activity, pharmacodynamics, and immunologic correlates. J Clin Oncol 2010;28(19):3167–75.
[97] Carbognin L, Pilotto S, Milella M, et al. Differential activity of nivolumab, pembrolizumab and mpdl3280a according to the tumor expression of programmed death-ligand-1 (pd-l1): sensitivity analysis of trials in melanoma, lung and genitourinary cancers. PLoS One 2015;10(6):e0130142.
[98] Weinstock M, McDermott D. Targeting PD-1/PD-L1 in the treatment of metastatic renal cell carcinoma. Ther Adv Urol 2015;7(6):365–77.
[99] Galon J, Costes A, Sanchez-Cabo F, et al. Type, density, and location of immune cells within human colorectal tumors predict clinical outcome. Science 2006; 313(5795):1960–4.
[100] Kim H, Jen J, Vogelstein B, et al. Clinical and pathological characteristics of sporadic colorectal carcinomas

with DNA replication errors in microsatellite sequences. Am J Pathol 1994;145(1):148–56.
[101] Alexander J, Watanabe T, Wu TT, et al. Histopathological identification of colon cancer with microsatellite instability. Am J Pathol 2001;158(2):527–35.
[102] Llosa NJ, Cruise M, Tam A, et al. The vigorous immune microenvironment of microsatellite instable colon cancer is balanced by multiple counter-inhibitory checkpoints. Cancer Discov 2015;5(1):43–51.
[103] Schwitalle Y, Kloor M, Eiermann S, et al. Immune response against frameshift-induced neopeptides in HNPCC patients and healthy HNPCC mutation carriers. Gastroenterology 2008;134(4):988–97.
[104] Dudley JC, Lin MT, Le DT, et al. Microsatellite instability as a biomarker for PD-1 blockade. Clin Cancer Res 2016;22(4):813–20.
[105] Le DT, Uram JN, Wang H, et al. PD-1 blockade in tumors with mismatch-repair deficiency. N Engl J Med 2015;372(26):2509–20.
[106] FDA grants accelerated approval to pembrolizumab for first tissue/site agnostic indication. U.S. Food & Drug Administration Web site. 2017. Available at: https://www.fda.gov/Drugs/InformationOnDrugs/ApprovedDrugs/ucm560040.htm. Accessed June 14, 2018
[107] FDA grants nivolumab accelerated approval for MSI-H or dMMR colorectal cancer. U.S. Food & Drug Administration Web site. 2017. Available at: https://www.fda.gov/Drugs/InformationOnDrugs/ApprovedDrugs/ucm569366.htm. Accessed June 14, 2018.
[108] Shin DS, Zaretsky JM, Escuin-Ordinas H, et al. Primary resistance to PD-1 blockade mediated by JAK1/2 mutations. Cancer Discov 2017;7(2):188–201.
[109] Seo HM, Chang YS, Joo SH, et al. Clinicopathologic characteristics and outcomes of gastric cancers with the MSI-H phenotype. J Surg Oncol 2009;99(3):143–7.
[110] Schwark AL, Srinivasan P, Kemel Y, et al. Pan-cancer microsatellite instability to predict for presence of Lynch syndrome. J Clin Oncol 2018;36(18_suppl):LBA1509.
[111] Okuda T, Kawakami K, Ishiguro K, et al. The profile of hMLH1 methylation and microsatellite instability in colorectal and non-small cell lung cancer. Int J Mol Med 2005;15(1):85–90.
[112] Ruemmele P, Dietmaier W, Terracciano L, et al. Histopathologic features and microsatellite instability of cancers of the papilla of Vater and their precursor lesions. Am J Surg Pathol 2009;33(5):691–704.
[113] Agaram NP, Shia J, Tang LH, et al. DNA mismatch repair deficiency in ampullary carcinoma: a morphologic and immunohistochemical study of 54 cases. Am J Clin Pathol 2010;133(5):772–80.
[114] Murphy MA, Wentzensen N. Frequency of mismatch repair deficiency in ovarian cancer: a systematic review this article is a US Government work and, as such, is in the public domain of the United States of America. Int J Cancer 2011;129(8):1914–22.
[115] Farris AB 3rd, Demicco EG, Le LP, et al. Clinicopathologic and molecular profiles of microsatellite unstable Barrett Esophagus-associated adenocarcinoma. Am J Surg Pathol 2011;35(5):647–55.
[116] Kawaguchi K, Oda Y, Takahira T, et al. Microsatellite instability and hMLH1 and hMSH2 expression analysis in soft tissue sarcomas. Oncol Rep 2005;13(2):241–6.
[117] Alldinger I, Schaefer KL, Goedde D, et al. Microsatellite instability in Ewing tumor is not associated with loss of mismatch repair protein expression. J Cancer Res Clin Oncol 2007;133(10):749–59.
[118] Glavac D, Volavsek M, Potocnik U, et al. Low microsatellite instability and high loss of heterozygosity rates indicate dominant role of the suppressor pathway in squamous cell carcinoma of head and neck and loss of heterozygosity of 11q14.3 correlates with tumor grade. Cancer Genet Cytogenet 2003;146(1):27–32.
[119] Hammerschmied C, Stoehr R, Walter B, et al. The role of elevated microsatellite alterations at selected tetranucleotides (EMAST) in renal cell carcinoma (RCC). Cancer Res 2007;67(9 Supplement):1934.
[120] Ninomiya H, Nomura K, Satoh Y, et al. Genetic instability in lung cancer: concurrent analysis of chromosomal, mini- and microsatellite instability and loss of heterozygosity. Br J Cancer 2006;94:1485.
[121] Warth A, Korner S, Penzel R, et al. Microsatellite instability in pulmonary adenocarcinomas: a comprehensive study of 480 cases. Virchows Arch 2016;468(3):313–9.
[122] Winkelmann R, Schneider M, Hartmann S, et al. Microsatellite instability occurs rarely in patients with cholangiocarcinoma: a retrospective study from a German tertiary care hospital. Int J Mol Sci 2018;19(5):1421.
[123] Catto JW, Xinarianos G, Burton JL, et al. Differential expression of hMLH1 and hMSH2 is related to bladder cancer grade, stage and prognosis but not microsatellite instability. Int J Cancer 2003;105(4):484–90.
[124] Anbazhagan R, Fujii H, Gabrielson E. Microsatellite instability is uncommon in breast cancer. Clin Cancer Res 1999;5(4):839–44.
[125] Kuligina E, Grigoriev MY, Suspitsin EN, et al. Microsatellite instability analysis of bilateral breast tumors suggests treatment-related origin of some contralateral malignancies. J Cancer Res Clin Oncol 2007;133(1):57–64.
[126] Adem C, Soderberg CL, Cunningham JM, et al. Microsatellite instability in hereditary and sporadic breast cancers. Int J Cancer 2003;107(4):580–2.
[127] Martinez R, Schackert HK, Appelt H, et al. Low-level microsatellite instability phenotype in sporadic glioblastoma multiforme. J Cancer Res Clin Oncol 2005;131(2):87–93.
[128] Laghi L, Beghelli S, Spinelli A, et al. Irrelevance of microsatellite instability in the epidemiology of sporadic pancreatic ductal adenocarcinoma. PLoS One 2012;7(9):e46002.

[129] Palmieri G, Ascierto PA, Cossu A, et al. Assessment of genetic instability in melanocytic skin lesions through microsatellite analysis of benign naevi, dysplastic naevi, and primary melanomas and their metastases. Melanoma Res 2003;13(2):167–70.

[130] Entz-Werle N, Schneider A, Kalifa C, et al. Genetic alterations in primary osteosarcoma from 54 children and adolescents by targeted allelotyping. Br J Cancer 2003; 88(12):1925–31.

[131] Reuschenbach M, Sommerer C, Hartschuh W, et al. Absence of mismatch repair deficiency-related microsatellite instability in non-melanoma skin cancer. J Invest Dermatol 2012;132(2):491–3.

[132] Mayer F, Gillis AJ, Dinjens W, et al. Microsatellite instability of germ cell tumors is associated with resistance to systemic treatment. Cancer Res 2002;62(10): 2758–60.

[133] Mitmaker E, Alvarado C, Begin LR, et al. Microsatellite instability in benign and malignant thyroid neoplasms. J Surg Res 2008;150(1):40–8.

[134] Cesinaro AM, Ubiali A, Sighinolfi P, et al. Mismatch repair proteins expression and microsatellite instability in skin lesions with sebaceous differentiation: a study in different clinical subgroups with and without extracutaneous cancer. Am J Dermatopathol 2007;29(4):351–8.

[135] Kruse R, Rutten A, Schweiger N, et al. Frequency of microsatellite instability in unselected sebaceous gland neoplasias and hyperplasias. J Invest Dermatol 2003; 120(5):858–64.

[136] Chiappini F, Gross-Goupil M, Saffroy R, et al. Microsatellite instability mutator phenotype in hepatocellular carcinoma in non-alcoholic and non-virally infected normal livers. Carcinogenesis 2004;25(4):541–7.

Identity/HLA

Advances in Molecular Pathology 1 (2018) 209–228
ADVANCES IN MOLECULAR PATHOLOGY

Tackling the Human Cell Line and Tissue Misidentification Problem Is Needed for Reproducible Biomedical Research

Christopher Korch, PhD*, Marileila Varella-Garcia, PhD
Division of Medical Oncology, University of Colorado, Anschutz Medical Campus, Mailstop 8117, Aurora, CO 80045, USA

KEYWORDS

- STR genotyping • SNP genotyping • Molecular karyotyping • Cell line misidentification
- Tissue misidentification • Cell line authentication • Xenograft authentication

KEY POINTS

- Description of various features, the scope, and causes of the cell line and tissue misidentification problems with examples from the literature.
- Comparison and utility of several molecular genotyping approaches for identifying imposter cell lines, including various short tandem repeat and single nucleotide polymorphism methods, next-generation sequencing, and karyotyping by Giemsa banding and different fluorescent in situ hybridization techniques.
- Outline methods for authentication of cell lines and xenograft (patient-derived xenograft and patient-derived organoid) tissue samples.
- Discussion of published articles that have been retracted or corrected because of using misidentified cell lines and various tactics for ameliorating the cell line misidentification problem.

INTRODUCTION

Historical Background of Cell Line Cross-Contamination, Misidentification, and Authentication

Sixty-seven years ago, in 1951, the first human cell line, HeLa, was established by George Gey and colleagues [1,2] from a robustly growing cervical adenocarcinoma. Human biologists were so excited by this fortuitous development that HeLa cells were shared widely around the world [2–5] and used to learn how to develop cell lines from human and other mammalian tissues.

Judging by karyotype analysis, in 1959 and 1962 there were reports that cross-contamination of cell lines by other cell lines, including HeLa, was a prevalent phenomenon resulting in transformed cells [6–8]. Between 1967 and 1971, Stanley Gartler used genetic variants of isozymes of glucose-6-phosphate dehydrogenase (G6PD) and phosphoglucomutase (PGM) to show that 19 widely used human cell lines were not from the purported original cells but were most likely derivatives of the human cervical adenocarcinoma HeLa cell line [9–11]. Table 1 lists many of these HeLa imposter cell lines with their purported origins and

Disclosure: The authors have nothing to disclose.

*Corresponding author, *E-mail address:* Christopher.Korch@UCDenver.edu

https://doi.org/10.1016/j.yamp.2018.07.003

TABLE 1
Alternative Disguises of HeLa Cells and Publication Rates

Cell Line	Cellosaurus CVCL Number	Claimed Tissue Origin	Articles Mentioning Cell Line in PubMed[a]	Articles Mentioning Cell Line in PubMed Central[a]
HeLa	CVCL_0030	Human adenocarcinoma of uterine cervix	92,883 (1953–2018)	107,253 (1953–2018)
Cells Identified by Gartler [9,10] to be Cross-contaminated Derivatives of HeLa				
AV_3	CVCL_1904	Human amnion	16 (1972–2011)	38 (1967–2018)
Chang Liver	CVCL_0238	Human normal liver	490 (1961–2017)	813 (1961–2018)
Detroit 6	CVCL_2436	Human sternal marrow	13 (1963–2009)	124 (1961–2018)
Detroit 98	CVCL_8188	Human sternal marrow	2 (1960–1991)	4 (1365–1991)
Embryonic lung = L-132	CVCL_1908	Human lung	74 (1969–2017)	124 (1966–2018)
Girardi heart	CVCL_2254	Human heart, normal cells	14 (1971–2008)	32 (1971–2017)
Girardi heart clone 2	CVCL_1815			
Girardi heart clone 7	CVCL_1816			
HEK (not HEK293)	CVCL_M624	Human embryonic kidney cells	[b]	[b]
HEp-2	CVCL_1906	Human carcinoma of larynx	4017 (1961–2018)	9563 (1957–2018)
Intestine 407, Henle 407, Int407	CVCL_1907	Human normal embryonic intestine	324 (1979–2017)	932 (1968–2018)
J-111	CVCL_2965	Human leukocytes	10 (1962–2011)	12 (1961–2017)
KB, KB-3-1, and other variants	CVCL_0372	Human epidermoid oral carcinoma	4035 (1956–2018)	4869 (1958–2018)
NCTC 2544	CVCL_0461	Human skin epithelium	34 (1976–2018)	36 (1993–2017)
WISH	CVCL_1909	Human amniotic cells	68 (1970–2017)	130 (1962–2018)
Other Commonly Used Cell Lines Cross-contaminated by HeLa Cells				
Clone 1-5c-4	CVCL_2260	Human conjunctiva	6 (1971–1983)	14 (1968–1977)
ED27	CVCL_8345	Human chorionic villus	6 (2000–2004)	5 (2000–2013)
FL	CVCL_1905	Human amnion	151 (1959–2016)	164 (1960–2018)
HES	CVCL_W635	Human normal endometrium	[c]	[c]
PC-93	CVCL_4888	Human prostate adenocarcinoma	19 (1983–2014)	9 (1983–2003)

These imposter cell lines are all HeLa cells that were identified by Gartler [9] (1967) and others. The numbers of publications using these lines under their false identities were determined using PubMed and PubMed Central. Many of these lines are still used.

[a] PubMed was searched for publications that mention the cell line and some variants of the cell line names in the title or abstract. The numbers of articles are considerable underestimates of the publications using these cell lines, because many earlier PubMed entries do not include article abstracts, and PubMed does not allow searching within the article (eg, in the Materials and Methods section) for mention of the cell line. PubMed Central can be searched for matches to text in those articles deposited with open access, but it does not include all of the articles found by using the same search algorithm on PubMed.

[b] HEK293 cells are also called HEK. Therefore, it is difficult to identify those publications that used the original HeLa-derived HEK cells.

[c] The cell line name HES is also used for other types of unrelated cells and therefore it is difficult to identify the publications using this cell line.

the frequency of publications using them. Today, there are more than 110 cell lines that are derived from HeLa [12,13], but many of them continue to be used under their false identities for biological studies. Box 1 defines several pertinent terms used throughout this article in the discussion of this problem.

The International Cell Line Authentication Committee (ICLAC; Website ICLAC.org) lists almost 500 cell lines

BOX 1
Definition of Terms as Used in This Article

CODIS, an abbreviation for the FBI's DNA database program entitled COmbined DNA Index System, is often used to indicate the STR loci that have been selected by the FBI for human identification. In the context of this review, it refers to those FBI-selected STR loci that are used for identification of human cell lines and tissues.

Cell line terms

Authenticated cell line is one that has had its identity confirmed or verified by genotyping to be derived from the correct species and donor.

Contaminated cell line is a culture of cells that have been contaminated by viruses, bacteria, yeast, or other organisms.

Cross-contaminated cell line is one that has been contaminated by cells from a different culture (of either human or nonhuman cells) than the original donor. In the mixed culture, if these cross-contaminating cells grow rapidly and vigorously, they may replace the authentic cells in the culture. For example, HeLa cells often took over many cultures in the early days of cell culturing, giving rise to cross-contaminated misidentified false cell lines, such as Intestine 407, KB, HEp-2, Chang Liver, and WISH cells.

Interspecies and intraspecies cross-contaminations arise frequently because of improper handling of cell lines, such as using poor sterile technique or the same bottle of medium for multiple cell lines, improper cleaning of sterile flow hood area between cell lines, or generation of aerosols droplets that infect culture flasks or media bottles.

False or imposter cell line is one that has been shown to be misidentified and generally for which no authentic sample is known to exist but continues to be used under its false or incorrect identity.

Misidentified cell line is one that does not correspond with its correct species or donor origin and is instead from a different donor. Such a culture can arise by either cross-contamination caused by improper handling or because of clerical errors, such as mislabeling of the sample.

Passaging is the process for maintaining actively growing cells in continuous culture by serially diluting aliquots of a cell culture (usually 10–20 fold) into fresh medium regularly.

STR genotyping is the process of determining which variants of STR sequences are present at selected STR loci in the genome of an individual or tissue sample.

SNP genotyping is the process of determining which variants of single nucleotide polymorphic alleles are present at selected single nucleotide polymorphism sites in the genome of an individual or tissue sample.

Tissue terms

Tissue samples are usually derived from tumors (in the context of this article) and are used to study the behavior of cell cultures, as a source for xenografts to study tumor in vivo behavior, or for establishing cell lines.

Xenograft tissues are samples of either normal tissue or cancerous tissue from patients, which are cultured often by implanting into immunodeficient mice.

Misidentified xenograft tissue samples can arise by mislabeling of mice, transplanting into the wrong mouse, or placing extracted samples of the xenograft into the wrong vial in preparation for subsequent analysis. This type of error is potentially the most serious in tissue handling because of the consequences for diagnosis and treatment of patient cancers.

Patient-derived xenografts or patient-derived tumor xenografts are xenografts, usually of cancerous cells or tumors, developed to serve as in vivo models (usually in mice) for studying the mechanisms of the tumor development and the development of therapies.

Patient-derived tumor organoids (PDOs) are tumor samples that are grown in vitro as miniature replicas of organs or tumors with the goal of recapitulating several features of the original sample and for the development of tumor treatments. PDOs are one type of three-dimensional (3D) culture as described by Aboulkheyr Es and colleagues [58] and Vlachogiannis and colleagues [59].

3D in vitro culture tumor models are in vitro cultures that grow into free-floating multicellular spheres of tumor cells. These models include many different types, including PDO cultures as described by Weiswald and colleagues [60].

described in the biomedical literature that are known to be misidentified. Horbach and Halffman [14] analyzed citations in Web of Science to show that ~250 of these cell lines have been used in more than 32,000 publications, which in turn have been cited more than 500,000 times. Between 2000 and 2014, for one of the HeLa-derived cell lines, KB (originally claimed to be from an oral epidermoid carcinoma), 574 publications described the cell line incorrectly versus 57 articles that described it correctly, a 10:1 ratio [15]. In this pool of 631 publications using KB cells with correct and incorrect descriptions, only 2 of the correct publications were found to have authenticated their samples of the cell line.

The Misidentified Cell Line Problem Is Enormous

In 1962, Lewis L. Coriell [16] showed that HeLa cells could survive and be dispersed in aerosols; namely, HeLa cells could "fly," cross-contaminate another cell line, and within 3 passages take over the culture leaving only debris of the original cells. It was in the 1960s that Dr Coriell pioneered the use of biosafety tissue culture hoods to address this contamination problem [17] and these are now a staple in the biomedical laboratory. However, cross-contamination between cultures of cell lines has persisted. Table 2 summarizes reports from the literature describing the frequency of cross-contaminated cell lines [18–33]. Three major studies of cell line authenticity by different repository collections of cell lines using short tandem repeat (STR) genotyping were published between 1999 and 2003 (first 3 entries in Table 2) and they reported between 15% and 36% contamination or mislabeling of cell line samples [18,19,24]. These studies served as an impetus for implementing cell line authentication. Other published studies and unpublished data of prostate, thyroid, ovarian and endometrial, breast, and head and neck cancer cell lines from the University of Colorado (see Table 2) showed that high incidences of misidentified cell lines are common. Recently, 3 reports from Chinese tissue culture facilities also revealed high frequencies of cross-contaminated cell lines in Chinese collections: 25%, 46%, 20%, respectively [30,32,33]. Among 71 cell lines developed in Chinese laboratories, about half of them (35 samples) were HeLa cells [33]. The potential dangers of using misidentified cell lines are shown by finding, for instance, that cell lines derived from melanoma and colon cancer were used to study thyroid cancer [25] and HeLa cells from a cervical carcinoma were used to study prostate cancer [23].

Cell line cultures can be contaminated with cells from various animal species and microorganisms. Drexler and colleagues [34] found that the incidence of mycoplasma contamination of human cell lines obtained from the originators' laboratories decreased from 23% to 0% between 1990 and 2014. However, during this same period, cell line contamination remained stable (14% vs 18%) for samples received from laboratories that had not developed the cell lines but had obtained them from other sources. The frequency of cross-contamination of human lines with cells from other mammalian species (usually mouse) has been lower (eg, 4%) [32]. Both cross-species and intra-species cross-contamination can give rise to mixtures of cells (see example in Raymond Whiting Nims' article, "Historical and Current Methods for Detecting Inter- and Intra-species Cell Mixtures and Thereby Assuring Cell Line Purity," in this issue). Furthermore, from cell mixtures, hybrid cells can be formed by cell fusion [35–40] which can be facilitated by different mechanisms, including the Epstein-Barr virus (EBV) membrane protein [41]. Several nasopharyngeal cell lines established originally from EBV-positive tissue have been reported to have evolved from a fusion between HeLa cells and an unidentified human cell [42,43]. Clearly, interspecies and intraspecies cross-contamination must be detected, especially in laboratories working with cell lines and tissues from multiple species. Methods for detecting mixtures of cell lines that are either of the same or different species are discussed in Raymond Whiting Nims' article, "Historical and Current Methods for Detecting Inter- and Intra-species Cell Mixtures and Thereby Assuring Cell Line Purity," in this issue.

Numerous publications have warned of this dire situation since 1967. Between 2001 and 2012, John Masters [19,44–46] at University College London described the problem and urged it be tackled vigorously. Roland Nardone [47] called for the eradication of cross-contaminated cell lines, which resulted in the National Institutes of Health (NIH) issuing a suggestion that cell lines be authenticated. An international collaboration that led to the development of the ASN-0002 (American National Standard) American National Standards Institute (ANSI) American Type Culture Collection (ATCC) standard [48,49] and the publication of a list of known misidentified cell lines by Capes-Davis and colleagues [50] resulted in 2012 in the establishment of the ICLAC, which maintains and updates this list [12,50]. Bairoch and colleagues [51] established Cellosaurus, an online annotated list of more than 100,000 cell lines with descriptions gleaned from the literature. The ICLAC and Cellosaurus lists are cross-linked. Supplementary Table 1 provides a detailed timeline for relevant events related to the efforts toward cell line authentication. Despite

TABLE 2
Frequencies of Cell Line Cross-Contamination from Published and Unpublished Studies

Cancer Cell Line Type	Year	Genotyping Assay Types	Sample Size	Number of Contaminated Cell Lines	Frequency of Cross-Contamination (%)	References
Various	1999	STR	252	45	18	MacLeod et al [18], 1999
Various	2001	STR	253	91	36	Masters et al [19], 2001
Prostate	2001–2003	STR	28	12	43	van Bokhoven et al [20], 2001; van Bokhoven et al [21], 2001; van Bokhoven et al [22], 2003; van Bokhoven et al [23], 2003
Leukemia and lymphoma	2003	STR	550	82	15	Drexler et al [24], 2003
Thyroid	2008	STR	44	21	48	Schweppe et al, [25], 2008
Adenoid cystic carcinoma	2009	STR and COI	6	6	100	Phuchareon et al [26], 2009
Esophageal adenocarcinoma	2010	STR and SNP	3	14	21	Boonstra et al [27], 2010
Head, neck cancer	2011	STR	122	37	30	Zhao et al [28], 2011
Endometrial	2012	STR	39	11	28	Korch et al [29], 2012
Ovarian	2012	STR	130	49	38	Korch et al [29], 2012
Various	2015	STR	380	113	30	Ye et al [30], 2015
Various	2016	SNP	907	87	9.6	Liang-Chu et al [31], 2015
Various	2017	STR	482	96	20	Bian et al [32], 2017
Various	2017	STR	278	128	46	Huang et al [33], 2017
Breast cancer	NA	STR	117	16	14	Korch, unpublished 2012
Head and Neck		STR	39	7	18	
Totals and overall average contamination (%)			3630	815	22.5	

The mean frequency of cross-contaminated cell lines of different purported cell types in 11 published reports and 2 unpublished studies is 22.5% (n = 3630 samples; range, 9.6%–100%).

Abbreviations: COI, Barcode of Life based on mitochondrial cytochrome C oxidase; SNP, single nucleotide polymorphism; STR, short tandem repeat.

all of these warnings and tools, this problem continues. Descriptions of numerous aspects of the problem and how they may be tackled are provided later.

Laboratory Causes of Misidentified and Cross-Contaminated Cell Lines

In the laboratory, cross-contamination between cultures can result in misidentified cell lines in many ways, including clerical errors (eg, mislabeling of samples); more than 1 person working in a hood at the same time; handling more than 1 cell line at the same time in a biosafety hood; handling the slower growing lines in the hood after handling the more robust, faster growing cultures; sharing reagents (media) between cell lines; maintaining a cluttered work space that is not cleaned between handling distinct cell lines; working hastily; and inadequate training in various techniques, including pipetting and aseptic cell line handling. With such poor techniques, a faster growing contaminant cell can take over a culture in as little as 2 or 3 passages [16,52]. Overgrowth of a faster growing contaminant is also favored if cultures are passaged infrequently or at lower densities [53]. Moreover, the common practice of sharing unauthenticated samples between researchers has been a decisive step in spreading the contaminated cell lines easily and rapidly.

In 2004, Buehring and colleagues [54] reported that more than 80% of researchers using cell lines never authenticated them by karyotyping, isozyme analysis, or STR genotyping. In 2015, Freedman and colleagues [55] reported that the situation had not improved, with 74% of researchers still not authenticating their cell lines by STR genotyping (the standard method, discussed later) because of cost, time constraints, or not seeing the necessity because they thought they were being careful. Clearly, detailed guidelines for handling cell lines, such as those described by Geraghty and colleagues [56], should be implemented in the laboratory to address this problem.

Misidentification of Tissue Samples May Be Less Likely but Riskier for Patient Diagnoses and Treatments

Human and other mammalian cell lines and xenograft tissues, including patient-derived xenografts (PDXs) [57] and patient-derived organoids (PDOs) [58–60] are used as preclinical biomedical research model systems to study different aspects of biological processes (infection, enzymes, gene structure and expression control), behavior of different types of human tissues and cells, diseases such as cancers and infection by microbes (eg, viruses, bacteria), and effects of drugs on normal and abnormal biological processes.

Tissue misidentification is also a problematic quality-control aspect of biomedical research. However, unlike cell line misidentification, it does not usually arise by cross-contamination of one tissue sample by another sample, but primarily occurs through mislabeling of samples. Two examples of this are described by Rebecca E. Schweppe and Christopher Korch's article, "Challenges and Advances in the Development of Cell Lines and Xenografts," in this issue. Although this mix-up may occur less frequently than cell line misidentification, the consequences may be more severe because tissue samples (such as xenografts and organoids) are more likely to be used for clinical diagnosis and treatment decisions. Therefore, compliance with authentication and other quality-control requirements is more critical because of the levels of potential risks for patients from whom the tissue was biopsied.

Warning Indicators of Cross-Contamination or Misidentification

Dramatic changes (indicated by observations of spontaneous transformation or altered cell lines) in culture phenotypes are common indicators of cell line cross-contamination [8]. The cell line M14 from a melanoma of a male patient cross-contaminated the breast cancer cell line MDA-MB-435 sometime between 1978 and 1981 to give rise to a spindle-shaped, faster growing MDA-MB-435S [61]. Since 1981, only the S variant was distributed by the MD Anderson Cancer Center and the ATCC to breast cancer researchers, who often did not realize the significance of the S (thus omitting it from the name) and used this line believing it was an excellent model of breast cancer. To rationalize why this purported breast cancer cell line MDA-MB-435S had some melanoma phenotypes, Sellappan and colleagues [62] invoked lineage infidelity to explain the unexpected phenotypes. Moreover, M14 cells have also been used to study uveal melanoma and thyroid carcinoma [25,61]. Fig. 1A shows how extensively the M14 cell line has infected the literature for melanoma, breast, and thyroid cancers. However, some researchers accepted that MDA-MB-435S was a melanoma cell line and used it in melanoma studies. The different imposters in the M14 family of misidentified cell lines continue to be investigated scientifically despite their identity being incorrect.

The WISH cell line, originally isolated at the Wistar Institute from the normal primary amnion epithelium (birth placenta of a family member, thus the name) was shown in 1967 by Gartler [9] to be derived from the robust and aggressive HeLa cells [9,10]. However, under its disguise, WISH continues to be used extensively to study amnion biology by the parturition community [63]. This cell line, under its disguise as a novel endometrial cell line, was used as a feeder cell for the pretreatment of human zygotes that were implanted in 316 women by in vitro fertilization treatment, 76 of whom gave birth to 111 children [64]. HES and its variants (eg, EM42) have since been shown to be WISH (ie, HeLa) cells ([5,29,65]; Korch unpublished data, 2015). There are some safety concerns with this experiment. For example, it is conceivable that the zygotes may have been contaminated with microbes (such as mycoplasma or viruses), which may have been present in the cultures of these HeLa cells that were used to feed the zygotes in culture that

A

False Cell Identity	Publications[b]
Breast Cancer MDA-MB-435(S) MDA-MB435[a] MDA-435[a] MDA435[a] MDA-MB-435-DTP MDA-MB-435-LCC M4A4 & derivatives NM2C5 & derivatives	1247 (1982–2018)
Melanoma[c] M14 Authentic Melanoma Cell Line)	242 (1976–2018)
MDA-MB-435 MDA-MB-435S MDA-MB435[a] MDA-435[a] MDA435[a] MDA-MB-435-DTP MDA-MB-435-LCC M4A4 & derivatives NM2C5 & derivatives	193 (1983–2018)
Thyroid Cancer BHP5–16 BHP14–9 BHP15–3 BHP17–10 NPA87	15 (1990–2010)
Uveal Melanoma MUM2C, OCM1	108 (1989–2017)

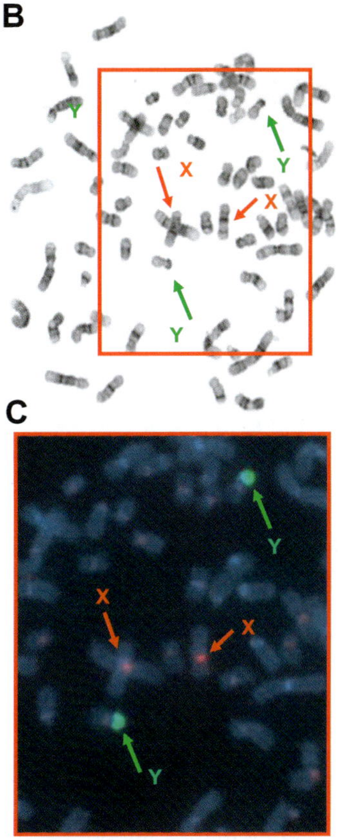

FIG. 1 The many false faces of the male melanoma M14 cell line. (**A**) List of the various derivatives of the M14 cell line from a man that had been misidentified as being from a breast cancer and its derivatives, 5 thyroid cancers, and 2 uveal melanomas. The number of publications listed for each cell line or tissue type was found in PubMed over the indicated periods using the cell line names and are minimum estimates. [a] Boolean wildcard used in searches. [b] Searched on March 1, 2018. [c] Cell lines used as melanoma models. Some samples of MDA-MB435S cells have been also used correctly as samples of the melanoma cell line M14. (**B**) M14 G-banding karyotype and (**C**) partial insert of FISH image showing 2 copies of X chromosomes (*red arrows*) + 2 copies of a derivative of chromosome 22 with Yq12 DNA sequences on its short arm (*green arrows*), which confirms that person from who the M14 cells were taken was male.

subsequently could have infected the zygotes or the maternal uterine cells during implantation. Because HeLa cells are easily dispersed in aerosols [16], they also could have cross-contaminated the zygotes during in vitro culturing and thus carried along with the implanted zygotes into the uteri of some of these women with unknown consequences. According to the report, the cell line in these experiments was neither genetically identified nor tested for microbes [64].

Retractions and Corrigenda of Publications Using False Cell Lines

The authors have identified only 25 published retractions in the literature because of cell line misidentification (Supplementary Table 2). From those, only 2 reports were republished after the work had been repeated with authenticated cell lines (cases R-5 and R-10ab in Supplementary Table 2) by Linger and colleagues [66–69] and Cai and colleagues [70–72]. More often what happens is that, when the investigators realize they have used a misidentified cell line in a published article, they acknowledge this information in a new publication (Supplementary Table 3, examples E-4 and E-5). Seldom is a corrigendum issued on the original article or the original article retracted by either the investigators or the journal, as shown for several examples in Supplementary Table 3. Furthermore, if the investigators submit an erratum, it can be difficult to find on the journal's Web site or in PubMed, because the erratum often is not clearly linked to the original article at either site. Even when it is clear that the results are incorrect, the journal does not seem to tackle the problem by linking the original article to the letter of concern as shown for examples E-6 and E-7 (Supplementary Table 3).

CURRENT TECHNOLOGIES FOR AUTHENTICATION OF HUMAN CELL LINES

Classical Cytogenetic Methods for Detecting Cell Line Cross-Contamination

As early as the 1950s, cytogenetic methodology was the first approach to authenticate the species origin of continuous cell lines and to identify cross-contamination between lines originating from different species. The number and morphology of metaphase chromosomes were, and still are, used to detect inter-species contamination of cell lines when different species had markedly dissimilar diploid content or when the distribution of different classes of chromosomes (telocentric, acrocentric, submetacentric, metacentric) were visibly distinct. Using these strategies, the species of mouse, monkey, and human cell lines were correctly determined [6,7] and, when coupled with immunologic analysis and tumorigenicity in mice, human cell lines were distinguished from mouse lines, and multiple lines of different purported origins were either from human (probably HeLa) cells or from the mouse line L929 [6,7,73].

It was in the late 1960s and early 1970s that the development of protocols for the Giemsa (G) and Quinacrine (Q) banding of chromosomes allowed the identification of abnormal, rearranged chromosomes and thus the detection of intraspecies cross-contamination. The G-banding technique allowed Nelson-Rees and colleagues [74–76] to identify marker chromosomes unique to HeLa cells and thereby confirm Gartler's [9] identification of the 19 HeLa imposters. They went on to identify 279 cases of intraspecific and interspecific misidentification of cell lines caused by contamination and mislabeling [47,77]. In 1978, Lavappa [78] reported analysis of early stocks of multiple cell lines at the ATCC. By G-banding and Q-banding, he confirmed the earlier reports of cell lines cross-contaminated by HeLa (sharing common marker chromosomes and lacking Y-chromosomal DNA) and found an additional 16 HeLa-derived misidentified cell lines.

Molecular Cytogenetic Methods Complement Short Tandem Repeat and Single Nucleotide Polymorphism Genotyping Methods

The development of various new molecular cytogenetic techniques in the 1990s dramatically increased the accuracy of karyotyping and their use for intraspecies cell line identification. Two of the most useful karyotyping technologies are multiplex fluorescence in situ hybridization (M-FISH) and spectral karyotyping (SKY). At the University of Colorado, the Miller–van Bokhoven group with Varella-Garcia and Korch studied prostate cell lines using a combination of M-FISH, SKY, G-banding, STR genotyping, mutation screening by DNA/cDNA sequencing, and different gene expression assays. They found that 43% (see Table 2) of cell lines of purported prostate origin were cross-contaminated [20–23,79]. One was from the cervical carcinoma cell line HeLa, adding to the list of 4 other HeLa-derived cell lines used to study prostate cancer [23]. Two lines were from the female-derived T24 bladder cancer cell line, and 8 lines had been cross-contaminated with other prostate cell lines [23]. The cell line PEAZ-1 was actually the fibrosarcoma cell line HT-1080 [80]. However, this finding led to only an erratum cited in PubMed but not to retraction of the original article describing PEAZ-1 or to a link between the original article and the erratum on the journal's Web site (see Supplementary Table 3) [81,82].

These investigative approaches were extended to other nonhuman species. For instance, Wiegant and colleagues [83] used a 21-color fluorescence in situ hybridization (FISH) strategy (COBRA [COmbined Binary RAtio labeling]) to karyotype 6 murine cell lines established from lymphoma and 3 from colon cancer cells. These investigators were able to show that 3 lymphoma cell lines had a common origin, having arisen by cross-contamination.

Another simple, but very efficient, molecular cytogenetic strategy for cell line identification was more recently used to study the relationship between the melanoma cell line UCLA-SO-M14 (also called M14) from a male donor and the breast cancer cell line MDA-MB-435 and its spindle-shaped derivative MDA-MB-435S from a female donor [61]. As mentioned earlier, MDA-MB-435S cell line (often labeled only as MDA-MB-435) has been used extensively in breast cancer studies up through 2018, as well as in studies of thyroid cancer and uveal melanoma (see Fig. 1A). Earlier STR genotyping had shown that both of these cell lines came from the same individual and did not have a copy of the Y-linked amelogenin gender-identifying locus, implying they were both derived from a female donor [84,85]. Expression analyses showed that they both expressed melanoma phenotypes [86], which was used to argue that MDA-MB-435(S) showed lineage infidelity [62]. Furthermore, G-banding karyotyping of metaphase chromosomes showed that the cell line carried 2 copies of the X chromosome and apparently no Y chromosome [87]. Korch and colleagues [42] decided to resolve this seeming conundrum by STR and single nucleotide polymorphism (SNP) genotyping samples of M14, a lymphoblastoid cell line (ML14) derived from the M14 patient's blood and DNA from serum of a UCLA-SO-M14 patient (which predated the establishment of MDA-MB-435S). DNA from the serum of UCLA-SO-M14 and from the ML14 cell line carried the Y-linked amelogenin locus [61] and thus showed that all of the samples came from the male patient with melanoma M14.

What had happened to the Y chromosome in M14 and MDA-MB-435S? Using a cytogenetic dual-color FISH assay, the authors confirmed that these cells carried 2 copies of the X chromosome as reported earlier [87], which we found by variable number tandem repeat genotyping to be homozygous, showing that they arose by duplication [61]. Furthermore, the Yq12 region (which did not contain the Y-linked allele of amelogenin) was found to have been retained in the genome by translocation to chromosome 22 (Fig. 1B, C). Thus, the FISH assay resolved the discordance between the male origin of the cell line and the lack of a Y-linked amelogenin locus, and showed definitively that this cell line was not a suitable model for studying cancers of the breast, thyroid, or uvea.

How the breast cancer cross-contamination probably arose is explained by Korch and colleagues [61]. The verification of the similarities between M14 and MDA-MB-435S might have been resolved by other technologies, such as next-generation SNP sequencing or transcriptome analysis. However, FISH is a simpler, faster, and less costly technology, and was able to show where the remnant of the Y chromosome was in the specimen's genome.

Cell Line Genotyping by Short Tandem Repeats on Capillary Sequencers

There are currently 3 principal technologies used to genetically authenticate cell lines and tissues: STR genotyping, SNP genotyping, and karyotyping by Giemsa banding (G-banding); molecular approaches (M-FISH, SKY); or combinations thereof. Two publications provide detailed guidelines of the methods for authenticating cell lines by STR DNA genotype analysis [49,88,89].

The reference standard protocol determines the number of microsatellite repetitive sequences with tetranucleotide or pentanucleotide repeats at STR loci, which are present at specific, highly polymorphic loci in the human genome. Each locus may contain from 5 to more than 50 tetranucleotide repeats and there may be 100 or more different alleles per locus (Fig. 2A). At present, STR genotyping is performed using an optimized, balanced multiplex polymerase chain reaction (PCR) to amplify selected STR loci with fluorescently labeled primers (1 labeled primer per locus) as shown in Fig. 2B. The amplicons are electrophoretically separated (Fig. 2C) and, from their sizes (see examples in Fig. 2B), the number of repeats at the various loci are deduced.

The forensic community has established a set of loci (which are not in exons to avoid using markers related to genetic diseases) to identify forensic samples from crime scenes, disasters, and missing persons. Some of these well-validated STR kits can be used for both forensic purposes and for genotyping of human cell lines, because the PCRs are robust, optimized with minimal artifacts, and most of the loci are highly polymorphic providing great discriminatory power to distinguish between both individuals and human cell lines. However, STR genotyping cannot distinguish between cell lines from different tissues from the same donor, because they are from the same genetic background.

The forensic market has driven the development of many kits by companies such as Promega Corporation, Applied Biosystems/Thermo Fisher Scientific, and Qiagen. The cell line authentication community has established as a standard the use of STR kits that test for the amelogenin locus, plus the 13 CODIS STR loci shown in Supplementary Table 4. Supplementary Table 5 lists the currently available capillary genetic analyzers and software needed for STR genotyping. The older kits Promega Powerplex 1.2 and Applied Biosystems Profiler Plus have been discontinued, but there is a great deal of data in the literature based on each of these kits. Besides being commercially available, an advantage of using the other newer kits listed in Supplementary Table 4 is that they test most of the same STR loci tested by the discontinued kits, allowing laboratories to compare data between new and old kits. Newer STR kits that test 25 to 30 STR loci (eg, Westen and colleagues [90]) may allow better resolution between related cell lines and provide additional information about any gross changes in the genomes arising in sublines of cells because of genetic drift and loss of heterozygosity (LOH).

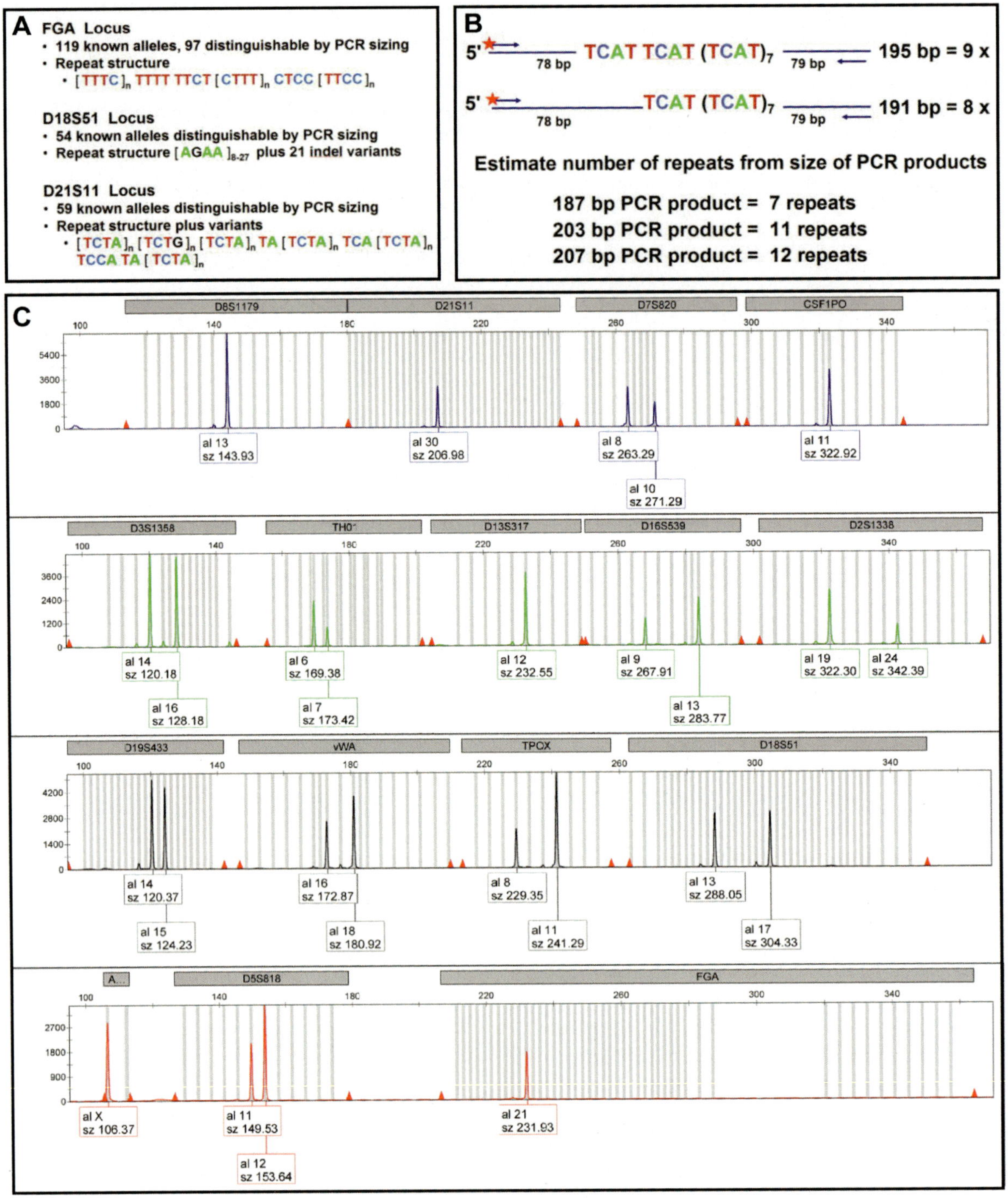

FIG. 2 STR methodology. (**A**) Examples of the sequence variability at 3 STR loci: FGA, D18S51, and D21S11. (**B**) Target STR loci with tetranucleotide or pentanucleotide repeat sequences are PCR amplified with 1 fluorescently labeled and 1 unlabeled primer per STR locus. From the size of the amplicons, the number of repeats are deduced as shown. For analysis of multiple STR loci, the PCR reactions are multiplexed in 1 reaction tube and different fluorescent labels and amplicon sizes are used to distinguish the products of the different STR loci. (**C**) Electropherogram of the STR profile for passage 15 of the melanoma cell line M14 illustrating the appearance of the data showing the sizes of the different alleles in number of repeats (al) and in nucleotides (sz).

Authentication of Cell Lines by Single Nucleotide Polymorphism Genotyping

Several different techniques are available for SNP genotyping of cell lines, including:

- Sanger sequencing of individual PCR amplicons containing a mutation or SNP of interest
- Screening for mutations and SNPs based using SNP microarrays
- Single base extension (SBE) assays (such as Thermo Fisher Scientific's SNaPshot kit, both single and multiplexed assay)
- Fluidigm's SNP Trace proprietary technology
- Thermo Fisher Scientific's TaqMan technology
- High-resolution melting analysis of PCR amplicons containing the SNP target

Castro and colleagues [91] used the high-throughput, medium-density microarray Illumina Luminex platform to develop a 24-SNP multiplex profiling (multiplex cell line authentication [MCA]) assay and screened 436 cell lines from the German Collection of Microorganisms and Cell Cultures (DSMZ) that had previously been STR genotyped. They reported excellent concordance between the two assays for most cell lines. In the case of cell lines showing microsatellite instability, they found the SNP-based MCA technique was more robust in distinguishing between cell lines than the STR genotyping assay. However, the genotyping results were not provided in the article and are not available online for comparison purposes.

In forensic settings, the primary SNP assay is the multiplexed SBE assay using the multiplex SNaPshot technology. In this technology, SNP targets are PCR amplified in short amplicons. Then an assay primer adjacent to the SNP site to be queried is extended by incorporating fluorescently tagged dideoxynucleotides complementary to the SNP base using multiple extension cycles (Fig. 3), as described in detail elsewhere [92]. The fluorescent color of the resulting products indicates which of the 4 bases was incorporated at the

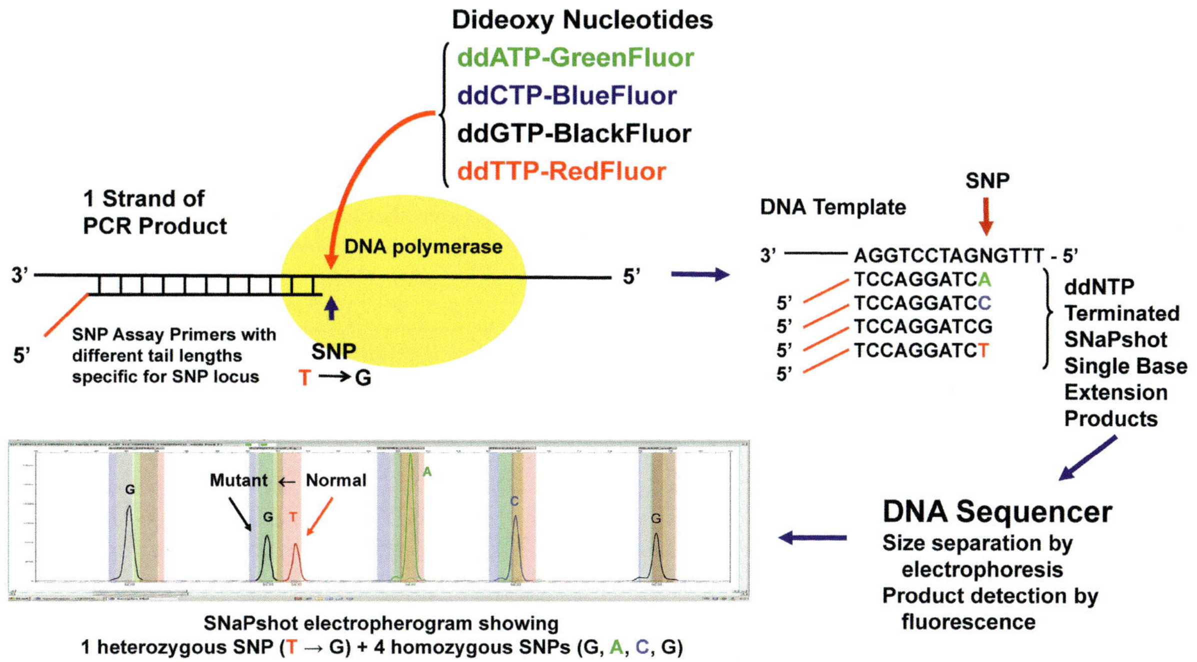

FIG. 3 SNaPshot SBE SNP methodology. Regions containing SNPs are PCR amplified and purified. A SNP assay primer is annealed adjacent to the SNP site and fluorescently labeled dideoxynucleotides (ddNTPs) and DNA polymerase extends the primer by 1 nucleotide across the SNP site, incorporating the complementary fluorescently labeled ddNTP, which prevents further extension. For each SNP site, primers of different lengths are used and, after incorporating the ddNTP, they are electrophoretically separated by size to produce an electropherogram. The different labeled ddNTPs may cause slight shifts in mobility of the primers, as shown in the electropherogram. From the color of the signals, the ddNTPs that were incorporated, and thus the sequences at the SNP locus, can be deduced.

SNP site. In the multiplex version of this assay, the assaying primers differ in length by 10 or so nucleotides so that, when the resulting reaction products are electrophoresed into the capillary array of a sequencer, they are distinguished by their different lengths. Both the initial PCR amplification and the SBE steps may be multiplexed with suitable optimization of primer design and concentrations. One set of reactions can query 30 to 40 targets; to query additional SNP targets, additional sets of SBE reactions are needed.

An important consideration for the implementation of the SNaPshot assay is the design of primers for the initial PCR and for the SBE assay primer; namely, some loci have both transition and transversion mutations. For example, in the KRAS DNA sequence for codon 12, coding nucleotide 34 can be mutated from G to T, C, or A and coding nucleotide 35 can be altered from G to C or T. As a consequence, the assay must be able to detect all 4 versions and the primer that queries nucleotide position 35 should not overlap nucleotide 34, and vice versa, because of potential inhibition of proper annealing of the assay primer adjacent to the test target. This requirement must be taken into consideration when designing SBE and other assays.

There are several advantages of the SNaPshot technology, including that (1) in laboratories or shared research facilities that already have a capillary sequencer, this technology can be used on it along with STR genotyping and Sanger sequencing; and (2) unlike most other SNP assays, which only consider 2 alternative sequences at a SNP (usually transition mutations A or C ↔ G or T), this SBE technology can distinguish between all 4 possible alleles, as described earlier for the KRAS codon for amino acid G12 (see Fig. 3). The SBE assay has also been developed for the Sequenom Sample ID Plus SNP genotyping kit, which differentiates between variants by mass spectrometry (Agena Bioscience iPLEX Pro Sample ID Panel with MassARRAY analysis system).

Another proprietary SNP technology applied to cell line authentication is the Fluidigm SNP Trace system in combination with Fluidigm's microfluidic instruments. This technology amplifies small amplicons by PCR, which are queried with fluorescent tagged assay probes and described by Fluidigm only as being "allele-specific PCR assays ... that use three primers and two universal probes to distinguish between two alleles" Available at: https://www.fluidigm.com/faq/gt-8. This technology was used to determine the SNP genotypes of DNA from almost 1000 cell lines that had also, in parallel, been SNP genotyped using Illumina HumanOmni2.5_4v1 arrays and STR genotyped [31]. To match the level of discrimination between cell lines obtained using STR genotyping of 15 autosomal STR loci required assaying a minimum of 48 SNP loci. Although this technology offers high-throughput capacity, in the case of cell lines with allelic imbalances, genetic rearrangements, and lack of reference normal DNA samples for each cell line, it can produce false-positives [61]. Also, some X-linked SNPs that were called heterozygous by the SNP Trace assay performed by Fluidigm personnel were found by PCR and Sanger DNA sequencing to be either homozygous or hemizygous and the assay detected Y-linked SNPs that were absent from the cell because of deletion of the corresponding segment of the Y chromosome [29]. Further validation of this assay and its software is needed for more reliable calling of SNPs in cell lines.

Short Tandem Repeat Genotyping by Next-Generation Sequencing

Next-generation sequencing (NGS) kits have been developed for several of the different NGS platforms in the forensic market, as listed in Supplementary Table 6. Several of the kits were designed by Illumina and Thermo Fisher Scientific to sequence a combination of STR, SNP, and mutation targets. Early Illumina kits (SNPforID 52-plex and so forth; Supplementary Table 6) intended for use on the Illumina MiSeq instrument were based on sequencing the initial PCR amplicons that had been originally designed for SNaPshot SNP assays (ie, before extension with dideoxynucleotides, as shown in Fig. 3).

Subsequent NGS approaches for forensic, cell line, and tissue identification determine the sequence of multiple STR and SNP targets as listed in Supplementary Table 6. The Illumina MiSeq FGx Forensic Genomics kit seems currently to be the most extensive kit for such analyses. Zaaijer and colleagues [93] have designed a novel approach using the Oxford Nanopore MinION sequencer, which is discussed in more detail by Amanda Capes-Davis' article, "Cell Line Detective Work: Basic Principles and Molecular Applications," in this issue. This sequencer is small and can be hooked up to a laptop computer to produce the sequence of 60 to 350 SNPs in short runs. Using a specifically designed bayesian algorithm, the data are checked for matching with a reference sample. The assay is intended for confirmation, by re-identification, that the samples in question have not become misidentified.

Recently, Shin and colleagues [94] describe their STR sequencing (STR-seq) protocol, which uses CRISPR-Cas9-targeted fragmentation of genomic DNA to sequence more than 2000 STR loci with nearby SNPs without needing to add unique bar codes to the library or to perform PCR amplification of the targets. The STR-SNP targets were selected for fitting within 150-bp read lengths and being polymorphic. An advantage of the high number of loci analyzed by STR-seq is that haplotype phasing and linkage information can be used to determine whether changes in heterozygosity of an STR locus are caused by loss of a chromosomal homologue or simply by a mutation under a primer site. Furthermore, NGS can differentiate between STR loci that have the same overall length but differ slightly in sequence.

These brute-force strategies provide far more data than are needed to identify a given cell line. However, as discussed later, in research, these extra data can be used to compare sublines that have undergone genetic drift in more detail than data based only on the 13 CODIS STR loci.

Authentication of Cell Lines by Next-Generation RNA Sequencing

Fasterius and colleagues [95] used next-generation RNA sequencing (whole-transcriptome sequencing) for cell line authentication by comparing single nucleotide variations (SNVs) and developed a computational pipeline for analyzing the data and comparing the results with SNV data for cell lines from the Catalogue of Somatic Mutations in Cancer (COSMIC) database. This approach is useful for validating that the cell line's RNA sequencing data match known data, (eg, those in the COSMIC database) and that the samples of a cell line from various stages in a set of experiments are the same, as discussed earlier for the MinION method. However, a premise of this approach is that, when comparing SNPs in complementary DNA (cDNA) sequences with genomic sequences, both/all copies of a gene are transcribed. In cases in which only 1 copy is transcribed, there may occur a discordance between cDNA and genomic DNA, as was observed in the Ishikawa cell line [29]. Another limitation of this approach is that it is not possible to search the COSMIC database for RNA sequence matches and identify other unknown cell lines that have identical or very similar SNP genotypes.

Inappropriate Methods for Cell Line Authentication: Phenotype Does Not Prove Genotype

Cell lines must be shown to be genetically related to the individual from which they were derived. Several inappropriate methods have been used to characterize cell lines, both genetically and phenotypically. Once a line has been associated with a specific tissue, it may continue to be used with that description, even when shown to be misidentified, because it is claimed to be a good, easy-to-use model and the phenotype is thought to match that expected for the original claimed tissue type. KB cells, purportedly from an oral epidermoid carcinoma, were shown in 1967 to be derived from HeLa, but their use under their false identity has continued to grow significantly over the past 50 years. During 2000 to 2014, there have been 10 times as many articles using this cell line describing it incorrectly than those describing it correctly [15]. However, a good, easy-to-use model does not make it a meaningful model.

Also, cell lines cannot be authenticated by morphologic observation under microscopy, as claimed by some investigators [96], although changes in cell morphology might be a warning of changes in the culture (eg, cross-contamination or a mix-up between cultures). Morphologic changes are subtle and difficult to interpret, and they can neither identify the cell genetically nor confirm they have not been cross-contaminated. Three of the cell lines (Bel7402, LO-2, SMMC7721) used for the major part of the report on liver cancer metastasis by Xu and colleagues [96] were purportedly of liver origin, but they have been shown to be HeLa cells [32,33]. Morphologic examination obviously missed identifying the 3 HeLa-derived cell lines. The applicability of the findings in studies using misidentified lines therefore must be seriously questioned.

The levels of expression of specific messenger RNAs (mRNAs), proteins, or enzymatic activities can be used to characterize the phenotypes of cell lines. For example, cDNA expression microarrays were used to characterize the NCI-60 cancer cell lines, with some cell lines being found not to show the phenotypes expected for their claimed tissues of origin [97]. The purported breast cancer cell line MDA-MB-435, which is included in the NCI-60 panel, does not group with the other breast cancer cell lines but with melanoma cell lines, including M14. Rae and colleagues [84] showed that these two cell lines shared the same STR genotype. Other phenotypic methods have been used to confirm a cell line's genetic origin, including semiquantitative Western blotting of specific proteins expressed by cell lines [98] or immunocytofluorescence to detect proteins expressed on the cell surface [99] to argue that the cells were authentic. Many factors influence gene expression, including media components; for example, different batches of serum [100], contamination by mycoplasma [101,102]), and even cell culture densities influenced which proteins were expressed by cells [103]. These approaches can only indicate tissue specificity, not genetic background.

Earlier, the expression of genetic variants of isoenzymatic proteins that differed in size, specific activity, or isoelectric properties were used to authenticate cell lines (eg, Gartler [9]). It is important to understand that, in contrast with the inappropriate phenotypic methods mentioned earlier, it is not their amounts but the genetic alterations to the genes for these isozymes that alter the behavior of isozymic proteins and thus allows genetic identification of cells.

Therefore, although different measures of expressed amounts of mRNA and proteins may help identify a specific cell type or tissue origin of a cell line, they are not valid for identity authentication because they only characterize the phenotype of cell lines and not their genetic origins. For cell line authentication, it is critical to understand that although a cell's genotype gives rise to its phenotype, the phenotype can be variable and does not prove a cell's genotype.

Searching for Matching Cell Lines in the Scientific Literature and Databases of Genotypes

Searching for publications using specific cell lines in different databases (for instance, PubMed) can be difficult because cell lines often have multiple names, slight variations in the spelling of their names, or even nonunique names. Therefore, for cell lines to be valid, reliable, and useful models, they must not only be authenticated, but also described accurately with unique names [104–106]. Standardization of cell line naming conventions will make it easier to find publications using specific cell lines.

of May 2018). The ATCC database is a collection of STR genotypes for only the ATCC cell lines. One relevant difference between the 2 databases is that the ATCC assumes single peaks are only entered once; whereas for the DSMZ search engine single peaks should be entered twice on the premise that it is homozygous. This second approach may bias the search results when comparing cell lines that have different degrees of heterozygosity. The CLIMA (Cell Line Integrated Molecular Authentication) database is a third approach for finding cell lines with matching STR genotypes [108]. All 3 databases contain the STR genotypes for 8 or more loci. Different institutions and laboratories have developed their own searchable databases of STR profiles from the literature and various databases, but they are proprietary and cannot be freely searched.

To search for cell lines with matching STR profiles, researchers need only enter the profiling results of a sample and the database automatically pulls forth any potential matching cell lines within the database and ranks them with a similarity score. The currently favored scoring algorithms are variants of the so-called Tanabe algorithm [109]. This formula was used by Yu and colleagues [13]) and Liang-Chu and colleagues [31]) for analyzing their collection of STR and SNP genotype profiles, respectively. The identity quotient or percentage match is calculated by multiplying by 2 the number of shared alleles at those loci examined in both the test sample and the database sample. This value is divided by the total number of alleles at the same loci:

$$\%\ \text{Identity} = \frac{2 \times (\text{number of shared alleles between samples at shared loci}) \times 100\%}{(\text{number of alleles in test sample}) + (\text{number of alleles in database sample})}$$

There are few sets of cell line genotyping data that allow searching for matches of a cell line of unknown origin to determine its identity and find related cell lines. The best-developed databases for authentication of cell lines comparing STR genotypes are the 2 publicly available at the DSMZ and ATCC Web sites [107] (Supplementary Box 1). The DSMZ database is a collection of STR profiles from the ATCC, DSMZ, Japanese Cancer Research Resources Bank (JCRB), and RIKEN cell repositories that have been consolidated into a single searchable database of 3274 samples (as

It is currently accepted that an 80% or greater STR genotype identity score for 2 cell lines shows that the cell lines are derived from the same person [13,109]. However, this does not prove that 2 samples of a cell line are genetically or phenotypically identical, because cell cultures are heterogeneous and can drift genetically [110–112]. Kleensang and colleagues [113] showed this problem when they studied 2 aliquots of the same batch of the breast cancer cell line MCF-7 that differed by only 4 passages (grown for only 3 and 7 passages after receipt from the ATCC). They controlled for many factors, such as using the same batches of media, and the assays were done by the same personnel on the same equipment. Although the samples had identical STR genotypes, they showed many phenotypic and genetic differences. See Rebecca E. Schweppe and Christopher Korch's article, "Challenges and Advances in the Development of Cell Lines and Xenografts," in this issue.

Single Nucleotide Polymorphism Genotyping Data Resources

At present (March, 2018), the authors are not aware of any publicly available online SNP database that can be searched like the STR databases of the ATCC, the DSMZ consolidation of STR profiles, or the CLIMA Web site (see Supplementary Box 1). The various SNP assays applied to cell lines have not used a consensus set of SNPs. A major collection of SNP genotyping data has been published for 907 cell lines [31] but has not been established with a searchable Web tool for identifying related cells. Based on the work of Castro and colleagues [91], Multiplexion maintains a private SNP database (http://www.multiplexion.de/en/cell-line-testing-service/multiplex-human-cell-line-authentication) and now offers a SNP genotyping service for cell lines. Their proprietary (not publicly available) database contains SNP genotypes for ~850 cell lines, which they offer to search for potential cell line matches for their customers on a fee basis.

Ethical Concerns of Genotyping Assays

Genotyping of cell lines and tissue samples raises several ethical concerns about donor privacy. The current STR standard uses only 8 or 9 autosomal loci for authenticating cell lines to minimize linkage of samples to specific donors. Cell lines can often undergo genetic drift because they are passaged extensively, which manifests as a LOH and results in STR profiles with fewer alleles. Such low-heterozygosity profiles can be inadequate for distinguishing between unrelated cell lines with similar genotypes. To improve the discriminatory power, the number of STR loci tested needs to be increased. However, this also increases the likelihood of being able to link a cell line to a specific person. Moreover, Edge and colleagues [114] have shown that, using extensive SNP data, it is possible to deduce by linkage the STR genotype of 90% to 98% of the tested samples, which in turn could link SNP data to STR profiles in collections of forensic and clinical genetic data sets.

SNaPshot-based assays have been developed to be used forensically to screen for 4 classes of SNPs: (1) identity informative SNPs for genetic identification of individuals; (2) lineage informative SNPs for inferring genealogies, kinships, blood types, and paternities; (3) ancestry informative SNPs for determining biographic and ethnic ancestry; and (4) phenotype informative SNPs for inferring phenotypes such as eye, skin, and hair color [92]. The lineage, ancestry, and phenotype SNP assays could allow determining the ethnicity, appearance, biogeographical origin, or the presence of ethnic-specific or race-specific mutations of the donors of cell lines. Furthermore, NGS genotyping would provide even more extensive genetic data that could readily identify individuals. Such information is not useful for authentication of cell lines and tissue samples, because it is not available for properly de-identified donor samples. However, as Erlich and Narayanan [115] described, there are multiple routes by which patient privacy can be breached and DNA samples could be re-identified using SNP data. The power of consumer DNA genealogy data was recently shown when it was used to identify a suspect in the Golden State Killer case [116].

Therefore, because these forensic and consumer DNA genotyping assays (especially the lineage, ancestry, and phenotype SNP assays) pose serious ethical issues that could breach patient confidentiality, they should not be used for authenticating cell lines and nor should such results ever be made publicly available. However, there still remains the dilemma of how extensive STR or SNP profiles may safely be published in the scientific literature without compromising patient privacy.

SUMMARY

Advantages of Different Genotyping Assays

Advantages and uses of different genotyping assays are summarized in Table 3. It is likely that STR genotyping assay by capillary electrophoresis will remain the most frequently used technique for cell line authentication until SNP genotyping cell line data are consolidated into a searchable format and all the cell lines in the STR databases have also been SNP genotyped. The SNP assay most likely to be used for cell lines will be a form of the SBE assay because of its design simplicity, the availability of capillary sequencers, and the development of NGS of standard SBE amplicons (Supplementary Table 6). Also, DNA sequencing and SBE SNP assays could be developed for the analysis of either isozymes or specific mutations so that newer SNP or STR genotypes of cell lines could be linked to the original identity tests of older cell lines. This ability would make it possible to confirm whether a current sample of a cell line has the genotype that was originally determined for older cell lines, as was done for the M14 melanoma cell line [61]).

TABLE 3
Advantages of Different Molecular Methods for Authentication of Human Cell Lines and Tissues

Assays	Advantage Explanation
Karyotyping	Karyotyping assays (G-banding, M-FISH, SKY) can reveal genomic changes and localize them (eg, translocations) unlike SNP, STR, or NGS assays
NGS	NGS of numerous variants can be examined, which permits evaluating causes of LOH by examining chromosome-specific sets of SNPs and/or STRs
NGS	NGS allows comparison with older STR data in established databases
NGS	NGS allows comparison with published SNP data
NGS STR-seq	Screens for both STR and linked SNP sequences, allowing determination of haplotypes and sequences of variant STR alleles of the same length but that differ in sequence of repeat units
NGS MinION	The MinION NGS SNP screening approach can provide quicker bench-side information about changes (mix-ups) of cell and tissue samples, but requires SNP array data as a reference
SNP	SNP assays use shorter PCR amplicons than STR assays and therefore are better for degraded DNA (from formalin-fixed paraffin-embedded sections, old samples)
SNP	SNP assays are better suited for determining identity of microsatellite instability (MSI) high samples
SNP	Multiple SNP assays per chromosome can be used to determine whether LOH of STR alleles caused by loss of the whole chromosome or localized alteration of the STR region (eg, loss vs mutation of primer sites vs mitotic gene conversion)
SNP	High number of SNP calls can compensate for poor-quality calls and still provide sufficient data to determine cell line identities
SNP	Various types of SNP assays can be used to authenticate cell lines samples with limited information about their provenance (eg, ABO blood types; isozymes [eg, G6PD variants])
SNP	Extensive SNP data that are not based on lineage, ancestry, and phenotype SNP assays may not have the same societal or privacy concerns in countries that do not allow the release of genetic information publicly (eg, the limit of 9 STR loci permitted by Japanese law)
SNP SBE	The SBE SNaPshot assay for identity-information-SNP kits based on 52, 55, or 57 SNPs are excellent choices for authentication of cell lines because they are well developed and tested for the forensic arena and meet the 48 SNP minimum criterion of Liang-Chu et al [31]
SNP SBE	SNaPshot SBE assays are not based on the assumption of only biallelic changes and can therefore be used for cases in which targets have 3 or 4 sequence variants (eg, KRAS codon for glycine 12)
SNP SBE	SBE SNP amplicons can be analyzed by Sanger and NGS
SNP and STR	Several newer kits for determining LOH and chromosomal duplication based on SNPs and STRs on the X and Y chromosomes are available commercially
SNP and STR	Unlike karyotyping data, STR or SNP data are readily searchable in a database format for identifying matching cell lines
SNP and STR	Karyotyping requires specialized equipment, high levels of expertise, and costs higher than standard SNP and STR assays. Core laboratories may be a useful resource to address these issues
STR	Fewer PCR reactions are needed for STR genotyping than for SNP assays, because the STR loci are highly polymorphic
STR	Commercial STR genotyping kits are well validated, use consensus sets of loci, and are accepted as the gold standard method by the cell line authentication community
STR	Searchable STR databases are freely available for authenticating cell lines; in contrast, searchable and freely available SNP-based databases remain to be established

Various approaches to authentication of human cell lines and tissues (original tumor, xenografts, and organoids) offer different advantages and can be complementary. The method of choice depends on available equipment, expertise, the level of discrimination and information required for the planned experiments, and whether the results are to be compared with previously published genotypes in the literature or databases.

Lessons Learned and Positive Advances from Tackling the Cell Line Problem

It is hoped that the evidence presented herein shows the magnitude of the problem of cell line and tissue misidentification. Clearly, complacency about this problem must be dispelled by rigorously authenticating these biological reagents in order for biomedical research to be reproducible and meaningful. Simply stating which cell lines or tissues were used, or checking them for their phenotype, is inadequate, even if the sample used is a robust one like HeLa cells, because it could have been taken over by an even more robust line. Without authentication, it will never be known which cell line or subclone was used in experiments. Detailed laboratory guidelines for the careful handling of authenticated cell lines and tissues during research to minimize cell line contaminations and for the implementation of a cell line authentication policy at research institutions are presented by Rebecca E. Schweppe and Christopher Korch's article, "Challenges and Advances in the Development of Cell Lines and Xenografts," in this issue.

The problem of cell line and tissue misidentification does not need to be only doom and gloom. There may be a boon to studying cell cross-contamination, as suggested by Rae and colleagues [84]). For example, in the case of the cell line M14 and its various imposters (see Fig. 1A), with the assumption that the cell lines listed are truly derivatives of M14, then the research done using the breast cancer, thyroid, and uveal melanoma variants of M14 can now be reinterpreted and perhaps applied profitably to understanding cutaneous melanoma. The Cellosaurus [51] and ICLAC (iclac.org) Web sites and the experiments in publications showing different cases of misidentification may provide new insights into specific biological conundrums once the data are reinterpreted in light of the true identities of the samples.

ACKNOWLEDGMENTS

The authors would like to thank Drs. Amanda Capes-Davis and Ferric Fang for sharing with us the identity of 10 and 6 retraction notices, respectively, that are listed in Supplementary Table 2. We are very grateful to Dr Capes-Davis for her detailed comments and suggestions on our article. This article is dedicated to the memory of Dr Roland M. Nardone (1928-2018). In 2007, he reignited the campaign to eliminate the widespread use of misidentified cell lines [47] and tissues [117] for biomedical research, a practice that has led to extensive questionable research and squandered research funds.

We also acknowledge financial support from the National Cancer Institute (NCI) Cancer Center Support Grant P30CA046934 (Molecular Pathology and DNA Sequencing & Analysis Shared Resources).

REFERENCES

[1] Gey GO, Coffman WD, Kubicek MT. Tissue culture studies of the proliferative capacity of cervical carcinoma and normal epithelium. Cancer Res 1952; 12(4):264–5.

[2] Lucey BP, Nelson-Rees WA, Hutchins GM. Henrietta Lacks, HeLa cells, and cell culture contamination. Arch Pathol Lab Med 2009;133(9):1463–7.

[3] Gold M. A conspiracy of cells - one woman's immortal legacy and the medical scandal it caused. Albany (NY): State University of New York Press; 1986.

[4] Skloot R. The immortal life of Henrietta Lacks. New York: Crown Publishers; 2010.

[5] Harris R. Rigor mortis - how sloppy science creates worthless cures, crushes hope, and wastes billions. New York: Basic Books; 2017.

[6] Rothfels KH, Parker RC. The karyotypes of cell lines recently established from normal mouse tissues. J Exp Zool 1959;142:507–20.

[7] Clausen JJ, Syverton JT. Comparative chromosomal study of 31 cultured mammalian cell lines. J Natl Cancer Inst 1962;28:117–45.

[8] Brand KG, Syverton JT. Results of species-specific hemagglutination tests on "transformed," nontransformed, and primary cell cultures. J Natl Cancer Inst 1962;28:147–57.

[9] Gartler SM. Genetic markers as tracers in cell culture. Natl Cancer Inst Monogr 1967;26:167–95.

[10] Gartler SM. Apparent Hela cell contamination of human heteroploid cell lines. Nature 1968;217(5130):750–1.

[11] Auersperg N, Gartler SM. Isoenzyme stability in human heteroploid cell lines. Exp Cell Res 1970;61(2):465–7.

[12] International Cell Line Authentication Committee (ICLAC). Database of cross-contaminated or misidentified cell lines. 2016. Available at: http://iclac.org/wp-content/uploads/Cross-Contaminations-v8_0.pdf. Accessed March 9, 2018.

[13] Yu M, Selvaraj SK, Liang-Chu MM, et al. A resource for cell line authentication, annotation and quality control. Nature 2015;520(7547):307–11.

[14] Horbach S, Halffman W. The ghosts of HeLa: how cell line misidentification contaminates the scientific literature. PLoS One 2017;12(10):e0186281.

[15] Vaughan L, Glanzel W, Korch C, et al. Widespread use of misidentified cell line KB (HeLa): incorrect attribution and its impact revealed through mining the scientific literature. Cancer Res 2017;77(11):2784–8.

[16] Coriell LL. Detection and elimination of contaminating organisms. Natl Cancer Inst Monogr 1962;7:33–53.

[17] Coriell LL. Laminar flow systems for sterile work. Natl Cancer Inst Monogr 1968;29:569–72.

[18] MacLeod RA, Dirks WG, Matsuo Y, et al. Widespread intraspecies cross-contamination of human tumor cell lines arising at source. Int J Cancer 1999;83(4):555–63.

[19] Masters JR, Thomson JA, Daly-Burns B, et al. Short tandem repeat profiling provides an international reference standard for human cell lines. Proc Natl Acad Sci U S A 2001;98(14):8012–7.

[20] van Bokhoven A, Varella-Garcia M, Korch C, et al. TSU-Pr1 and JCA-1 cells are derivatives of T24 bladder carcinoma cells and are not of prostatic origin. Cancer Res 2001;61(17):6340–4.

[21] van Bokhoven A, Varella-Garcia M, Korch C, et al. Widely used prostate carcinoma cell lines share common origins. Prostate 2001;47(1):36–51.

[22] van Bokhoven A, Caires A, Maria MD, et al. Spectral karyotype (SKY) analysis of human prostate carcinoma cell lines. Prostate 2003;57(3):226–44.

[23] van Bokhoven A, Varella-Garcia M, Korch C, et al. Molecular characterization of human prostate carcinoma cell lines. Prostate 2003;57(3):205–25.

[24] Drexler HG, Dirks WG, Matsuo Y, et al. False leukemia-lymphoma cell lines: an update on over 500 cell lines. Leukemia 2003;17(2):416–26.

[25] Schweppe RE, Klopper JP, Korch C, et al. Deoxyribonucleic acid profiling analysis of 40 human thyroid cancer cell lines reveals cross-contamination resulting in cell line redundancy and misidentification. J Clin Endocrinol Metab 2008;93(11):4331–41.

[26] Phuchareon J, Ohta Y, Woo JM, et al. Genetic profiling reveals cross-contamination and misidentification of 6 adenoid cystic carcinoma cell lines: ACC2, ACC3, ACCM, ACCNS, ACCS and CAC2. PLoS One 2009;4(6):e6040.

[27] Boonstra JJ, van Marion R, Beer DG, et al. Verification and unmasking of widely used human esophageal adenocarcinoma cell lines. J Natl Cancer Inst 2010;102(4):271–4.

[28] Zhao M, Sano D, Pickering CR, et al. Assembly and initial characterization of a panel of 85 genomically validated cell lines from diverse head and neck tumor sites. Clin Cancer Res 2011;17(23):7248–64.

[29] Korch C, Spillman MA, Jackson TA, et al. DNA profiling analysis of endometrial and ovarian cell lines reveals misidentification, redundancy and contamination. Gynecol Oncol 2012;127(1):241–8.

[30] Ye F, Chen C, Qin J, et al. Genetic profiling reveals an alarming rate of cross-contamination among human cell lines used in China. FASEB J 2015;29(10):4268–72.

[31] Liang-Chu MM, Yu M, Haverty PM, et al. Human biosample authentication using the high-throughput, cost-effective SNPtrace™ system. PLoS One 2015;10(2):e0116218.

[32] Bian X, Yang Z, Feng H, et al. A combination of species identification and STR profiling identifies cross-contaminated cells from 482 human tumor cell lines. Sci Rep 2017;7(1):9774.

[33] Huang Y, Liu Y, Zheng C, et al. Investigation of cross-contamination and misidentification of 278 widely used tumor cell lines. PLoS One 2017;12(1):e0170384.

[34] Drexler HG, Dirks WG, MacLeod RA, et al. False and mycoplasma-contaminated leukemia-lymphoma cell lines: time for a reappraisal. Int J Cancer 2017;140(5):1209–14.

[35] Jacobsen BM, Harrell JC, Jedlicka P, et al. Spontaneous fusion with, and transformation of mouse stroma by, malignant human breast cancer epithelium. Cancer Res 2006;66(16):8274–9.

[36] Willkomm L, Bloch W. State of the art in cell-cell fusion. Methods Mol Biol 2015;1313:1–19.

[37] Bastida-Ruiz D, Van Hoesen K, Cohen M. The dark side of cell fusion. Int J Mol Sci 2016;17(5) [pii:E638].

[38] Ephrussi B, Weiss MC. Interspecific hybridization of somatic cells. Proc Natl Acad Sci U S A 1965;53(5):1040–2.

[39] Hussain T, Mulherkar R. Lymphoblastoid cell lines: a continuous in vitro source of cells to study carcinogen sensitivity and DNA repair. Int J Mol Cell Med 2012;1(2):75–87.

[40] Duelli D, Lazebnik Y. Cell-to-cell fusion as a link between viruses and cancer. Nat Rev Cancer 2007;7(12):968–76.

[41] Wang D, Liebowitz D, Kieff E. An EBV membrane protein expressed in immortalized lymphocytes transforms established rodent cells. Cell 1985;43(3 Pt 2):831–40.

[42] Chan SY, Choy KW, Tsao SW, et al. Authentication of nasopharyngeal carcinoma tumor lines. Int J Cancer 2008;122(9):2169–71.

[43] Strong MJ, Baddoo M, Nanbo A, et al. Comprehensive high-throughput RNA sequencing analysis reveals contamination of multiple nasopharyngeal carcinoma cell lines with HeLa cell genomes. J Virol 2014;88(18):10696–704.

[44] Masters JR. False cell lines: the problem and a solution. Cytotechnology 2002;39(2):69–74.

[45] Masters JR. HeLa cells 50 years on: the good, the bad and the ugly. Nat Rev Cancer 2002;2(4):315–9.

[46] Masters JR. Cell-line authentication: end the scandal of false cell lines. Nature 2012;492(7428):186.

[47] Nardone RM. Eradication of cross-contaminated cell lines: a call for action. Cell Biol Toxicol 2007;23(6):367–72.

[48] Barallon R, Bauer SR, Butler J, et al. Recommendation of short tandem repeat profiling for authenticating human cell lines, stem cells, and tissues. In Vitro Cell Dev Biol Anim 2010;46(9):727–32.

[49] American Type Culture Collection Standards Development Organization Workgroup ASN-0002. Cell line misidentification: the beginning of the end. Nat Rev Cancer 2010;10(6):441–8.

[50] Capes-Davis A, Theodosopoulos G, Atkin I, et al. Check your cultures! A list of cross-contaminated or misidentified cell lines. Int J Cancer 2010;127(1):1–8.

[51] Bairoch A. The Cellosaurus: a cell line knowledge resource. 2018; version 25: Available at: https://web.expasy.org/cellosaurus/. Accessed September 15, 2018.

[52] Nims RW, Shoemaker AP, Bauernschub MA, et al. Sensitivity of isoenzyme analysis for the detection of interspecies cell line cross-contamination. In Vitro Cell Dev Biol Anim 1998;34(1):35–9.

[53] Jordan I, Munster VJ, Sandig V. Authentication of the R06E fruit bat cell line. Viruses 2012;4(5):889–900.

[54] Buehring GC, Eby EA, Eby MJ. Cell line cross-contamination: how aware are mammalian cell culturists of the problem and how to monitor it? In Vitro Cell Dev Biol Anim 2004;40(7):211–5.

[55] Freedman LP, Gibson MC, Wisman R, et al. The culture of cell culture practices and authentication–results from a 2015 Survey. Biotechniques 2015;59(4):189–90, 92.

[56] Geraghty RJ, Capes-Davis A, Davis JM, et al. Guidelines for the use of cell lines in biomedical research. Br J Cancer 2014;111(6):1021–46.

[57] Morton JJ, Bird G, Keysar SB, et al. XactMice: humanizing mouse bone marrow enables microenvironment reconstitution in a patient-derived xenograft model of head and neck cancer. Oncogene 2016;35(3):290–300.

[58] Aboulkheyr Es H, Montazeri L, Aref AR, et al. Personalized cancer medicine: an organoid approach. Trends Biotechnol 2018;36(4):358–71.

[59] Vlachogiannis G, Hedayat S, Vatsiou A, et al. Patient-derived organoids model treatment response of metastatic gastrointestinal cancers. Science 2018;359(6378):920–6.

[60] Weiswald LB, Bellet D, Dangles-Marie V. Spherical cancer models in tumor biology. Neoplasia 2015;17(1):1–15.

[61] Korch C, Hall EM, Dirks WG, et al. Authentication of M14 melanoma cell line proves misidentification of MDA-MB-435 breast cancer cell line. Int J Cancer 2018;142(3):561–72.

[62] Sellappan S, Grijalva R, Zhou X, et al. Lineage infidelity of MDA-MB-435 cells: expression of melanocyte proteins in a breast cancer cell line. Cancer Res 2004; 64(10):3479–85.

[63] Yao JL, He QZ, Liu M, et al. Effects of Delta(9)-tetrahydrocannabinol (THC) on human amniotic epithelial cell proliferation and migration. Toxicology 2018;394:19–26.

[64] Desai N, Abdelhafez F, Bedaiwy MA, et al. Live births in poor prognosis IVF patients using a novel non-contact human endometrial co-culture system. Reprod Biomed Online 2008;16(6):869–74.

[65] Kniss DA, Summerfield TL. Discovery of HeLa cell contamination in HES cells: call for cell line authentication in reproductive biology research. Reprod Sci 2014; 21(8):1015–9.

[66] Linger RM, DeRyckere D, Brandao L, et al. Mer receptor tyrosine kinase is a novel therapeutic target in pediatric B-cell acute lymphoblastic leukemia. Blood 2009; 114(13):2678–87.

[67] Linger RMA, DeRyckere D, Brandao L, et al. Retraction. Linger RMA, DeRyckere D, Brandao L, Sawczyn KK, Jacobsen KM, Liang X, Keating AK, Graham DK. Mer receptor tyrosine kinase is a novel therapeutic target in pediatric B-cell acute lymphoblastic leukemia. Blood. 2009;114(13):2678–87. Blood 2012;120(7):1533.

[68] Linger RM, Lee-Sherick AB, DeRyckere D, et al. Mer receptor tyrosine kinase is a therapeutic target in pre-B-cell acute lymphoblastic leukemia. Blood 2013;122(9):1599–609.

[69] Linger RM, Graham DK. A common case of cell line misidentification. 2014. Available at: https://thewinnower.com/discussions/9-a-common-case-of-cell-line-misidentification. 2018. Accessed September 15, 2018.

[70] Cai C, Rodepeter FR, Rossmann A, et al. Nef from SIV(-mac239) decreases proliferation and migration of adenoid-cystic carcinoma cells and inhibits angiogenesis. Oral Oncol 2011;47(9):847–54.

[71] Cai C, Rodepeter FR, Rossmann A, et al. SIVmac(2)(3)(9)-Nef down-regulates cell surface expression of CXCR4 in tumor cells and inhibits proliferation, migration and angiogenesis. Anticancer Res 2012;32(7):2759–68.

[72] Cai C, Rodepeter FR, Rossmann A, et al. Retraction notice to "Nef from SIVmac239 decreases proliferation and migration of adenoid-cystic carcinoma cells and inhibits angiogenesis" [OO 47 (2011) 847-854]. Oral Oncol 2012;48(1):95.

[73] Defendi V, Billingham RE, Silvers WK, et al. Immunological and karyological criteria for identification of cell lines. J Natl Cancer Inst 1960;25:359–85.

[74] Nelson-Rees WA, Flandermeyer RR. HeLa cultures defined. Science 1976;191(4222):96–8.

[75] Nelson-Rees WA, Hunter L, Darlington GJ, et al. Characteristics of HeLa strains: permanent vs. variable features. Cytogenet Cell Genet 1980;27(4):216–31.

[76] Nelson-Rees WA, Daniels DW, Flandermeyer RR. Cross-contamination of cells in culture. Science 1981; 212(4493):446–52.

[77] Buehring GC. In memoriam. Walter Anthony Nelson-Rees, research geneticist, UC Berkeley, 1929 – 2009. 2010; Obituary for Walter Nelson-Rees. Available at: http://senate.universityofcalifornia.edu/_files/inmemoriam/html/walteranthonynelson-rees.html. Accessed March 9, 2018.

[78] Lavappa KS. Survey of ATCC stocks of human cell lines for HeLa contamination. Vitro 1978;14(5):469–75.

[79] Varella-Garcia M, Boomer T, Miller GJ. Karyotypic similarity identified by multiplex-FISH relates four prostate adenocarcinoma cell lines: PC-3, PPC-1, ALVA-31, and ALVA-41. Genes Chromosomes Cancer 2001;31(4):303–15.

[80] van Bokhoven A. Models of prostate cancer. Molecular characterization and critical appraisal of human prostate carcinoma cell lines. Doctoral Dissertation, University Medical Centre St Radboud, Nijmegen, The Netherlands. Self published, 2004.

[81] Schmelz M, Cress AE, Barrera J, et al. PEAZ-1: a new human prostate neoplastic epithelial cell line. Prostate 2001;48(2):79–92.

[82] Schmelz M, Cress AE, Barrera J, et al. Erratum: PEAZ-1: a new human prostate neoplastic epithelial cell line. Prostate 2001;48:79–92. Prostate 2004;61(4):375.

[83] Wiegant J, van Hall T, van der Burg M, et al. Application of multicolor fluorescence in situ hybridization analysis for detection of cross-contamination and in vitro progression in commonly used murine tumor cell lines. Cancer Genet Cytogenet 2002;139(2): 126–32.

[84] Rae JM, Creighton CJ, Meck JM, et al. MDA-MB-435 cells are derived from M14 melanoma cells–a loss for breast cancer, but a boon for melanoma research. Breast Cancer Res Treat 2007;104(1):13–9.

[85] Lorenzi PL, Reinhold WC, Varma S, et al. DNA fingerprinting of the NCI-60 cell line panel. Mol Cancer Ther 2009;8(4):713–24.

[86] Ellison G, Klinowska T, Westwood RF, et al. Further evidence to support the melanocytic origin of MDA-MB-435. Mol Pathol 2002;55(5):294–9.

[87] Chambers AF. MDA-MB-435 and M14 cell lines: identical but not M14 melanoma? Cancer Res 2009;69(13):5292–3.

[88] ATCC Standards Development Organization. ASN-0002. Authentication of human cell lines: standardization of STR Profiling. ANSI eStandards Store. 2011. Available at: https://webstore.ansi.org/RecordDetail.aspx?sku=ANSI%2FATCC+ASN-0002-2011. Accessed September 15, 2018.

[89] Reid Y, Storts D, Riss T, et al. Authentication of human cell lines by STR DNA profiling analysis. Assay Guidance Manual 2013. Available at: https://www.ncbi.nlm.nih.gov/books/NBK144066/. Accessed September 15, 2018.

[90] Westen AA, Kraaijenbrink T, Robles de Medina EA, et al. Comparing six commercial autosomal STR kits in a large Dutch population sample. Forensic Sci Int Genet 2014;10:55–63.

[91] Castro F, Dirks WG, Fahnrich S, et al. High-throughput SNP-based authentication of human cell lines. Int J Cancer 2013;132(2):308–14.

[92] Mehta B, Daniel R, Phillips C, et al. Forensically relevant SNaPshot® assays for human DNA SNP analysis: a review. Int J Legal Med 2017;131(1):21–37.

[93] Zaaijer S, Gordon A, Speyer D, et al. Rapid re-identification of human samples using portable DNA sequencing. eLife 2017;6 [pii:e27798].

[94] Shin G, Grimes SM, Lee H, et al. CRISPR-Cas9-targeted fragmentation and selective sequencing enable massively parallel microsatellite analysis. Nat Commun 2017;8:14291.

[95] Fasterius E, Raso C, Kennedy S, et al. A novel RNA sequencing data analysis method for cell line authentication. PLoS One 2017;12(2):e0171435.

[96] Xu HT, Lai WL, Liu HF, et al. PAK4 phosphorylates p53 at serine 215 to promote liver cancer metastasis. Cancer Res 2016;76(19):5732–42.

[97] Ross DT, Scherf U, Eisen MB, et al. Systematic variation in gene expression patterns in human cancer cell lines. Nat Genet 2000;24(3):227–35.

[98] Marlowe TA, Lenzo FL, Figel SA, et al. Oncogenic receptor tyrosine kinases directly phosphorylate focal adhesion kinase (FAK) as a resistance mechanism to FAK-kinase inhibitors. Mol Cancer Ther 2016;15(12):3028–39.

[99] Wang M, Wu C, Guo Y, et al. The primary growth of laryngeal squamous cell carcinoma cells in vitro is effectively supported by paired cancer-associated fibroblasts alone. Tumour Biol 2017;39(5):1010428317705512.

[100] Sikora MJ, Johnson MD, Lee AV, et al. Endocrine response phenotypes are altered by charcoal-stripped serum variability. Endocrinology 2016;157(10):3760–6.

[101] Olarerin-George AO, Hogenesch JB. Assessing the prevalence of mycoplasma contamination in cell culture via a survey of NCBI's RNA-seq archive. Nucleic Acids Res 2015;43(5):2535–42.

[102] Drexler HG, Uphoff CC. Mycoplasma contamination of cell cultures: Incidence, sources, effects, detection, elimination, prevention. Cytotechnology 2002;39(2):75–90.

[103] Nerlich AG, Bachmeier BE. Density-dependent lineage instability of MDA-MB-435 breast cancer cells. Oncol Lett 2013;5(4):1370–4.

[104] Sarntivijai S, Ade AS, Athey BD, et al. A bioinformatics analysis of the cell line nomenclature. Bioinformatics 2008;24(23):2760–6.

[105] International Cell Line Authentication Committee (ICLAC). Naming a cell line. 2015. Available at: iclac.org/wp-content/uploads/Naming-a-Cell-Line_v1_6.pdf. Accessed September 15, 2018.

[106] Kurtz A, Seltmann S, Bairoch A, et al. A standard nomenclature for referencing and authentication of pluripotent stem cells. Stem Cell Reports 2018;10(1):1–6.

[107] Dirks WG, MacLeod RA, Nakamura Y, et al. Cell line cross-contamination initiative: an interactive reference database of STR profiles covering common cancer cell lines. Int J Cancer 2010;126(1):303–4.

[108] Romano P, Manniello A, Aresu O, et al. Cell line data base: structure and recent improvements towards molecular authentication of human cell lines. Nucleic Acids Res 2009;37(Database issue):D925–32.

[109] Capes-Davis A, Reid YA, Kline MC, et al. Match criteria for human cell line authentication: where do we draw the line? Int J Cancer 2013;132(11):2510–9.

[110] Hughes P, Marshall D, Reid Y, et al. The costs of using unauthenticated, over-passaged cell lines: how much more data do we need? Biotechniques 2007;43(5): 575, 7-8, 81–2 passim.

[111] Nishida M. The Ishikawa cells from birth to the present. Hum Cell 2002;15(3):104–17.

[112] Parson W, Kirchebner R, Muhlmann R, et al. Cancer cell line identification by short tandem repeat profiling: power and limitations. FASEB J 2005;19(3):434–6.

[113] Kleensang A, Vantangoli MM, Odwin-DaCosta S, et al. Genetic variability in a frozen batch of MCF-7 cells invisible in routine authentication affecting cell function. Sci Rep 2016;6:28994.

[114] Edge MD, Algee-Hewitt BFB, Pemberton TJ, et al. Linkage disequilibrium matches forensic genetic records to disjoint genomic marker sets. Proc Natl Acad Sci U S A 2017;114(22):5671–6.

[115] Erlich Y, Narayanan A. Routes for breaching and protecting genetic privacy. Nat Rev Genet 2014;15(6):409–21.

[116] Fuller T. How a genealogy site led to the front door of the Golden State Killer suspect. New York Times; Available at: https://www.nytimes.com/2018/04/26/us/golden-state-killer.html. Accessed September 16, 2018

[117] Nardone RM, MacLeod RA, Capes-Davis A. Cancer: Authenticate new xenograft models. Nature 2016; 532(7599):313.

Advances in Molecular Pathology 1 (2018) 229–238
ADVANCES IN MOLECULAR PATHOLOGY

Cell Line Detective Work

Basic Principles and Molecular Applications

Amanda Capes-Davis, MB BS, BSc(Med), PhD
CellBank Australia, Children's Medical Research Institute, The University of Sydney, 214 Hawkesbury Road, Westmead, New South Wales 2145, Australia

KEYWORDS

• Authentication • Cell line • Characterization • Genotyping • Misidentification • Provenance

KEY POINTS

- A misidentified cell line fails to correspond to its correct species or donor origin, corresponding instead to a cell line from a different donor.
- Misidentified cell lines can be detected through authentication testing. For human cell lines, short tandem repeat (STR) genotyping is a consensus method that allows comparison between laboratories.
- Cell line investigation requires assessment of cell line provenance, including reported information and authentication data. A test sample is authenticated and compared with reference samples from the reported donor, or to cell line datasets to help exclude misidentification with other cell lines.
- Genotype-based methods, including single nucleotide polymorphism (SNP) genotyping, offer new opportunities for authentication.
- Proteome-based methods allow better understanding of tissue origin and disease diagnosis, which is useful for cell line investigations.

WHY DO CELL LINES NEED DETECTIVE WORK?

Cell Lines Are Valuable Models

Cell lines are essential resources for biomedical research, clinical diagnostics, and clinical translation. A cell line is typically established from a tissue sample, placed into culture because an ongoing supply of cells is considered desirable. Once established as a continuous cell line, the culture will proliferate indefinitely and becomes an inexhaustible source of material. Although cell cultures can be replaced by in vitro cell-free systems in some fields, cell lines continue to be used for diagnostic assays, therapeutic screens, and biomedical research. For example, animal cell culture was used to generate an estimated 65% of biopharmaceuticals used in 2012 [1].

The first human cell line, HeLa, was established in the 1950s [2]. Over time, genetic modification and manipulation of growth conditions have increased rates of cell line establishment, making this process easier and more accessible for research laboratories [3]. As a result, the research community now has an abundance of cell line models. Cellosaurus, which acts as a cell line knowledge resource, lists more than 107,000 cell lines, with approximately 80,000 of human origin (https://web.expasy.org/cellosaurus/).

Disclosure: The author is self-funded as a consultant in the areas of good cell culture practice and laboratory safety. No conflicts of interest are declared.
E-mail address: acapdav@gmail.com

https://doi.org/10.1016/j.yamp.2018.06.011
2589-4080/18/

Cell Lines Can Have Uncertain Origins

Although cell lines are widely used, they are subject to quality concerns. Misidentified cell lines (terminology: see Box 1) fail to correspond to the correct donor origin and instead correspond to a cell line from a different donor. Misidentified cell lines can arise through mislabeling of cultures or through cross-contamination, where cells from another culture are accidentally introduced without the scientist's knowledge. Cross-contamination initially results in a mixture of cells from different sources, as described in an article by Raymond Nims, "Historical and Current Methods for Detecting Inter- and Intra-species Cell Mixtures and Thereby Assuring Cell Line Purity", elsewhere in this issue. However, a faster growing contaminant can replace the original, authentic material after only a few passages [4–6]. In most cases, it is unclear how the misidentification occurred. An early study of contamination demonstrated that HeLa cells (the commonest cause of misidentification) are readily spread via droplets during handling procedures [4].

BOX 1
Terminology

Authentication: testing performed to confirm or verify the identity of a cell line, demonstrating that it is derived from the correct species and donor.

Characterization: testing performed to confirm or verify the characteristics of a cell line, demonstrating that it is a representative model for research or in vitro assays.

Misidentification: the finding that a cell line fails to correspond to its correct species or donor origin and corresponds instead to a cell line from a different donor.

Originator, Originating Laboratory: the scientist or laboratory that establishes a cell line.

Primary Reference: the first publication to describe a cell line and its establishment, handling, and validation.

Primary Source: an originator or reference repository that provides a cell line for use.

Provenance: the records that provide information on the origin, source, handling, and validation of a cell line.

Reference Repository: a laboratory or organization that receives a cell line from a depositor (typically the originator), documents its provenance, and prepares low-passage, authenticated stocks of the cell line for distribution. Reference repositories include cell banks, culture collections, and core facilities that specialize in this work.

Reference Sample: a physical sample of a cell line that is held by a primary source. Reference samples include donor tissue or blood, early passages of the same cell line, or synonymous cell lines. Reference samples also include datasets of widely used classic tumor cell lines to pick up unexpected matches.

Research Resource Identifier (RRID): a unique identifier that can be applied to the cell line regardless of its source; used to unambiguously identify the cell line in publications.

Secondary Source: any individual, laboratory, or organization that provides a cell line for use, provided it is not a primary source (originator or reference repository).

Synonymous: cell lines established from the same donor.

Test Sample: a physical sample of a cell line used for authentication or characterization.

A recent survey of cell line quality concerns showed that misidentified cell lines are common. The risk of encountering a misidentified cell line from a secondary source was estimated at 1:6 [7]. Misidentified cell lines are also widely used in publications. The International Cell Line Authentication Committee (ICLAC) curates a register of misidentified cell lines (http://iclac.org/databases/cross-contaminations/). These misidentified cell lines have been used in an estimated 32,755 scientific publications [8].

Misidentified cell lines can be detected through authentication, defined here as the testing performed to confirm or verify the identity of a cell line, demonstrating that it is derived from the correct species and donor. "Authentication" can be defined more broadly, to encompass all testing used to examine a cell line's validity [9]. However, a broader definition would mean that authentication requirements would vary with tissue type and disease diagnosis. In this article, "authentication" refers to genotype-based methods used to detect misidentified cell lines, and "characterization" to the broader testing used to determine that a cell line is a valid model.

In some cases, it is difficult to prove that a cell line is misidentified after authentication has been performed. This is usually because the origin of the cell line is unclear. Problems with the origin of a cell line typically relate to its age and the quality of cell line samples and information. Most cell lines in widespread use were established in the past century [10]. As laboratories close and researchers retire, it becomes increasingly difficult to contact the originating laboratory to ask for assistance when problems are discovered. Early samples become increasingly difficult to access, unless the cell line was deposited at a reference repository. Early samples are also important because cell lines may experience genetic drift with passaging, particularly loss of heterozygosity (LOH). If a cell line is serially passaged as it is passed from one investigator to another, genetic drift becomes more evident and authentication data can become more difficult to interpret.

When the origins of a cell line are unclear, scientists must use a process of investigation to determine if the cell line is authentic or misidentified. This is best demonstrated by the work of Jørgen Fogh, MD, who established a pioneering reference repository at Sloan-Kettering Institute (Fig. 1). Fogh [11] used the molecular methods of his time, primarily isoenzyme analysis, for authentication. Dracopoli and Fogh [12] were the first to recognize that cell line genotypes were subject to LOH, resulting in the need to increase the number of loci tested to improve discriminatory power. Their meticulous approach solved cases of uncertain origin that would still be challenging today. For example, Fogh investigated a set of 8 cell lines that shared a common donor origin, working with the originator to show that 2 of these cell lines were authentic and the remaining 6 were misidentified (summary: Box 2). The 2 authentic cell lines, SW480 and SW620, were established from primary and secondary tumors in the same patient and are now well-characterized models of tumor progression [13,14].

This article describes a workflow for cell line investigation that is used by the author as a member of ICLAC (http://iclac.org/). The overall aim of this workflow is to illustrate how to investigate a problematic cell line and decide if it is authentic or misidentified. In some cases, cell line information and samples are insufficient to reach a decision. Recent advances are discussed to see how molecular applications might improve the investigative workflow.

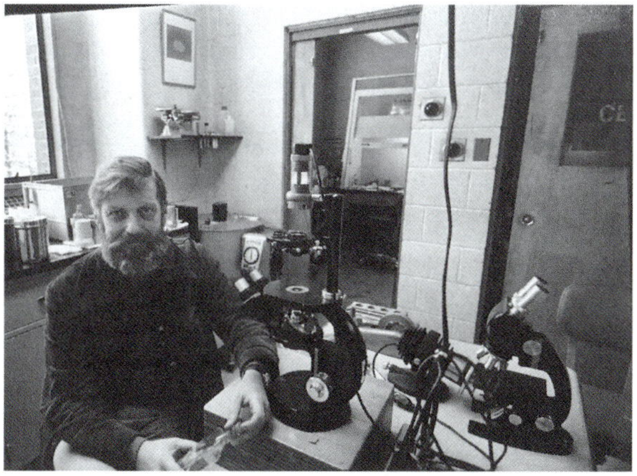

FIG. 1 Jørgen Fogh. Jørgen Fogh was a pioneer of cell line authentication. His laboratory at the Sloan-Kettering Institute for Cancer Research focused on the development and characterization of cell lines for more than 20 years, performing authentication and characterization on their collection of approximately 500 human tumor cell lines. Fogh's approach to cell line investigation acts as a foundation for the basic principles described in this review. (*Courtesy of* Jens and Peter Fogh, Stockholm, Sweden.)

WORKFLOW FOR CELL LINE INVESTIGATION

Step 1: Cell Line Information

There is an increasing focus on molecular techniques for cell line analysis, which may lead scientists to jump straight to these molecular techniques to investigate cell lines. However, scientists who succumb to that temptation can easily misinterpret their data. Two cell lines, SW480 and SW620, show the importance of cell line provenance if authentication data are to be interpreted correctly (summary: Box 2).

Cell line provenance can be defined as the records that provide information on a cell line's origins, source, handling, and validation [15]. The term used may vary, with some investigators preferring "history" or "background information." Regardless of the term used, the importance of cell line provenance for research and clinical translation is widely acknowledged [6,16].

Table 1 sets out a dataset of information that the author has found helpful to investigate the origins of a cell line. Cell line investigations can rely on unusual information. For example, the physical location of the originator's laboratory may be relevant. If 2 cell lines have a shared donor origin, but were established by different laboratories on different continents, it is unlikely that the donor traveled from one continent to the other; it is more likely that one of the cell lines will be misidentified.

Recent publications and resources have made cell line information easier to find [6]. For example, Cellosaurus (https://web.expasy.org/cellosaurus/) is a cell line knowledge resource that aims to describe all cell lines used in biomedical research. Research Resource Identifiers (RRIDs) are generated using Cellosaurus and can be cited in publications [17], making it easier for researchers to unambiguously identify cell lines despite duplication and similarities in cell line names [6].

There are limits to the donor-specific information that may be publicly accessible. Personal identifiers, such as donor names and dates of birth, carry a risk to privacy and should always be treated as confidential information, unless the donor consents to release of information [18]. Personal identifiers should be retained by a data custodian, who may be a member of the patient's clinical care team or the cell line's originator. A minimal dataset of information (sex, age, tissue type, disease

BOX 2
Investigation of SW480 and SW620

SW480 and SW620 cell lines were established in the laboratory of Albert Leibovitz, who sent approximately 100 of his cell lines to Jørgen Fogh for characterization and storage [13]. Isoenzyme analysis in Fogh's laboratory demonstrated that an unexpectedly high number of these cell lines shared a rare isoenzyme variant (peptidase D phenotype 2). Further testing by isoenzyme and cytogenetic analysis showed that 8 cell lines shared a common donor origin: SW480, SW527, SW598, SW608, SW613, SW620, SW732, and SW733. Looking at cell line information, a timeline was established for handling of the 8 cell lines. The earliest cell line, SW480, was in its sixth passage before the other cell lines were passaged. Cytogenetic analysis of SW480 was performed at passage 6 and demonstrated that it was authentic. SW620 was derived from a later metastasis in the same donor; after further characterization, Fogh concluded that SW620 was authentic but the other 6 cell lines were misidentified [13]. SW480 and SW620 continue to be widely used as models for colorectal carcinoma and tumor progression [14].

Images show SW480 (*A*, ATCC CCL-228) and SW620 (*B*, ATCC CCL-227) in culture. Cell lines were deposited by Albert Leibovitz. Scale bar represents 100 μm.

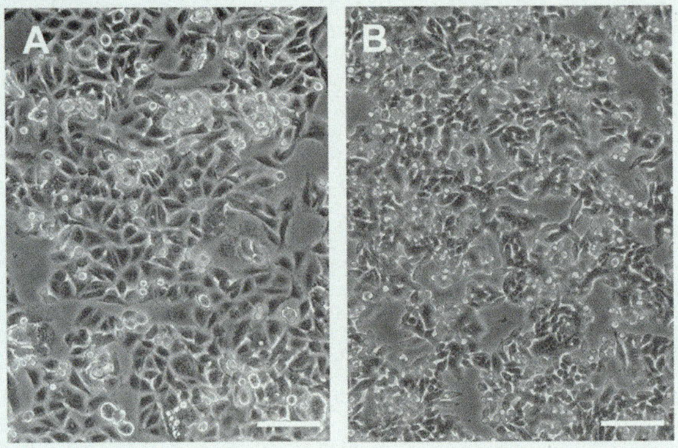

Courtesy of ATCC, Manassas, VA; with permission.

diagnosis) is valuable for cell line provenance and should be reported in the primary reference.

Step 2: Authentication Data

Cell line authentication relies on data comparison. Typically, a laboratory tests a sample from its own stocks (the "test sample") and compares their data to samples from primary sources ("reference samples"). Reference samples may include tissue or blood from the original donor, early passage samples of the cell line, or synonymous cell lines. It is possible for reference samples to be misidentified; for example, widely used stocks of U-87 MG were recently discovered to be misidentified when compared with samples held by the originator [19]. To reduce this risk, a dataset of classic tumor cell lines is used to detect misidentification from a large group of likely contaminants [20].

For comparison of samples between laboratories, we need a consensus method for authentication. A number of test methods have been used for authentication, including isoenzyme analysis, cytogenetic analysis, HLA analysis, short tandem repeat (STR) genotyping, and single nucleotide polymorphism (SNP) genotyping [5,6,11]. Most methods are donor-specific, based on genomic sequence variants that are inherited by the individual but vary at the population level. Donor-specific methods will not detect problems if cell lines were established from the same individual (eg, from different tissues or tumor stages); however, these methods are effective for all other cell lines and, provided sufficient loci are used to discriminate between samples from different individuals, donor-specific testing can give unambiguous results.

Currently, STR genotyping is the consensus method for authentication of human cell lines [2]. Early sharing of STR profiles by primary sources [20] and broad uptake by the international research community have generated a treasure trove of data from 20 years of testing. Genetic drift in culture can lead to variations in STR profiles across samples from the same donor, making some data more difficult to interpret. Match criteria have been developed to guide interpretation of STR profiles from cell line samples

TABLE 1
Dataset of Information for Cell Line Investigation

Type of Information	Item of Information
Cell line	Cell line name Research Resource Identifier (RRID) Primary reference Synonymous cell lines Misidentification status if known Source of authentic stock if known Contaminating/Parental cell line name Contaminating/Parental RRID Misidentification reference
Donor	Species Strain or pedigree (for nonhuman species) Sex Age Tissue type Disease diagnosis for example, tumor type
Establishment	Originator Location of originating laboratory Date of first culture Date of first publication Method of immortalization (also note if spontaneous transformation occurred) Growth curve during and after immortalization
Authentication	Species data available Short tandem repeat profile available Additional authentication data available; for example, single nucleotide polymorphism genotype, cytogenetic data, isoenzyme data
Characterization	Culture images available Genomic data available; for example, mutations, viral integration Phenotypic data available; for example, expression profiling
Test sample	Source; for example, reference repository, originator, colleague Catalog number (for reference repository or supplier) Sample passage or population doubling level Sample date

and can resolve most difficult cases, provided a sufficient number of loci are examined [6].

Step 3: Discrepancies in Cell Line Information and Authentication Data

Now that we have assembled relevant cell line information and authentication data, we are ready to look for discrepancies: unexpected or unusual findings that do not fit with the reported origins of the cell line. Discrepancies may arise when looking at cell line information; for example, "spontaneous transformation" in tissues where cell lines are difficult to establish can be a sign that cross-contamination has occurred [21]. Discrepancies usually become more obvious when cell line information is brought together with authentication data; for example, an STR profile may show that a cell line has a shared donor origin with HeLa, which is an important discrepancy if the cell line was reported to have been established from a different donor.

Fig. 2 sets out a workflow that the author finds helpful for investigating discrepancies in cell line information and authentication data. It is particularly important to assess discrepancies, asking if they can be explained by known variations in culture. For example, loss of Y-chromosomal material has been reported in 331 of 974 male cell lines, and gain of Y-chromosomal material in only 10 of 872 female cell lines [6]. Loss of the Y chromosome in male cell lines is therefore a common cell culture artifact; gain of the Y chromosome in female cell lines is more informative, suggesting that the cell line is misidentified and might have arisen from a male donor.

Once discrepancies are found, how are they resolved? Discrepancies are typically resolved through comparison with reference samples as sources of reliable information. For example, widely used stocks of the U-87 MG cell line were recently found to be misidentified when STR profiles from those stocks were compared with early reference samples held by the originator [19]. It is still possible to find reference samples dating back to the 1960s and 1970s, thanks to the vision and organizational skills of some early investigators [19,22] and their willingness to deposit cell lines in reference repositories [10]; however, early samples are becoming increasingly rare as laboratories close and their frozen stocks are discarded. When early samples are not available, comparison with other cell lines is essential to detect unexpected matches [20].

Additional clues may be present in authentication data apart from donor origin. For example, cell line STR profiles display LOH that becomes increasingly evident as the cell line is passaged. The degree of LOH can indicate

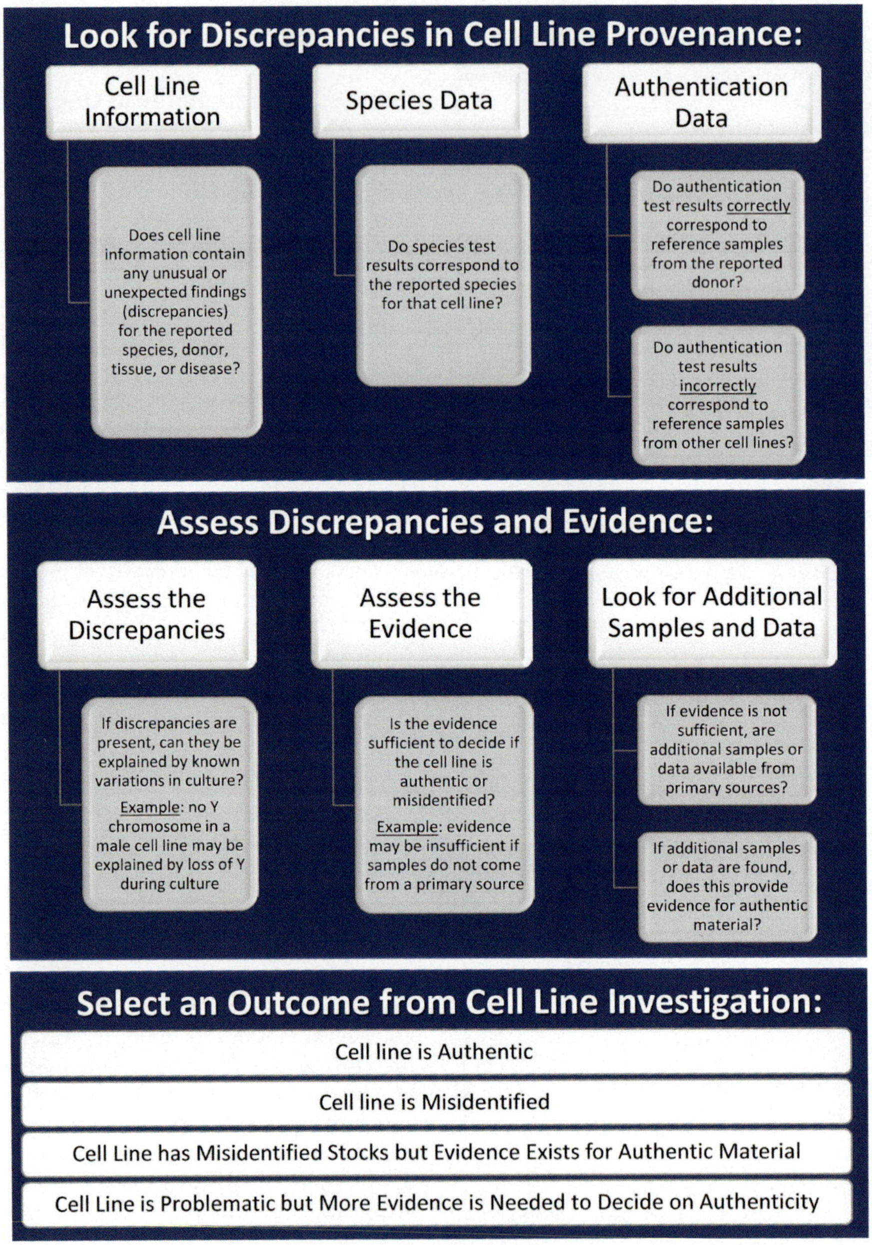

FIG. 2 Investigation of cell line information and authentication data. This workflow can be used for investigation of cell line information and authentication data. The workflow requires the user to look for discrepancies in cell line provenance, assess those discrepancies and the quality of the available evidence, and reach a final conclusion by selecting an outcome from cell line investigation. A broad approach is taken here, rather than setting out a detailed and structured workflow; the approach will vary with each cell line investigation, depending on the amount of cell line information and authentication data that are available.

whether one cell line is more extensively passaged than another from the same donor. Close observation of STR profiles from cell lines with a common donor origin, such as the M14 melanoma cell line and its family of derivatives [22], indicates which cell line has the least amount of LOH and is most likely to be the parental cell line; cell lines with higher levels of LOH are likely to be derivatives. However, this type of evidence relies on consistent approaches to culture handling, including freezing cell lines at early passage and recording passage numbers or population doubling levels. If the parental cell line is extensively used, it may be stored at a higher passage compared with other derivative cell lines and relative levels of LOH may be misleading.

There is a need for additional molecular techniques to resolve discrepancies, particularly when reference samples are not available or may be unreliable. For example, cytogenetic analysis can detect chromosomal rearrangements that are disease-specific or cell line–specific [23]. Unfortunately, the level of expertise required for cell line cytogenetic analysis means that STR genotyping is preferred as the consensus for comparison between laboratories. Although STR profiles can include rare variants, for example, the HeLa cell line has a rare allelic variant at D13S317 [5], most alleles are present at high frequency within the population and are not cell line–specific.

NEW MOLECULAR APPLICATIONS FOR CELL LINE INVESTIGATION

Genome-Based Methods Give New Opportunities for Cell Line Authentication

SNP analysis is emerging as a complementary method for authentication, with potential use for human and nonhuman cell lines [6,24,25]. SNP-based methods are already used to test laboratory animals, allowing detection of misidentification in rodent strains [25,26]. SNP genotyping is also a useful technique for forensic genetics, particularly for automated workflows and samples in which STR profiling is unsuccessful [27]. SNP markers can be used for analysis of identity, lineage (eg, via kinship analysis), ancestry, and phenotype [27]. SNP genotyping can also offer disease-specific information, providing a better understanding of disease predisposition and drug susceptibility [28].

For cell lines, SNP genotyping offers some clear advantages for authentication. SNP loci appear to be less prone to genetic instability [29,30], although this conclusion needs to be examined at greater depth in the subset of cell lines in which more pronounced genetic drift has been observed. SNP loci can be analyzed using multiple platforms, reducing reliance on any one platform or kit and allowing more than 1 type of analysis to be performed simultaneously. Many SNP analysis platforms allow rapid, high-throughput workflows. For example, SNP genotyping can be performed using matrix-assisted laser desorption/ionization time-of-flight mass spectrometry and combined with expression profiling [28].

Despite these advantages, SNP genotyping is not yet ready to overtake STR analysis as a consensus method for cell line authentication. Artifacts have been demonstrated with some SNP genotyping platforms [22], which is not surprising considering that cell lines have complex karyotypes and may carry multiple copies of SNP loci. Consensus has not yet been reached on a minimal SNP marker set for comparison between laboratories. Publications with cell line SNP genotyping data have used different marker sets, making comparison across datasets impossible [6,24,29,30]. A minimal marker set is important for both STR and SNP loci because of potential privacy concerns. SNP genotyping can be used to analyze the lineage, ancestry, phenotype, and disease susceptibility of the donor from whom the cell line was established [27]. Although this risk applies to all genomic data, the degree of risk may vary depending on the amount of data that is shared. A minimal dataset can reduce the amount of data shared per sample and the associated privacy risks.

An alternative approach to SNP genotyping would minimize such privacy concerns [31]. "MinION sketching" uses a portable DNA sequencing device that can be connected to any computer with a USB port (Fig. 3A). The test sample is subjected to shotgun sequencing at low coverage, and SNP variants compared with sequence data from reference samples to look for matches. This approach does not require agreement on a shared SNP marker set. A Bayesian algorithm is used to detect SNP markers in common between test and reference samples. The random DNA marker set can be queried against a private database, reducing the need for data sharing. MinION sketching offers a rapid and compact approach to authentication that researchers can perform in-house (Fig. 3B); however, widespread adoption of the method for this purpose will require a suitable database of reference samples and further validation. Any new test method must be able to discriminate between cell lines with different donor origins; detect cell lines with shared donor origin; and do so consistently in the presence of genetic instability, prolonged passaging, allelic imbalances, and variable culture conditions.

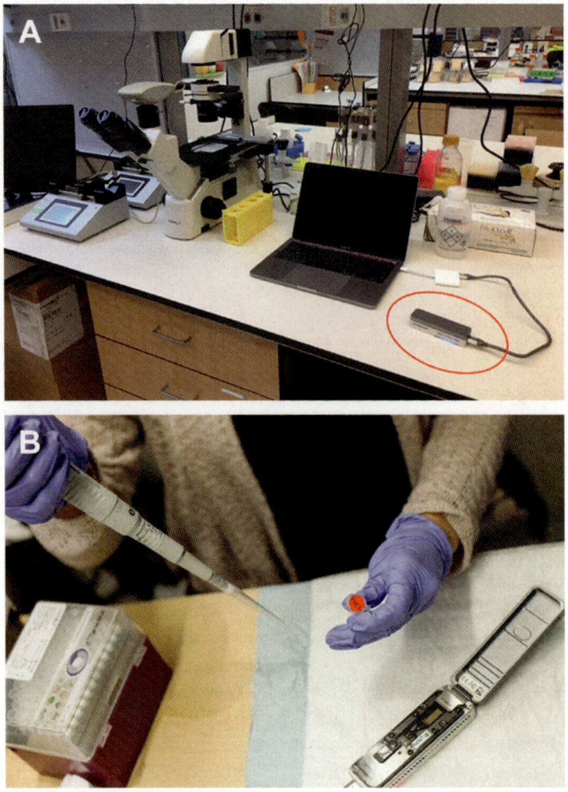

FIG. 3 Authentication using MinION sketching. (**A**) Typical laboratory set-up for MinION sketching. The MinION sequencer (Oxford Nanopore Technologies, Oxford, United Kingdom) shown here (circled) is a portable real-time sequencing device connected to a laptop via USB. Note the small size of the MinION sequencer compared with nearby laboratory equipment. (**B**) Loading of MinION sequencer with DNA. Sequencing data are generated in real-time; authentication requires comparison to a reference sequence library using a Bayesian algorithm [31]. (*Courtesy of* Sophie Zaaijer, New York, NY.)

Proteome-Based Methods Give New Opportunities for Cell Line Characterization

Cell lines are often used as models for specific tissues or disease states. Tissue origin and disease diagnosis can be highly relevant for cell line investigations; for example, when misidentification involves cells from a different tissue type. If reference samples are not available, tissue origin may be one of the only clues available to decide on discrepancies. For example, in the case of U-87 MG, we know that widely used stocks of this cell line are misidentified, but the origin of those stocks is not yet known. The only clue published to date relates to tissue origin, with expression profiling demonstrating that cells are likely to come from the central nervous system [19].

Most cell lines are representative of their tissues of origin when assessed using expression profiling [32,33]. For example, 51 cell lines in the NCI-60 panel are congruent with their reported tumors of origin [32]. This leaves a minority of cell lines that are not representative of their tissues of origin. Tissue-specific or disease-specific markers may be lost or gained with passaging; atypical markers may be present, through transdifferentiation or other mechanisms [22]. For example, MDA-MB-435 "breast" cells cluster with melanoma cell lines by expression profiling but can express breast-specific and epithelial-specific markers under some culture conditions [34,35]. STR profiling shows conclusively that the MDA-MB-435 cell line is not from breast as originally reported and is a misidentified derivative of melanoma cell line M14 [22]. Cell lines must undergo detailed characterization and assessment before a decision can be made regarding tissue origin. Large datasets are more likely to be reliable, compared with a small number of "tissue-specific" markers in which expression may vary in cell lines. Controlled culture conditions must also be used to minimize variation [33].

Despite these challenges, the advent of transcriptomic and proteomic analysis offers new opportunities for cell line characterization. Mass spectrometry can be used for species determination and rapid characterization of cell lines [36]. Reverse-phase protein assays have been used to assess cancer-related proteins in more than 700 cell lines, allowing a stronger focus on mutated signaling pathways [37]. It remains to be seen whether proteomic data will vary when different stocks from a cell line are passaged and grown using different culture conditions. Initial validation work has shown that species determination is not affected by variation in culture medium or cell density [36].

Analysis of the full proteome has particular promise for cell line characterization. Sequential window acquisition of all theoretic mass spectra (SWATH) analyzes the proteome in a data-independent fashion, resulting in a single, permanent digital file that can be explored in more depth at any time following data acquisition [38]. Work is now under way to use SWATH in high-throughput workflows, establishing libraries of data from tumor biopsies [39]. This work is likely to be undertaken in specialized facilities, enabling precisely controlled conditions for mass spectrometry. However,

SWATH files can be accessed at any location for data mining, allowing a personalized approach to cancer management. Increasing precision in cancer management will benefit cell lines, either directly through analysis of cell line panels, or indirectly through improved classification of tissue type and disease diagnosis.

SUMMARY

Cell lines are valuable models, but their continuing proliferation and extended history mean that they can have uncertain origins. Misidentified cell lines are detected through authentication using STR genotyping or other molecular techniques. New molecular techniques offer exciting opportunities for cell line authentication. However, the same basic principles apply regardless of technique. Provenance information and authentication data must be assessed, looking for discrepancies and considering whether those discrepancies can be explained by known variations in culture. In some cases, the evidence is not sufficient to decide if a cell line is authentic or misidentified, and additional samples or data are required. Cell line information, reference samples, and molecular applications are all required to ensure that cell lines are valid models for diagnostic assays, therapeutic screens, and biomedical research.

ACKNOWLEDGMENTS

All members of the International Cell Line Authentication Committee (ICLAC) are warmly thanked for their commitment, expertise, and willingness to share their various approaches to cell line authentication. I particularly thank Ian Freshney, Ray Nims, and Christopher Korch for their feedback on the manuscript draft, and American Type Culture Collection (ATCC; Manassas, VA) for its contribution of the cell morphology images. I am delighted to acknowledge Jens and Peter Fogh for sharing photographs of Jørgen Fogh, and Sophie Zaaijer for photographs and helpful discussion on MinION sketching and its use in authentication. Apologies to the authors of many excellent studies that I was unable to cite due to space limitations.

REFERENCES

[1] Kremkow BG, Lee KH. Sequencing technologies for animal cell culture research. Biotechnol Lett 2015;37(1): 55–65.

[2] ASN-0002 ATCC Standards Development Organization Workgroup. Cell line misidentification: the beginning of the end. Nat Rev Cancer 2010;10(6):441–8.

[3] Liu X, Krawczyk E, Suprynowicz FA, et al. Conditional reprogramming and long-term expansion of normal and tumor cells from human biospecimens. Nat Protoc 2017;12(2):439–51.

[4] Coriell LL. Detection and elimination of contaminating organisms. Natl Cancer Inst Monogr 1962;7:33–53.

[5] Nims RW, Sykes G, Cottrill K, et al. Short tandem repeat profiling: part of an overall strategy for reducing the frequency of cell misidentification. In Vitro Cell Dev Biol Anim 2010;46(10):811–9.

[6] Yu M, Selvaraj SK, Liang-Chu MM, et al. A resource for cell line authentication, annotation and quality control. Nature 2015;520(7547):307–11.

[7] Drexler HG, Dirks WG, MacLeod RA, et al. False and mycoplasma-contaminated leukemia-lymphoma cell lines: time for a reappraisal. Int J Cancer 2017;140(5): 1209–14.

[8] Horbach SPJM, Halffman W. The ghosts of HeLa: how cell line misidentification contaminates the scientific literature. PLoS One 2017;12(10):e0186281.

[9] Nims RW, Reid Y. Best practices for authenticating cell lines. In Vitro Cell Dev Biol Anim 2017;53(10): 880–7.

[10] MacLeod RA, Dirks WG, Drexler HG. Where have all the cell lines gone? Int J Cancer 2013;132(5):1232–4.

[11] Fogh J. Human tumor lines for cancer research. Cancer Invest 1986;4(2):157–84.

[12] Dracopoli NC, Fogh J. Loss of heterozygosity in cultured human tumor cell lines. J Natl Cancer Inst 1983;70(1): 83–7.

[13] Leibovitz A, Wright WC, Pathak S, et al. Detection and analysis of a glucose 6-phosphate dehydrogenase phenotype B cell line contamination. J Natl Cancer Inst 1979; 63(3):635–45.

[14] Ahmed D, Eide PW, Eilertsen IA, et al. Epigenetic and genetic features of 24 colon cancer cell lines. Oncogenesis 2013;2:e71.

[15] Freshney RI. Cell line provenance. Cytotechnology 2002; 39(2):55–67.

[16] Gazdar AF, Girard L, Lockwood WW, et al. Lung cancer cell lines as tools for biomedical discovery and research. J Natl Cancer Inst 2010;102(17):1310–21.

[17] Bandrowski AE, Martone ME. RRIDs: a simple step toward improving reproducibility through rigor and transparency of experimental methods. Neuron 2016;90(3):434–6.

[18] Beskow LM. Lessons from HeLa cells: the ethics and policy of biospecimens. Annu Rev Genomics Hum Genet 2016;17:395–417.

[19] Allen M, Bjerke M, Edlund H, et al. Origin of the U87MG glioma cell line: good news and bad news. Sci Transl Med 2016;8(354):354re353.

[20] Dirks WG, MacLeod RA, Nakamura Y, et al. Cell line cross-contamination initiative: an interactive reference database of STR profiles covering common cancer cell lines. Int J Cancer 2010;126(1):303–4.

[21] Torsvik A, Røsland GV, Svendsen A, et al. Spontaneous malignant transformation of human mesenchymal stem

cells reflects cross-contamination: putting the research field on track—letter. Cancer Res 2010;70(15):6393–6.

[22] Korch C, Hall EM, Dirks WG, et al. Authentication of M14 melanoma cell line proves misidentification of MDA-MB-435 breast cancer cell line. Int J Cancer 2018; 142(3):561–72.

[23] Macleod RA, Kaufmann M, Drexler HG. Cytogenetic analysis of cancer cell lines. Methods Mol Biol 2011; 731:57–78.

[24] Demichelis F, Greulich H, Macoska JA, et al. SNP panel identification assay (SPIA): a genetic-based assay for the identification of cell lines. Nucleic Acids Res 2008; 36(7):2446–56.

[25] Didion JP, Buus RJ, Naghashfar Z, et al. SNP array profiling of mouse cell lines identifies their strains of origin and reveals cross-contamination and widespread aneuploidy. BMC Genomics 2014;15:847.

[26] Nitzki F, Kruger A, Reifenberg K, et al. Identification of a genetic contamination in a commercial mouse strain using two panels of polymorphic markers. Lab Anim 2007; 41(2):218–28.

[27] Budowle B, van Daal A. Forensically relevant SNP classes. Biotechniques 2008;44(5):603–8, 610.

[28] Tang K, Oeth P, Kammerer S, et al. Mining disease susceptibility genes through SNP analyses and expression profiling using MALDI-TOF mass spectrometry. J Proteome Res 2004;3(2):218–27.

[29] Castro F, Dirks WG, Fähnrich S, et al. High-throughput SNP-based authentication of human cell lines. Int J Cancer 2013;132(2):308–14.

[30] Liang-Chu MM, Yu M, Haverty PM, et al. Human biosample authentication using the high-throughput, cost-effective SNPtrace(TM) system. PLoS One 2015;10(2): e0116218.

[31] Zaaijer S, Gordon A, Speyer D, et al. Rapid re-identification of human samples using portable DNA sequencing. Elife 2017;6 [pii:e27798].

[32] Wang H, Huang S, Shou J, et al. Comparative analysis and integrative classification of NCI60 cell lines and primary tumors using gene expression profiling data. BMC Genomics 2006;7:166.

[33] Mohseny AB, Machado I, Cai Y, et al. Functional characterization of osteosarcoma cell lines provides representative models to study the human disease. Lab Invest 2011; 91(8):1195–205.

[34] Ross DT, Scherf U, Eisen MB, et al. Systematic variation in gene expression patterns in human cancer cell lines. Nat Genet 2000;24(3):227–35.

[35] Nerlich AG, Bachmeier BE. Density-dependent lineage instability of MDA-MB-435 breast cancer cells. Oncol Lett 2013;5(4):1370–4.

[36] Karger A, Bettin B, Lenk M, et al. Rapid characterisation of cell cultures by matrix-assisted laser desorption/ionisation mass spectrometric typing. J Virol Methods 2010;164(1–2):116–21.

[37] Li J, Zhao W, Akbani R, et al. Characterization of human cancer cell lines by reverse-phase protein arrays. Cancer Cell 2017;31(2):225–39.

[38] Liu Y, Hüttenhain R, Collins B, et al. Mass spectrometric protein maps for biomarker discovery and clinical research. Expert Rev Mol Diagn 2013;13(8):811–25.

[39] Guo T, Kouvonen P, Koh CC, et al. Rapid mass spectrometric conversion of tissue biopsy samples into permanent quantitative digital proteome maps. Nat Med 2015;21(4):407–13.

Advances in Molecular Pathology 1 (2018) 239–251
ADVANCES IN MOLECULAR PATHOLOGY

Challenges and Advances in the Development of Cell Lines and Xenografts

Rebecca E. Schweppe, PhD[a,*], Christopher Korch, PhD[b]
[a]Division of Endocrinology, Metabolism, and Diabetes, University of Colorado Cancer Center, University of Colorado Anschutz Medical Campus, 12801 East 17th Avenue, Aurora, CO 80045, USA; [b]Division of Medical Oncology, University of Colorado Cancer Center, University of Colorado Anschutz Medical Campus, 12801 East 17th Avenue, Aurora, CO 80045, USA

KEYWORDS
• Misidentified cell lines • Authentication policy • Genetic drift • Patient derived xenografts (PDX) • Feeder cell • ROCK inhibitor • Xenotransplantation • Chemically defined media

KEY POINTS

- Cell line integrity is critical to ensure the integrity and reproducibility of biomedical research, as illustrated by several examples of how the use of unauthenticated cell lines and tissues has compromised biomedical research.
- New approaches to generate cell lines are being developed, which are increasing the success rate of cell line establishment and providing a key resource of new low-passage cell lines.
- A 12-step cell line authentication policy is proposed as a mechanism for safeguarding the integrity and reproducibility of biomedical research at research institutions.

INTRODUCTION

The Cell Line Authentication Problem

Cell lines are the most widely used preclinical tool in cancer research. The use of cell lines has clearly advanced our understanding of how distinct cellular mechanisms contribute to tumorigenesis and how to target these deregulated mechanisms in the clinic. Importantly, clinically relevant genomic changes and gene expression alterations present in tumor samples have also been identified in cancer cell lines. Thus, cell lines represent an excellent model to study tumor signaling mechanisms and the development of new therapies. Despite the success of using cell lines to advance cancer research, the widespread misidentification of cell lines remains a major problem and has hampered progress. It is also critical to ensure that cell lines represent the tissue of origin phenotypically and genomically. In addition to the well-known cross-contamination with the HeLa cell line, numerous other cell line misidentifications and cross-contaminations have occurred with other established and faster growing cell lines. For example, misidentifications of cell lines thought to be derived from prostate, breast, head and neck squamous cell cancers, ovarian, endometrial, and adenoid cystic carcinomas have been reported [1–7]. In 2008, we reported the comprehensive characterization of a panel of approximately 40 thyroid cancer cell lines, in which 40% of cell lines were either cross-contaminated or misidentified with cell lines from other tumor types [8]. Specifically, using short tandem

American Cancer Society RSG-13-060-01-TBE (RES) and National Institutes of Health (NCI) R01CA164193 (RES) and 1R01CA222299 (RES).

*Corresponding author, *E-mail address:* Rebecca.Schweppe@ucdenver.edu

https://doi.org/10.1016/j.yamp.2018.07.004
2589-4080/18/

repeat (STR) profiling, we showed that 6 of 40 of the thyroid cancer cell lines were redundant (eg, identical to other thyroid cancer cell lines: TPC1, BHP 2–7, BHP 10–3, and BHP 7–13; K1 and K2; Fig. 1 and [8]). In addition, 10 were misidentified with colon cancer or melanoma cell lines (ARO81, MRO87, KAT5, KAT10, KAT4, KAT7, KAT50, KAK1 derived from HT-29 colon cancer cell line; NPA87, BHP 5–16, BHP 17–10, and BHP 14–9 derived from the M14 melanoma cell line; and DRO 90 derived from the A-375 melanoma cell line; see Fig. 1 and [8]). We found that the 23 remaining cell lines were unique based on STR profiling. Because many of these cell lines were established more than 20 years ago, we have been unable to genetically link the unique cell lines to the corresponding patient tumors, because patient tissue samples are no longer available. Given that STR profiling does not provide information on the tissue of origin, we characterized the expression of the thyroid-specific transcription factors, PAX8 and NKX2.1, and found that all papillary and follicular thyroid cancer cell lines expressed either PAX8 and/or NKX2.1, supporting the thyroid origin of these cell lines [8]. Of note, only one-half of the anaplastic thyroid cancer cell lines expressed these thyroid-specific markers, likely owing to the poorly differentiated nature of these tumors [8]. To further characterize the origin of these cell lines, we have performed comprehensive gene expression profiling of the panel of 40 unique thyroid cancer cell lines. Using hierarchical clustering across a panel of more than 1000 cancer cell lines, we found that the majority of thyroid cancer cell lines cluster together, further supporting the thyroid origin of these unique cell lines (Schweppe, unpublished, 2018). Although promising, the unique cell lines have not been matched to their tumor of origin; thus, the development of new thyroid cancer cell lines that can be matched to their tissue of origin is needed to accurately study thyroid cancer biology and response to therapy. Recent progress in developing new, authenticated thyroid cancer cell lines, which have been linked to their corresponding patient tissue samples, is promising. Several new cell lines have been developed since our 2008 cell line misidentification study, which will provide new models to accurately study different stages of disease [9–15].

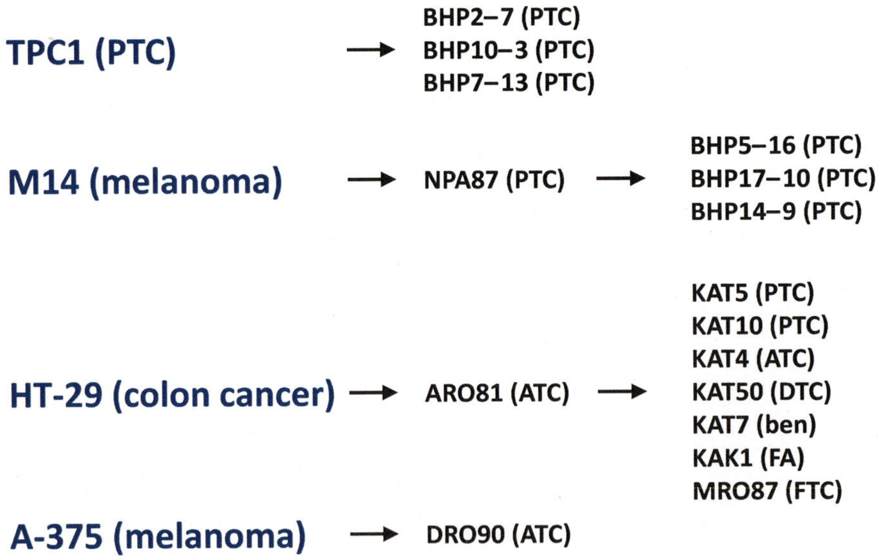

FIG. 1 Summary of the origin of misidentified thyroid cancer cell lines. Short tandem repeat (STR) profiling revealed that the papillary thyroid cancer (PTC) cell lines, BHP 2-7, BHP 10-3, and BYP 7-13, are redundant (identical to each other) and likely derived from the TPC1 PTC cell line. In addition, the BHP 5-16, BHP 17-10, and BHP 14-9 PTC cell lines are identical to each other and the NPA87 PTC cell line, which are all misidentified with the M14 melanoma cell line. The KAT5, KAT10, KAT4, KAT50, KAT7, KAK1, and MRO87 thyroid cancer cell lines are identical to each other and the ARO81 thyroid cancer cell line, which were all identical to the HT-29 colon cancer cell line. Finally, the DRO90 anaplastic thyroid cancer cell line genetically matches the A-375 melanoma cell line.

Passaging and Genetic Drift Pose Challenges to Establishing Reliable In Vitro Cell Line Models

An underappreciated aspect of cell line and tissue authenticity is the clonal evolution and genetic drift that continuous cultures undergo when serially passaged over time. Because human cell lines and xenografts (eg, patient-derived xenografts [PDX]) initially grow slowly, they are usually not grown up from single cells. Instead, they are cultured in vitro and in vivo by passaging either through dilution of cell suspensions (approximately 10-fold) or by mechanically disrupting the tissue and transplanting a portion of it into the next "incubator" (mouse).

A commonly held underlying assumption when passaging cells is that the established lines are stable, unchanging genetic and physiologic models that reliably represent the original tissue or tumor. Inherently, the more often a culture is passaged, the more likely it may be mixed up or cross-contaminated with a different culture. Passaging also increases the chances of selective loss of the intratumoral genetic diversity that was present in the original donor sample, thus, making these cell lines no longer a reliable model systems. Furthermore, during passaging of established cell lines, widespread numerical and structural abnormalities of chromosomes may arise and change in frequency [16,17]. Therefore, it may not be straightforward to determine whether 2 samples faithfully represent the original tissue sample. Moreover, those changes may not be detected by STR analyses [18–20].

The selection of clonal changes may occur by some known process(es). For instance, in studying how immunoresistant cells might escape alloreactive cytotoxic T lymphocytes, Gomez and colleagues [21] showed how immunoresistant human glioma cell clones with different chromosomal rearrangements and levels of aneuploidy arose after selection with alloreactive cytotoxic T lymphocytes.

Selective processes may also occur unplanned or unbeknownst to the investigator as a consequence of random genetic drift during long-time in vitro culturing. Although cell lines can be authenticated by molecular platforms such as STR analyses, these technologies may not provide sufficiently precise genetic information about the appropriateness of these resources for specific experiments. Some changes may only be detectable by single cell analysis strategies, such as those using molecular cytogenetics techniques. For example, the cell line KG-1, which was established in 1978 from bone marrow of a patient with erythroleukemia that evolved into acute myelogenous leukemia (reviewed in Mrozek and colleagues [22]), evolved into a much less differentiated leukemic pattern (subline KG-1a). A decade later, Pelliccia and colleagues [23] found the KG-1a karyotype had changed further.

Nishida [24] established in 1980 the vigorously growing Ishikawa cell line from a large endometrial tumor and shared the cell line widely. After exhausting his supplies of the original culture, he isolated 18 subclones from single cells and reported that their genotypes varied greatly and differed from the original cell line (Table 1). As Korch and colleagues [5] showed, this was likely due to the cell line being defective in DNA mismatch repair, which resulted in it being microsatellite unstable. Kasai and colleagues [25] showed that within 13 passages for one of these subclones (3-H-12), which had been distributed widely, the cell line's single nucleotide polymorphism (SNP), STR, and chromosomal genotypes had changed considerably through loss of heterozygosity and chromosomal rearrangements. Korch and colleagues [5] analyzed samples of the Ishikawa cell line that were claimed to have been passaged more than 700 times showing extensive variation in their STR profiles. To avoid this genetic drift, Kasai and colleagues [25], like Hughes and colleagues [16], strongly recommended only using cell lines with minimal passaging.

Kleensang and colleagues [20] reported that different sublines of the MSI stable cell line MCF-7, which differed by only 4 passages (150 vs 154), had several different phenotypes and yet there were no detectable alterations in their STR genotypes. These differences are partly explained by the findings of Wang and colleagues [26], who showed by SNP analysis that MCF-7 had a significantly lower frequency of homozygous SNPs (13.3%) than either a control cell line or in 24 normal human individuals. This finding supports the proposition that samples of MCF-7 cells are genetically heterogeneous and explains the reported phenotypic heterogeneity in a single batch of MCF-7 cells that had serious consequences for reproducibility and primary outcomes of the Human Toxome Project experiments [20].

Similarly, Torsvik and colleagues [27] found that the original U-251MG glioblastoma cell line and 3 subclones differed phenotypically Table 2. Intriguingly, with passaging and the resulting genetic drift, they observed that the cell line underwent numerous genomic and phenotypic changes, becoming more tumorigenic and thus less like the original tumor.

It would, therefore, be interesting to study whether in tumor cell line cultures, a specific subline derived

TABLE 1
Ishikawa Sublines Derived from Passage 25 of Original Culture by Dilution to Single Cells

Clone Code	Differentiation In Vivo	Differentiation In Vitro	Estradiol Binding Capacity (fmol/mg)	Progesterone Binding Capacity (fmol/mg)	Time from Inoculation to Subculture (d)	Population Doubling Time (h)	Saturation Density ($\times 10^4/cm^2$)	Colony Formation Rate (%)	Distribution Periods of Ishikawa Clones
Ishikawa passage 9	Well-differentiated adenocarcinoma	Became poorly differentiated by the 45th generation	238	50	6	36	NR	NR	Original cell line 1982–1993
3-H-4	Well	Moderately	365	325	20	31.6	31.0	39.6	1993–1995
3-H-12	Moderately	Poorly	146	574	69	24.0	37.9	34.7	1996–2002
1-A-12	Adenosquamous carcinoma	Well	23	59	52	40.8	34.9	13.7	NA
1-D-9	Adenosquamous carcinoma	Poorly	172	457	52	35.0	64.0	30.6	NA
2-B-12	Poorly	Poorly	155	74	20	36.5	77.7	11.8	NA
2-C-3	Moderately	Moderately	61	1000	69	26.4	64.6	28.4	NA
3-D-7	Well	Moderately	0	319	20	25.2	35.5	24.4	NA
3-D-9	Well	Well	0	NT	20	40.8	25.0	7.2	NA
3-H-7	Well	Moderately	36	251	20	26.4	44.5	18.9	NA

Only data for 9 of 18 subcultures shown. The sublines of Ishikawa differed in phenotypic characteristics. Of special importance are the phenotypic differences between the 3 sublines that were distributed (passage 9, 3-H-4, and 3-H-12).

Abbreviations: NA, not applicable, because it is not known to have been distributed; NR, not reported.

Data from Nishida M. The Ishikawa cells from birth to the present. Hum Cell 2002;15(3):104–17.

TABLE 2
Phenotypes of Different Sublines of the Glioblastoma Cell Line U-251MG

	Cell Lines			
Phenotype	**U-251MG**	**U-251-4q12**	**U-251N**	**U-251-FGAgain**
LOH in STR profile	Reference	1 allele @ 1 locus	3 alleles @ 3 loci	5 alleles at 5 loci
Karyotypic changes	Reference	Numerous	Numerous	Numerous
Additional homozygous deletions	Reference	2	5	5
PDGFRα expression	1.0	~31	~24	~36
Cell growth on plates	Dispersed growth	Dispersed growth	Clumpy	Clumpy
Median number of chromosomes	66	59	50	50
Cytoskeleton (α-tubulin)	Dispersed	Dispersed	Condensed	Condensed
Expression of surface markers	"Normal"	High	High	High
Cell size	Normal large	Normal large	Small	Small
Growth rate in vitro (h)	33.05	33.63	23.79	21.09
Cell morphology	Most are dendritic like	Slightly condensed	Condensed	Condensed
Colony size and morphology	Large and flat	Large/intermediate and flat	Small and not as flat	Small and not as flat
Growth pattern	Dispersed	Dispersed	Clustered and clonogenic	Clustered and clonogenic
Radiation sensitivity (LD50)	ND Reference	~2.5 Gy	~4.7 Gy	~4.5 Gy
In vivo tumorigenicity intracranial implantation (half-life of mouse)	Least (~100 d)	Intermediate (~80 d)	High (~37.5 d)	Highest (~31 d)

This information on 15 phenotypic characteristics of the U-251MG glioblastoma cell lines was compiled from descriptions reported by Torsvik and colleagues [27]. Different subclones of this cell line had evolved in several of their properties including loss of chromosomes and heterozygosity, growing faster, and becoming more tumorigenic as evident by shorted half-lives of mice with intracranial xenografts.

Abbreviations: LOH, loss of heterozygosity; STR, short tandem repeat.

Data from Torsvik A, Stieber D, Enger PO, et al. U-251 revisited: genetic drift and phenotypic consequences of long-term cultures of glioblastoma cells. Cancer Med 2014;3(4):812–24.

from a single cell faithfully models the disease as well as genetically heterogeneous subcultures or whether the tumorigenicity of the culture required multiple different subpopulations to be present. Clearly, proper cytogenetic and molecular characterization and authentication of cell lines, even established ones, are needed before using cell samples for research to exclude misidentification and unsuitability for the study. Even 20 passages, as recommend by Hughes and colleagues [16], may be too many, especially for the usefulness of microsatellite instability-high cell lines.

Cell Line Xenografts, Patient-Derived Tumor Xenografts, and Patient-Derived Organoids Can Also Be Misidentified

Different types of xenografts and organoids of patient samples offer exciting promises for understanding organ development, tumor biology, and treatments of cancers [28–31]. However, the great potential uses of these types of tissues can be compromised just as easily as cell lines by mislabeling or cross-contamination, as Nardone and colleagues [32] warned the xenograft research community. Clearly, a tool such as STR or SNP genotyping is needed to ensure that tissue samples are also verifiably derived from their original patient source so that results reliably reflect the original tissue state and are not due to laboratory errors.

TABLE 3
Examples of Cross-Contaminated or Mislabeled Human Xenografts Grown in Mice

Xenograft Label	Sample Date or Passage Number	D3S1358	vWA	D19S433
Example 1: Cross-contaminated EnCa101 tumor passaged as xenograft in mice since 1987				
EnCa101-1a	1988	12 20	18 21 22	14 14.2
EnCa101-397	2009	15 21	18 24	13.2 15
EnCa101-398	2009	15 21	18 23	13.2 14 15
EnCa101-399	2009	15 21	17 18 23	13.2 15
Example 2: Labeling mistakes of PDX samples				
PDX-120	F?	16	14	13
PDX-120	F3	16	14	13
PDX-271	***F4***	***16***	***14***	***13***
PDX-102	***F1***	***15***	***15 18***	***14 16.2***
PDX-265	***F1***	***15***	***15 18***	***14 16.2***
PDX-271	F1	15	15 18	14 16.2
PDX-271	F2	15	15 18	14 16.2
PDX-271	F3 p3	15	15 18	14 16.2

Example 1: Comparison of STR profiles of 4 samples of the EnCa101 tumor maintained by xenografting in mice from 1988 and 2009 shows that they are not related and sometime in this interval the tumor samples were mixed up or mislabeled. This mix-up raises questions about the validity of ≥23 publications identified in PubMed.

Example 2: From the STR profiles at 3 STR loci, it is evident that 4 samples of PDX tumors were mixed up or mislabeled samples (sample in bold italics font): namely, 2 Xeno271 F4 samples are actually Xeno 120 samples; 2 other samples (Xeno102 and Xeno265) have profiles matching those of Xeno271.

Korch, unpublished data.

Abbreviations: PDX, patient-derived xenograft; STR, short tandem repeat.

Table 3 shows partial STR profiles for 2 sets of xenograft samples, which illustrate how easily such mix-ups can occur. Example 1 involves EnCa101, an endometrial tumor, that was originally isolated in 1985 and was perpetuated by passaging in mice since the mid-1980s [33,34]. Korch and colleagues [5] STR profiled 3 samples of the tumor from 2009 and found that, although the profiles were from the same patient, differing only slightly among themselves, they did not match profiles of the ECC-1 cell line that was purportedly derived from EnCa101. Moreover, on analysis of a 1988 sample of the EnCa101 tumor in 2012, the STR profile differed from those of the 2009 samples (Korch, unpublished, 2012). It is not clear when the mix up might have occurred nor whether any of these profiles are from the original tumor because no original patient sample remains; however, this mix-up raises questions about the validity of at least 23 publications identified in PubMed. In example 2, several other PDX samples being passaged in mice were found by STR genotyping to have been mixed-up or mislabeled (samples in bold italics; Korch, unpublished data, 2017).

Alternative methods for authenticating PDX samples include those by Alkema and colleagues [35], who compared various approaches for establishing PDX tumors in mice and used a 900,000-SNP bead chip assay to determine the profiles of matched pairs of normal versus tumor samples and the 32-SNP genotyping assay developed by El-Hoss and colleagues [36].

Unfortunately, as currently designed, these protocols do not screen for the presence of mouse DNA in the sample, which may be important for subsequent analyses of the samples, for example, next-generation sequencing (NGS). Long read NGS, in combination with SNP analytical pipelines similar to those described by Cibulskis and colleagues [37], may provide better resolution of complex genetic rearrangements. These authors found that in The Cancer Genome Atlas (TCGA) Ovarian database, there were low levels of cross-individual contamination in approximately 10% of the samples. Furthermore, when performing SNP assays or NGS on human-in-mouse PDX samples, it is critical to test whether any observed SNPs are due contamination of human tumor samples with mouse DNA. The contamination of highly similar orthologous sequences from mice can give rise to false-positive changes in the SNP profile at positions where there is minimal differences between human and mouse sequences and a SNP may actually be a mouse sequence variant.

Clearly, xenograft samples need to be tested for authenticity just like cell lines. Using these techniques, especially NGS, it may be possible to detect mix-ups of samples and low levels of cross-contamination caused by carry-over during handling of cell lines, PDX, and patient-derived organoid samples. One can thus avoid the situation of tumors being mislabeled or one tumor overgrowing cells from another tumor, resulting in the misinterpretation of a tumor's phenotype and any associated genetic implications. Moreover, these approaches may be able to identify PDX or patient-derived organoid samples that are chimeras, have complex karyotypes, or even have undergone cell fusions, as has been reported by Jacobsen and colleagues [38].

ADVANCES IN CELL LINE DEVELOPMENT

Despite the importance of cell line models, the success rate of establishing new cell lines remains low. Although cell lines isolated from more aggressive tumors have a higher success rate, the success rate from less aggressive or indolent tumors is poor. Thus, the spectrum of disease for many tumor types is not accurately represented in the cell lines that are available currently. Given the low success rates, there has been long-standing interest in developing methods to enhance the ability to establish cell lines. In support of this, several new methods have been developed in recent years, including passaging of tumor cells on feeder cells, in the presence or absence of antiapoptotic agents [39–41], passaging of tumor cells through mice [42], and the use of chemically defined tissue culture media approaches [43,44].

Feeder Cell Approach

A feeder cell approach, which uses a layer of nondividing irradiated mouse fibroblast cells, was first developed in the 1970s and was shown to extend the growth of primary cells from 5 or 6 passages to between 30 and 50 passages, by delaying the onset of senescence [45,46]. More recently, the feeder cell approach was optimized by Dr Richard Schlegel's laboratory through the addition of a Rho kinase (ROCK) inhibitor (Y-27632), which is thought to suppress apoptosis and conditionally reprogram cells to a highly proliferative state [39]. Using this approach, epithelial colonies derived from different tumor types (prostate, breast, lung, and liver) developed rapidly, within 2 days, and reached confluence within 5 days [39]. The average success rate, as defined by the ability of cultured cells to reach 50 population doublings, was between 88% and 100% [39]. The mechanism by which the feeder cell/ROCK inhibitor approach promotes a proliferative phenotype is not clear, but may involve the induction of TERT expression. Importantly, this approach was also shown to result in the maintenance of a normal karyotype for up to 33 passages of normal prostate cells [39]. This approach clearly has the potential to rapidly establish normal and tumor cell lines from small amounts of material, but has some limitations. These limitations include the presence of feeder cells that can complicate downstream assays, difficulties involved in the eventual removal of the feeder cells, and understanding exactly how the conditional reprogramming with the ROCK inhibitor affects the biology of the cells.

The effects of conditional reprogramming on tumor genetic heterogeneity were recently addressed using a collection of non–small cell lung cancer cell lines developed using the conditional reprogramming approach [47]. Using whole exome sequencing and copy number variation analysis of normal, tumor tissue, and cell lines developed using the conditional reprogramming method, Correa and colleagues [47] showed that the cell lines largely maintained the tumor heterogeneity of their corresponding tumor by more than 90%. However, it was also shown that normal cells could grow alongside the tumor cells, which may comprise 50% of these cultures [47]. Nonetheless, this is an exciting approach for the development of new low-passage cell lines and a number of cell lines in different tumor types are successfully being established using this approach [48–50]. Future advancements will include the development of matched patient-derived fibroblasts to more accurately recapitulate the tumor microenvironment.

Xenotransplantation Approaches

Since the 1970s, xenografts of human cell lines and tumors have been transplanted into immunocompromised mice for studying tumor biology. More recently, Dangles-Marie and colleagues [42] tested whether this technique could be used to increase the success rate of establishing colon cancer cell lines by engrafting tumor samples directly in immunocompromised mice before culturing cells in vitro. Using this approach, the authors demonstrated a 77% success rate, in which 20 of 26 tumor samples were established in mice and, of these, 9 cell lines (47%) were then established in vitro. In comparison, only 3 of 31 tumor samples (9.7%) were established through direct in vitro culturing. Of interest, all 3 cell lines that were established using in vitro approaches were derived from primary tumors, and no cell lines derived from metastases were successfully established through direct in vitro culturing, indicating that cell lines from metastatic sites may be more difficult to establish using conventional in vitro approaches.

The authors further characterized 2 pairs of cell lines that were established by direct in vitro versus in vivo passaging. Interestingly, no differences in morphology or global gene expression profiles were noted. However, changes in karyotype, growth rates, and chemosensitivity were observed. Of note, chromosomal alterations were observed at early passages, and therefore were not due to selection owing to long-term culturing [42]. Importantly, this study also demonstrated that heterogeneity at different tumor sites is maintained in their corresponding cell lines in vitro [42]. Overall, this study demonstrated the ability to establish a large panel of colon cancer cell lines through a xenotransplantation approach. Although promising, this approach may be limited to tumor types that have high take rates in immunocompromised mice. However, recently Kiseljak-Vassiliades and colleagues [48] reported the establishment of new adrenocortical cancer cell lines, which have been historically difficult to establish, using a xenotransplantation approach followed by establishment in vitro using the feeder cell + ROCK inhibitor approach.

Chemically Defined Media Approaches

A major challenge with the establishment of cell lines is the long doubling times before the first cell passage. For instance, Tomlinson and colleagues [51] reported that it took 11 months of culturing with weekly changes of medium before the cell line HCC1937, from a primary breast carcinoma, started to grow and establish itself. Although upon in vitro culturing HeLa cells established themselves in 4 days [52] and Ishikawa cells in 6 days [24], Ince and colleagues [43] reviewed this process and concluded it could often take much longer (between 4 and 44 months) before cell lines could be established. Such long lag times can lead to the selective outgrowth of subclones that may not necessarily represent the tumor of origin or could even be unrelated cross-contaminating cells. As discussed elsewhere in this article, a conditional reprogramming approach with feeder cells in combination with a ROCK inhibitor shows promising results; however, there are concerns regarding the effects of the ROCK inhibitor on cellular phenotypes and the presence of feeder cells may complicate the interpretation of downstream assays.

Another emerging approach is the optimization of chemically defined cell culture media, because it is clear that standard tissue culture media are not optimal for cell line establishment. A recent multiinstitutional study reported testing many different cell culture conditions over a period of 10 years and developing a cell culture media (OCMI), which contains more than 80 ingredients, that enabled the generation of a panel of 25 new ovarian cancer cell lines in 26 attempts [43]. According to the authors, this process involved trial and error, along with the theoretic deduction of the importance of metabolic pathways [53]. The OCMI media allowed for the immediate and rapid proliferation of cells, thus avoiding clonal selection and genomic/epigenetic changes that commonly occur with cell line establishment. In fact, 14 of 16 cell lines showed a strong similarity to their corresponding tissue samples with a greater than 95% identity between their loss of heterozygosity patterns [43]. Significantly, the gene expression and proteomic profiles of the ovarian cancer cell lines matched their corresponding tumor of origin and the xenografts established from these cell lines reproduced the human tumor histology [43]. The authors further observed that 60 to 300 population doublings were possible in this medium, with no decrease in growth rate [43]. Interestingly, none of the ovarian cancer cell lines that were established in the OCMI medium were able to grow in standard media or the conditional reprogramming medium in the presence of a ROCK inhibitor, suggesting that the conditional reprogramming approach may actually negatively affect the growth of ovarian and other cancer cell lines [39,43,54–56]. The authors noted that colon and lung cancer cells were also successfully cultured in the OCMI medium, but importantly, do not recommend this as a universal culture medium because other tumor types were not as successfully cultured. Overall, this chemically defined media approach represents a breakthrough for the establishment of ovarian cancer cell lines, and other selected cancer models, resulting in the establishment of cell lines that phenotypically match their tissue of origin. It will be of great interest to see whether modifying this approach for other tumor types will be as fruitful.

Novel Approaches to Developing Cell Lines That Model Their Corresponding Tissue of Origin

There is a need to choose cell lines that most closely recapitulate their corresponding tumor of origin to increase the value and translatability of research using cell lines. Recent progress in the genomic and molecular characterization of patient tissue samples and cell lines has enabled an unbiased evaluation of how closely cell lines resemble their corresponding tumor type and, therefore, more guidance on choosing the appropriate cell line models. Gene expression and genomic data for more than 500 tissues samples per tumor type from more than 11,000 tumor and matched normal samples are now available through the TCGA, in addition to other large-scale studies [57]. In addition, the Cancer Cell Line Encyclopedia contains (as of March 2018) genomic and gene expression profiles for more than 1400 cell lines [58].

In 2013, Domcke and colleagues [59] were the first to perform a systematic analysis on how genomic and gene expression profiles of high-grade serous ovarian cancer tumors (HGSOC) from the TCGA (316 tumors) compared with a panel of 47 ovarian cancer cell lines. As with many cell lines, the histopathologic origin of many of the ovarian cancer cell lines is not clear [60,61]. Of the 1451 genes that were profiled, the median frequency of mutations was higher in the cell lines (4.3 mutations/Mb) versus the HGSOC tumors (1.6 mutations/Mb) [59]. Potential reasons for a higher mutation rate in the cell lines include (1) cell lines are purer populations, therefore low-frequency mutations may be selected for during culturing; (2) the TCGA only tested for *BRCA1/2* germline mutations, whereas the Cancer Cell Line Encyclopedia included both somatic and germline mutations; and (3) mutations may be acquired during in vitro culturing. Further, the authors performed a gene-by-gene analysis of copy number data, comparing each cell line with the original tumor samples, and ranked the cell lines by suitability as HGSOC models according to the following criteria: (1) correlation between copy number profile of cell line and tumors; (2) the lower frequency of nonsynonymous mutations in protein-coding genes; (3) the presence of a *TP53* mutation; and (4) the absence of mutations in non-HGSOC genes [59]. Using this approach, they found that the top 12 cell lines as HGSOC models only account for only 1% of current PubMed citations of the 47 cell lines at the time this study was published [59]. Strikingly, the most commonly used HGSOC cell lines (90% of PubMed citations) were not ranked as the most suitable models for HGSOC and two of the most commonly used cell lines, SK-OV-3 and A2780, which account for 60% of PubMed citations, were ranked as poorly suited HGSOC models owing to their stable copy-number alterations (CNA) profile, lack of *TP53* mutations, and expression of key mutations found in non-HGSOC tumors [59].

Consistent with this study, by Zhao and colleagues [62] used a similar approach, which integrated genomic features with functional annotation data to identify suitable cell lines for 8 cancer models (breast, ovarian, colon, kidney, glioblastoma multiforme, rectum adenocarcinoma, and brain lower grade glioma), and found that many of the commonly used cancer cell lines may not be suitable models for their corresponding tumor types. Thus, the analysis of the genomic and molecular features of cell lines and tumors represents a viable approach to accurately identify cell lines that closely resemble their corresponding tumors. These studies are important, because it is critical that cell line models accurately represent their tissue of origin. For example, BRAF-mutant melanoma is responsive to BRAF-directed therapies, whereas thyroid cancer is more resistant [63]. These tissue-specific responses can be recapitulated in cell lines and, in general, melanoma cell lines are more sensitive to BRAF or MEK inhibition versus thyroid cancer [64,65]. With the proper cell line models, mechanisms mediating sensitivity or resistance in melanoma versus thyroid cancer are beginning to be dissected [64,65].

PROPOSAL AND GUIDELINES FOR THE DEVELOPMENT OF RELIABLE IN VITRO MODELS OF MAMMALIAN TISSUE CULTURES (CELL LINES AND XENOTRANSPLANTS)

Much biomedical research is not reproducible [18,66,67]. Contamination or misidentification of cell cultures (cell lines, stem cells, and xenografts, both of tissue samples and cell suspensions) occurs frequently (10%–50% of cultures are misidentified; see Christopher Korch and Marileila Varella-Garcia's article, "Tackling the Human Cell Line and Tissue Misidentification Problem Is Needed for Reproducible Biomedical Research," in this issue), which can seriously compromise research using these cells to model diseases, biological phenomena, and drug testing in preclinical trials. There are at least approximately 500 known misidentified cell lines listed on the website of the International Cell Line Authentication Committee (available from: http://iclac.org/databases/cross-contaminations/). The National Institutes of Health requires authentication of cell lines, tissues, and other biological reagents (NIH-OD-16–011 and −012). Journals have also begun requiring, to different degrees, authentication of biological reagents. Wrong or mixed up cell lines and tissue samples can jeopardize research validity and reproducibility and increase potential risks for patients. The use of inappropriate reagents can result in retractions of publications, which cost on average about US$300,000 each; damaged reputations and careers of scientists and research facilities; reduced laboratory productivity; loss of research funding; and legal actions and risks at many levels [68]. To ameliorate this aspect of irreproducible biomedical research, we suggest that institutions adopt a cell line authentication policy for biomedical research, as was done by the MD Anderson Cancer Center in 2011 and in 2015 by the University of Colorado Cancer Center.

The goals of such a policy should be to:

- Ensure the validity and reproducibility of research based on cell and tissue cultures;
- Avoid noncompliance with research requirements of funding agencies that might cause eventual loss of research funding;
- Avoid legal risks and damaged reputations of all members of research teams;
- Avoid retractions of publication owing to use of inappropriate cell and tissue cultures; and
- Avoid having to repeat research owing to using the wrong cell lines with the associated additional time and expenses.

These policy guidelines should apply to all laboratory members of research teams using cell lines, xenografts, organoids, and tissue samples where the

BOX 1

A Cell Line Authentication Policy Proposal: Twelve Steps for Safeguarding Biomedical Research Using Cell Lines and Tissue Samples

1. Implement good cell culture practices and techniques in the laboratory as described by Geraghty and colleagues [70].
2. Before starting a project, check that the cell line or tissue culture to be used is not on the current International Cell Line Authentication Committee lists of misidentified cell lines are available from: http://iclac.org/databases/cross-contaminations [71] and whether there are any warnings about the cell line on the Cellosaurus list (https://web.expasy.org/cellosaurus/).
3. Obtain cell lines and tissue samples from reputable sources that provide STR genotype and mycoplasma testing data with the sample, such as the cell line repositories (eg, ATCC, DSMZ, ECACC, RIKEN, or JCRB cell banks) or from the originators of the cell line.
4. New cell lines or tissue cultures received by a laboratory should be quarantined in a separate incubator, authenticated by STR or SNP genotyping, and tested for mycoplasma contamination as soon as possible and before being used in the laboratory. The only allowed exception is if the cell line has been received directly from a repository that authenticates cell lines and it provides an STR profile made from the same batch of cells, and certification the sample is mycoplasma-free.
5. STR or SNP genotyping must be used for human samples, and for those organisms where available, and checked that they match published genotypes and designated species. Cell lines and xenograft tissues should be regularly genotyped and checked for mycoplasma to verify there has not occurred a mix up or contamination.
6. When establishing new cell lines from tissue samples, a portion should be kept as a reference source of DNA for authentication that the cell line and tissue are from the same individual.
7. A large batch of the cell line should be grown up and aliquoted into standard freezer vials. One aliquot of the batch (seed stock) should be STR genotyped to confirm the authenticity of the batch.
8. Cell lines or tissue cultures that have been subjected to biological selections (eg, after stable transfection/transduction or drug selection) should be authenticated by STR or SNP profiling before further use in the laboratory to avoid sample switching or other errors.
9. Whenever during a project the cell line or tissue seems to behave abnormally or shows abnormal morphology, it should be authenticated before further use or the experiments should be repeated with a new aliquot of the authenticated seed stock.
10. Avoid passaging cell lines more than 20 times for MSI stable cell lines and less than 10 times for MSI unstable cell lines. Use a new aliquot of the seed stock for the next set of experiments.
11. As part of grant applications and manuscript submissions, all cell lines or tissue cultures must be authenticated at the end of the experiments and before submission.
12. Troubleshoot questionable cell line and tissue samples using methods described in Raymond Whiting Nims' article, "Historical and Current Methods for Detecting Inter- and Intra-species Cell Mixtures and Thereby Assuring Cell Line Purity," and Christopher Korch and Marileila Varella-Garcia's article, "Tackling the Human Cell Line and Tissue Misidentification Problem Is Needed for Reproducible Biomedical Research," in this issue.

Abbreviations: MSI, microsatellite instability; SNP, single nucleotide polymorphism; STR, short tandem repeat.

identity of the samples is specified or named because its identity is considered critical for the research; otherwise, the experiments may not be reproducible. Box 1 lists 12 steps in research that can minimize misidentification of cell lines and tissue samples.

The implementation of such a policy by the MD Anderson Cancer Center reduced the incidence of misidentified cell lines from more than 10% to less than 3% [67] and the implementation of an authentication policy by the International Journal of Cancer eliminated the use of misidentified cell lines in their journal articles [69], although it increased in overall use in other journals tracked by PubMed. Hopefully, such positive changes will spread throughout the biomedical research endeavor to ensure the rigor and reproducibility of research.

REFERENCES

[1] van Bokhoven A, Varella-Garcia M, Korch C, et al. Widely used prostate carcinoma cell lines share common origins. Prostate 2001;47(1):36–51.

[2] van Bokhoven A, Varella-Garcia M, Korch C, et al. Molecular characterization of human prostate carcinoma cell lines. Prostate 2003;57(3):205–25.

[3] Zhao M, Sano D, Pickering CR, et al. Assembly and initial characterization of a panel of 85 genomically validated cell lines from diverse head and neck tumor sites. Clin Cancer Res 2011;17(23):7248–64.

[4] Phuchareon J, Ohta Y, Woo JM, et al. Genetic profiling reveals cross-contamination and misidentification of 6 adenoid cystic carcinoma cell lines: ACC2, ACC3, ACCM, ACCNS, ACCS and CAC2. PLoS One 2009; 4(6):e6040.

[5] Korch C, Spillman MA, Jackson TA, et al. DNA profiling analysis of endometrial and ovarian cell lines reveals misidentification, redundancy and contamination. Gynecol Oncol 2012;127(1):241–8.

[6] Korch C, Hall EM, Dirks WG, et al. Authentication of M14 melanoma cell line proves misidentification of MDA-MB-435 breast cancer cell line. Int J Cancer 2018; 142(3):561–72.

[7] Liscovitch M, Ravid D. A case study in misidentification of cancer cell lines: MCF-7/AdrR cells (re-designated NCI/ADR-RES) are derived from OVCAR-8 human ovarian carcinoma cells. Cancer Lett 2007;245(1–2): 350–2.

[8] Schweppe RE, Klopper JP, Korch C, et al. Deoxyribonucleic acid profiling analysis of 40 human thyroid cancer cell lines reveals cross-contamination resulting in cell line redundancy and misidentification. J Clin Endocrinol Metab 2008;93:4331–41.

[9] Marlow LA, D'Innocenzi J, Zhang Y, et al. Detailed molecular fingerprinting of four new anaplastic thyroid carcinoma cell lines and their use for verification of RhoB as a molecular therapeutic target. J Clin Endocrinol Metab 2010;95(12):5338–47.

[10] Henderson YC, Ahn SH, Ryu J, et al. Development and characterization of six new human papillary thyroid carcinoma cell lines. J Clin Endocrinol Metab 2015;100(2): E243–52.

[11] Onoda N, Nakamura M, Aomatsu N, et al. Establishment, characterization and comparison of seven authentic anaplastic thyroid cancer cell lines retaining clinical features of the original tumors. World J Surg 2014;38(3):688–95.

[12] Pozdeyev N, Pike LA, Zhou Q, et al. Establishment and characterization of two novel PTC cell lines expressing the RET/PTC1 rearrangement and BRAF V600E mutation respectively. Abstract from 15TH International Thyroid Congress Program And Meeting Abstracts, Thyroid 25, S1, A-372. Short Call Poster 39. https://www.liebertpub.com/doi/full/10.1089/thy.2015.29006.abstracts?src=recsys&mobileUi=0.

[13] Morrison JA, Pike LA, Lund G, et al. Characterization of thyroid cancer cell lines in murine orthotopic and intracardiac metastasis models. Horm Cancer 2015;6(2–3): 87–99.

[14] Schweppe RE. Thyroid cancer cell lines: critical models to study thyroid cancer biology and new therapeutic targets. Front Endocrinol (Lausanne) 2012;3:81.

[15] Pozdeyev N, Gay L, Sokol ES, et al. Genetic analysis of 779 advanced differentiated and anaplastic thyroid cancers. Clin Cancer Res 2018;24(13):3059–68.

[16] Hughes P, Marshall D, Reid Y, et al. The costs of using unauthenticated, over-passaged cell lines: how much more data do we need? Biotechniques 2007;43(5):575, 577-578, 581-572 passim.

[17] Saito S, Morita K, Kohara A, et al. Use of BAC array CGH for evaluation of chromosomal stability of clinically used human mesenchymal stem cells and of cancer cell lines. Hum Cell 2011;24(1):2–8.

[18] Freedman LP, Gibson MC, Ethier SP, et al. Reproducibility: changing the policies and culture of cell line authentication. Nat Methods 2015;12(6):493–7.

[19] Capes-Davis A, Reid YA, Kline MC, et al. Match criteria for human cell line authentication: where do we draw the line? Int J Cancer 2013;132(11):2510–9.

[20] Kleensang A, Vantangoli MM, Odwin-DaCosta S, et al. Genetic variability in a frozen batch of MCF-7 cells invisible in routine authentication affecting cell function. Sci Rep 2016;6:28994.

[21] Gomez GG, Varella-Garcia M, Kruse CA. Isolation of immunoresistant human glioma cell clones after selection with alloreactive cytotoxic T lymphocytes: cytogenetic and molecular cytogenetic characterization. Cancer Genet Cytogenet 2006;165(2):121–34.

[22] Mrozek K, Tanner SM, Heinonen K, et al. Molecular cytogenetic characterization of the KG-1 and KG-1a acute myeloid leukemia cell lines by use of spectral karyotyping and fluorescence in situ hybridization. Genes Chromosomes Cancer 2003;38(3):249–52.

[23] Pelliccia F, Ubertini V, Bosco N. The importance of molecular cytogenetic analysis prior to using cell lines in research: the case of the KG-1a leukemia cell line. Oncol Lett 2012;4(2):237–40.
[24] Nishida M. The Ishikawa cells from birth to the present. Hum Cell 2002;15(3):104–17.
[25] Kasai F, Hirayama N, Ozawa M, et al. Changes of heterogeneous cell populations in the Ishikawa cell line during long-term culture: proposal for an in vitro clonal evolution model of tumor cells. Genomics 2016;107(6):259–66.
[26] Wang HY, Greenawalt D, Cui X, et al. Identification of possible genetic alterations in the breast cancer cell line MCF-7 using high-density SNP genotyping microarray. J Carcinog 2009;8:6.
[27] Torsvik A, Stieber D, Enger PO, et al. U-251 revisited: genetic drift and phenotypic consequences of long-term cultures of glioblastoma cells. Cancer Med 2014;3(4):812–24.
[28] Clevers H. Modeling development and disease with organoids. Cell 2016;165(7):1586–97.
[29] Aboulkheyr Es H, Montazeri L, Aref AR, et al. Personalized cancer medicine: an organoid approach. Trends Biotechnol 2018;36(4):358–71.
[30] Vlachogiannis G, Hedayat S, Vatsiou A, et al. Patient-derived organoids model treatment response of metastatic gastrointestinal cancers. Science 2018;359(6378):920–6.
[31] Webb SP. Taking it to the gut. Biotechniques 2018;64(3):91–4.
[32] Nardone RM, MacLeod RA, Capes-Davis A. Cancer: authenticate new xenograft models. Nature 2016;532(7599):313.
[33] Gottardis MM, Robinson SP, Satyaswaroop PG, et al. Contrasting actions of tamoxifen on endometrial and breast tumor growth in the athymic mouse. Cancer Res 1988;48(4):812–5.
[34] Patel RR, Sengupta S, Kim HR, et al. Experimental treatment of oestrogen receptor (ER) positive breast cancer with tamoxifen and brivanib alaninate, a VEGFR-2/FGFR-1 kinase inhibitor: a potential clinical application of angiogenesis inhibitors. Eur J Cancer 2010;46(9):1537–53.
[35] Alkema NG, Tomar T, Duiker EW, et al. Biobanking of patient and patient-derived xenograft ovarian tumour tissue: efficient preservation with low and high fetal calf serum based methods. Sci Rep 2015;5:14495.
[36] El-Hoss J, Jing D, Evans K, et al. A single nucleotide polymorphism genotyping platform for the authentication of patient derived xenografts. Oncotarget 2016;7(37):60475–90.
[37] Cibulskis K, McKenna A, Fennell T, et al. ContEst: estimating cross-contamination of human samples in next-generation sequencing data. Bioinformatics 2011;27(18):2601–2.
[38] Jacobsen BM, Harrell JC, Jedlicka P, et al. Spontaneous fusion with, and transformation of mouse stroma by, malignant human breast cancer epithelium. Cancer Res 2006;66(16):8274–9.
[39] Liu X, Ory V, Chapman S, et al. ROCK inhibitor and feeder cells induce the conditional reprogramming of epithelial cells. Am J Pathol 2012;180(2):599–607.
[40] Wang CS, Goulet F, Tremblay N, et al. Selective culture of epithelial cells from primary breast carcinomas using irradiated 3T3 cells as feeder layer. Pathol Res Pract 2001;197(3):175–81.
[41] Cobleigh MA, Kennedy JL, Wong AC, et al. Primary culture of squamous head and neck cancer with and without 3T3 fibroblasts and effect of clinical tumor characteristics on growth in vitro. Cancer 1987;59(10):1732–8.
[42] Dangles-Marie V, Pocard M, Richon S, et al. Establishment of human colon cancer cell lines from fresh tumors versus xenografts: comparison of success rate and cell line features. Cancer Res 2007;67(1):398–407.
[43] Ince TA, Sousa AD, Jones MA, et al. Characterization of twenty-five ovarian tumour cell lines that phenocopy primary tumours. Nat Commun 2015;6:7419.
[44] Drost J, Karthaus WR, Gao D, et al. Organoid culture systems for prostate epithelial and cancer tissue. Nat Protoc 2016;11(2):347–58.
[45] Agarwal S, Rimm DL. Making every cell like HeLa a giant step for cell culture. Am J Pathol 2012;180(2):443–5.
[46] Taylor-Papadimitriou J, Shearer M, Stoker MG. Growth requirements of human mammary epithelial cells in culture. Int J Cancer 1977;20(6):903–8.
[47] Correa BRS, Hu J, Penalva LOF, et al. Patient-derived conditionally reprogrammed cells maintain intra-tumor genetic heterogeneity. Sci Rep 2018;8(1):4097.
[48] Kiseljak-Vassiliades K, Zhang Y, Bagby SM, et al. Development of new preclinical models to advance adrenocortical carcinoma research. Endocr Relat Cancer 2018;25(4):437–51.
[49] Crystal AS, Shaw AT, Sequist LV, et al. Patient-derived models of acquired resistance can identify effective drug combinations for cancer. Science 2014;346(6216):1480–6.
[50] Liu X, Krawczyk E, Suprynowicz FA, et al. Conditional reprogramming and long-term expansion of normal and tumor cells from human biospecimens. Nat Protoc 2017;12(2):439–51.
[51] Tomlinson GE, Chen TT, Stastny VA, et al. Characterization of a breast cancer cell line derived from a germ-line BRCA1 mutation carrier. Cancer Res 1998;58(15):3237–42.
[52] Gold M. A conspiracy of cells. Albany (NY): State University of New York Press; 1986.
[53] Ince TA, Richardson AL, Bell GW, et al. Transformation of different human breast epithelial cell types leads to distinct tumor phenotypes. Cancer Cell 2007;12(2):160–70.

[54] Bueno C, Montes R, Menendez P. The ROCK inhibitor Y-27632 negatively affects the expansion/survival of both fresh and cryopreserved cord blood-derived CD34+ hematopoietic progenitor cells: Y-27632 negatively affects the expansion/survival of CD34+HSPCs. Stem Cell Rev 2010;6(2):215–23.

[55] Lamas NJ, Serra SC, Salgado AJ, et al. Failure of Y-27632 to improve the culture of adult human adipose-derived stem cells. Stem Cells Cloning 2015;8:15–26.

[56] Routhier A, Astuccio M, Lahey D, et al. Pharmacological inhibition of Rho-kinase signaling with Y-27632 blocks melanoma tumor growth. Oncol Rep 2010;23(3):861–7.

[57] Tomczak K, Czerwinska P, Wiznerowicz M. The Cancer Genome Atlas (TCGA): an immeasurable source of knowledge. Contemp Oncol (Pozn) 2015;19(1A):A68–77.

[58] Barretina J, Caponigro G, Stransky N, et al. The cancer cell line encyclopedia enables predictive modelling of anticancer drug sensitivity. Nature 2012;483(7391):603–7.

[59] Domcke S, Sinha R, Levine DA, et al. Evaluating cell lines as tumour models by comparison of genomic profiles. Nat Commun 2013;4:2126.

[60] Berns EM, Bowtell DD. The changing view of high-grade serous ovarian cancer. Cancer Res 2012;72(11):2701–4.

[61] Vaughan S, Coward JI, Bast RC Jr, et al. Rethinking ovarian cancer: recommendations for improving outcomes. Nat Rev Cancer 2011;11(10):719–25.

[62] Zhao N, Liu Y, Wei Y, et al. Optimization of cell lines as tumour models by integrating multi-omics data. Brief Bioinform 2017;18(3):515–29.

[63] Shah MH, Wei L, Wirth LJ, et al. Results of randomized phase II trial of dabrafenib versus dabrafenib plus trametinib in BRAF-mutated papillary thyroid carcinoma. J Clin Oncol (Meeting Abstracts) 2017;35(suppl) [abstract: 6022]. Available at: http://ascopubs.org/doi/abs/10.1200/jco.2017.35.15_suppl.6022.

[64] Montero-Conde C, Ruiz-Llorente S, Dominguez JM, et al. Relief of feedback inhibition of HER3 transcription by RAF and MEK inhibitors attenuates their antitumor effects in BRAF-mutant thyroid carcinomas. Cancer Discov 2013;3(5):520–33.

[65] Sos ML, Levin RS, Gordan JD, et al. Oncogene mimicry as a mechanism of primary resistance to BRAF inhibitors. Cell Rep 2014;8(4):1037–48.

[66] Begley CG, Ioannidis JP. Reproducibility in science: improving the standard for basic and preclinical research. Circ Res 2015;116(1):116–26.

[67] Eterovic K. Getting the best data from your cells: from tissue culture to final analysis. 2017. Available at: http://www.sciencemag.org/custom-publishing/webinars/getting-best-data-your-cells-tissue-culture-final-analysis. Accessed May 3, 2017.

[68] Stern AM, Casadevall A, Steen RG, et al. Financial costs and personal consequences of research misconduct resulting in retracted publications. Elife 2014;3:e02956.

[69] Fusenig NE, Capes-Davis A, Bianchini F, et al. The need for a worldwide consensus for cell line authentication: experience implementing a mandatory requirement at the International Journal of Cancer. PLoS Biol 2017;15(4):e2001438.

[70] Geraghty RJ, Capes-Davis A, Davis JM, et al. Guidelines for the use of cell lines in biomedical research. Br J Cancer 2014;111(6):1021–46.

[71] Capes-Davis A, Theodosopoulos G, Atkin I, et al. Check your cultures! A list of cross-contaminated or misidentified cell lines. Int J Cancer 2010;127(1):1–8.

Advances in Molecular Pathology 1 (2018) 253–264
ADVANCES IN MOLECULAR PATHOLOGY

Historical and Current Methods for Detecting Interspecies and Intraspecies Cell Mixtures and Thereby Assuring Cell Line Purity

Raymond Whiting Nims, PhD
RMC Pharmaceutical Solutions, Inc, 1851 Lefthand Circle, Suite A, Longmont, CO 80501, USA

KEYWORDS

- Cell purity • Interspecies cell mixture • Intraspecies cell mixture • Karyotyping • Multiplex PCR
- SNP profiling • STR profiling • Next-generation sequencing

KEY POINTS

- Cell purity, defined in this article as absence of cross-contaminating cell types in a culture as opposed, for instance, to freedom from contamination by adventitious agents (eg, viruses, mycoplasma, yeast, bacteria) is a necessary aspect of cell line characterization.
- Methods of assuring cell line identity may not be capable of establishing cell line purity.
- The capabilities and limitations of historical and current methods for establishing cell line mixtures as part of assuring cell line purity are discussed.

INTRODUCTION

Cross-contamination of a cell culture with another can occur during routine manipulation of the separate cell cultures within the same laminar flow hood or when reagents, such as medium, trypsin, or buffers, are shared between different cell cultures. A transient or stable interspecies or intraspecies cell mixture can result from such a cross-contamination. Are actual intraspecies or interspecies cell mixtures ever detected during cell line authentication? The answer is yes, on rare occasions [1,2]. Unless the doubling times for the 2 cell types composing the mixture are the same (a rare case), the cell type with the shorter doubling time will rapidly overgrow and replace the slower growing cell type [3]. Given sufficient time, such a transient cell mixture will be replaced with a pure culture of the faster growing cell type (Fig. 1). This event may result in a cell line misidentification. This is likely the reason that so many continuous human cell lines thought to be unique model systems for various tumor types or tissues have, especially in the early days of cell culture, turned out to be HeLa cultures [2,4]. Many cell culture laboratories maintained HeLa cell cultures, and these cells easily dominated primary cell cultures being developed, given the opportunity through cross-contamination.

In the very early stages of any cross-contamination, when the culture consists of a mixture of 2 different cell types, it may be possible to detect the presence of the contaminating cell through light microscopic

Conflict Statement: The author declares that he does not have any commercial or financial conflicts of interest regarding this work, for which he received no funding.
E-mail address: rnims@rmcpharma.com

https://doi.org/10.1016/j.yamp.2018.07.005
2589-4080/18/

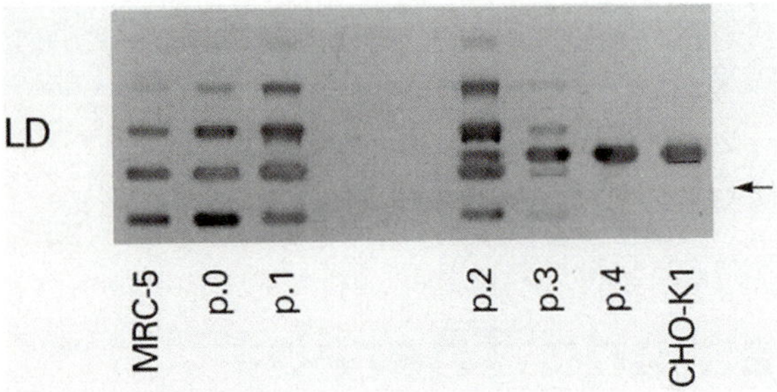

FIG. 1 Isoenzyme analysis of lactate dehydrogenase (LD) provides evidence of an interspecies cell mixture in which a faster-growing cell (CHO-K1) replaces a slower-growing cell (MRC-5). A small number of CHO-K1 cells were added to a confluent MRC-5 culture and the culture was then passaged 4 times, with cells analyzed for LD at the time of each passage (p). The CHO-K1 isoenzyme first became visible at passage 2, and only this isoenzyme is visible in the electropherogram by passage 4. The arrow indicates the location of the origin of the gel. (Reprinted by permission from Springer Nature: Nims RW, Shoemaker AP, Bauernschub MA, et al. Sensitivity of isoenzyme analysis for the detection of interspecies cell line cross-contamination. In Vitro Cell Dev Biol Anim 1998;34(1):38.)

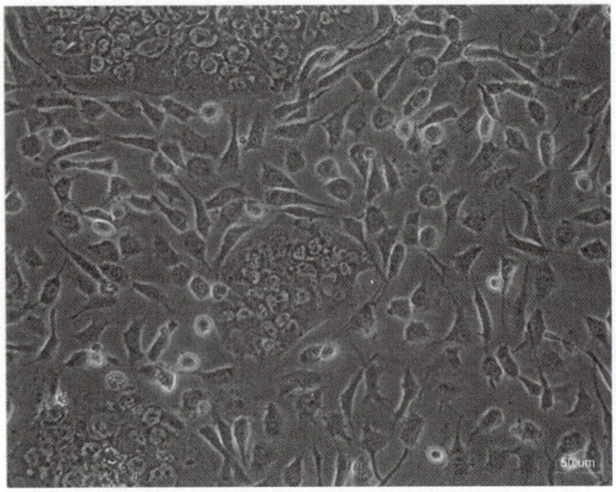

FIG. 2 Example of an interspecies cell mixture with a fibroblast-like component (mouse origin) and an epithelioid component (human [BeWo] origin). In this case, the cell mixture is evident because the 2 cell types have differing morphologies. The dual species of origin was confirmed using a multiplex PCR method that included primers targeting the genes encoding cytochrome *c* oxidase subunit 1 of a set of animal species. (Reprinted by permission from Springer Nature: Bian X, Yang Z, Feng H, et al. A combination of species identification and STR profiling identifies cross-contaminated cells from 482 human tumor cell lines. Sci Rep 2017;7(1):9774.)

inspection of cell morphology [1,2,5] (Fig. 2). For this to be possible, however, the 2 cell types in the mixture must have differing morphologies (eg, fibroblast vs epithelioid) and this is not always the case [2,5]. At the very earliest stages of cross-contamination, when the percentage of the contaminating cells may be relatively low, and at the end stages of a cross-contamination if 1 cell type predominates over the other, detection of the lower (as a percentage) population of the 1 cell type becomes increasingly difficult through visual inspection alone [2,5,6]. Inspection of cell morphology alone cannot, therefore, be relied on for detection of a mixed culture.

The determination of cell purity (defined here as absence of cross-contaminating cell types in a culture, as opposed, for instance, to freedom from contamination by adventitious agents) is considered to be a necessary component of cell line characterization. In this context, cell line characterization refers to the panel of assays used to fully characterize a cell culture. Such a panel typically includes methods for establishing identity to the species or donor level, morphology, growth characteristics (eg, doubling time, adherence to substrate), ploidy (diploid vs polyploid), immortality (continuous vs primary), freedom from adventitious agents (viral, yeast and fungi, and bacterial; including Mollicutes; eg, *Mycoplasma* and *Acholeplasma*), cell purity, and finally phenotype (eg, transformability, differentiation status, receptor status, secretion of proteins).

Identity testing for cell lines can determine identity to the species level, strain-level, or individual donor level. Species-level identity testing confirms that the cell line is derived from a given animal species (eg, mouse, human, pig). For a limited number of animal species, such as the mouse (*Mus musculus*), there are methods that allow determination of the specific strain of animal from which a cell line has been derived. For a few animal species (eg, mouse, human) there are methods that allow determination of the cell to the individual donor level (ie, to the specific individual from whom the cells were originally derived). The species-level and donor-level identity testing methods currently available for cell line authentication are not really designed for, or very sensitive for, detecting interspecies or intraspecies cell mixtures. (see Christopher Korch and Marileila Varella-Garcia's article, "Tackling the Human Cell Line and Tissue Misidentification Problem Is Needed for Reproducible Biomedical Research," in this issue.) Therefore, there is always a risk that a

TABLE 1
Attributes of Historical Cell Purity Methods

Method	Means of Discrimination	Detection Sensitivity	Limitations
Detection primarily of intraspecies cell mixtures			
G-banding	Chromosomal markers	~1%[a]	Number of metaphase spreads examined Presence of markers in the expected cell or contaminant
Detection primarily of interspecies cell mixtures			
Karyotyping	Modal chromosomal number and telocentricity	~1%[a]	Number of metaphase spreads examined
Isoenzyme analysis	Electrophoretic mobility of isoenzymes on agarose gels	~10%[b]	Depends on isoenzymes evaluated and the species of cells in the mixture

Abbreviations: G-banding, banding analysis of giemsa-stained chromosomes.
[a] Theoretic sensitivity, assuming 100 metaphase spreads are evaluated and at least 1 spread with unexpected attributes is observed [8,9].
[b] Very limited intraspecies discrimination is possible, based on polymorphisms for the enzymes evaluated (eg, glucose 6-phosphate dehydrogenase types A and B among human cell lines) [3,6].

small population of an interspecies or intraspecies cross-contaminant will escape detection during routine identity testing of cell lines. Complementary orthogonal analytical methods may, therefore, need to be used to detect the presence of cell mixtures. In this article, the capabilities and limitations of the historical and current (primarily molecular) methods for determining interspecies and intraspecies cell mixtures are discussed.

CLASSIC METHODS FOR DETERMINING CELL PURITY

The primary methods that have been used in the past for examining cell cultures for the presence of contaminating cells have been isoenzyme analysis and karyotyping [7]. The detection sensitivities and limitations of these methods are shown in Table 1.

Isoenzyme Analysis

The examination of electrophoretic mobility, on agarose gels, of a selection of cytoplasmic enzymes has been used for evaluating cell purity for decades. Indeed, this method has been used as the standard against which some of the newer cell purity methods have been compared and validated. An unexpected (extra) band or bands in a gel for 1 or more isoenzymes is the clue to the presence of a second cell type in the mixture. Gels indicating mixtures of Chinese hamster and human, Chinese hamster and mouse, bovine and African green monkey, and human and African green monkey cells have been described in the literature [1] and the gels displaying the human and African green monkey cell mixture are reproduced as Fig. 3. Nims and colleagues [3] demonstrated that isoenzyme analysis could detect interspecies cell mixtures containing approximately 10% of contaminating cells. On the other hand, Ramya and colleagues [6] found that interspecies cell mixtures containing only 1% of contaminating cells could not routinely be detected using this method. Nims and Herbstritt [1] detected, using isoenzyme analysis, only 2 instances of interspecies cell mixtures among nearly 900 cell submissions.

Several factors affect the sensitivity of this method for detecting cell mixtures, including the specific isoenzymes evaluated and the specific animal species comprising the cell mixture [1,3,6]. Unfortunately, the reagents required for performing isoenzyme analysis are no longer commercially available; therefore, this method is currently less commonly used.

Karyotypic (Cytogenetic) Analysis

Karyotypic or cytogenetic analysis reveals both modal chromosome number and chromosomal morphology (eg, the presence of characteristic markers and telocentricity or acrocentricity) [2,8,10,11]. For instance, mouse chromosomes may be telocentric (ie, the centromere is located at 1 end of the chromosome), whereas the centromeres of human chromosomes are never telocentric. Due to possible ploidy differences (differences in chromosomal complement) among cell lines of a given species and differences in telocentricity among differing animal species, karyotyping can detect both intraspecies and interspecies cell mixtures. As shown in Table 1, the sensitivity of karyotyping for detecting an interspecies or intraspecies cell mixture is determined by the number of metaphase spreads evaluated. If, for instance, 100 spreads are evaluated, the presence of a contaminant at the 1% level may theoretically be detected [8]. This level of sensitivity was confirmed by White and Sweeney [9] in detecting male versus female human cells in artificial intraspecies mixtures of peripheral blood cells through microscopic examination of 100 metaphase chromosomal spreads using banding analysis of giemsa-stained chromosomes (G-banding).

MOLECULAR METHODS FOR DETERMINING CELL PURITY

The evolution of molecular (DNA sequence-based) methods has resulted in the introduction of more specific, rapid, and (in most cases) more sensitive analytical approaches for evaluating cell line purity (see later discussion). Their detection sensitivities and limitations are shown in Table 2. In the case of polymerase chain reaction (PCR)-based assays, numerous reaction aspects (eg, primer design and concentrations, amounts of DNA loaded onto a gel, thermocycling conditions) can affect these detection sensitivities. Only very brief descriptions of the methods themselves have been included here due to constraints on article length. For a more complete discussion on methodologies, see references [12–14] and later discussion.

Mitochondrial DNA Analysis

The detection of interspecies cell mixtures by PCR methods using primers targeting mitochondrial genes, including those encoding cytochrome *b* and/or cytochrome *c* oxidase, is based on the relatively higher mutation rates for mitochondrial genes relative to nuclear

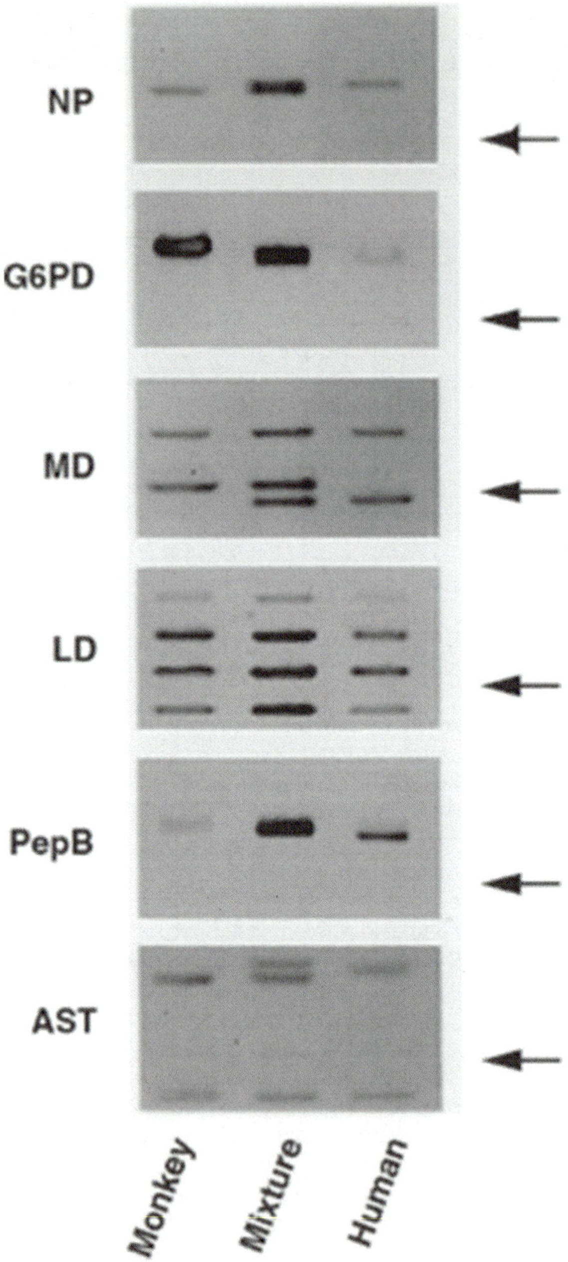

FIG. 3 Detection of an interspecies cell mixture by isoenzyme analysis. The mixture containing African green monkey (Vero) and human (MRC-5) cells is apparent as doublet bands in the case of the gels stained for malate dehydrogenase (MD) and aspartate aminotransferase (AST). The arrows indicate the approximate location of the gel origins. LD, lactate dehydrogenase; NP, nucleoside phosphorylase; G6PD, glucose 6-phosphate dehydrogenase; PepB, peptidase B. (*From* Nims RW, Herbstritt CJ. Cell line authentication using isoenzyme analysis. Strategies for accurate speciation and case studies for the detection of cell line cross-contamination using a commercial kit. BioPharm Int 2005;18(6):3; with permission.)

TABLE 2
Attributes of Molecular Cell Purity Methods

Method	Means of Discrimination	Detection Sensitivity	Limitations
Detection primarily of intraspecies cell mixtures			
STR profiling	Hypervariable genomic content	10%[a]	Designed primarily as a donor-level identity test
SNP Profiling	Multiplex for many targets	2%–50%	Designed primarily as a donor-level identity test Sensitivity displayed depends on copy number at locus of interest
Detection primarily of interspecies cell mixtures			
DNA barcoding	Mitochondrial genes	10%	Designed primarily as a species-level identity test
Cytochrome *b* RFLP	Mitochondrial genes	1%–33%	Depends on amplification efficiency of primers
Multiplex PCR	Mitochondrial genes	1%–50%	Depends on use of species-specific primers
Next-generation sequencing	Mitochondrial genes	0.1%	–

Abbreviations: PCR, polymerase chain reaction; SNP, single nucleotide polymorphism; STR, short tandem repeat.

[a] As typically performed, the technology is not designed to detect interspecies contamination. This may be overcome through inclusion of a few species-specific loci (eg, mouse-specific loci for detection of mouse feeder cells in human stem cell preparations).

genes and the low intraspecies variation in coding sequences for mitochondrial genes.

PCR–restriction fragment length polymorphism (RFLP) methods targeting cytochrome *b* have been characterized for sensitivity for detecting interspecies cell mixtures. For instance, Losi and colleagues [15] evaluated goat cell DNA intentionally contaminated with cat, duck, or horse cell DNA in different ratios of goat DNA to contaminating DNA. The presence of an additional DNA fragment following digestion by 1 or more restriction enzymes, with size corresponding to another animal species, indicated a cell mixture. Fig. 4 displays the results obtained by these investigators when examining the various goat or cat DNA mixtures following digestion only with *Hinf*I. Sensitivity of detection of the contaminating DNA depended on the amplification efficiency of the primer used for the contaminating species. It was 10% for cat as contaminant and 33% for duck or horse as contaminant [15].

Mohammadi and colleagues [16] used a PCR-RFLP assay to evaluate mixtures of DNA from human [MRC-5] and rhesus monkey [RMK-2] cells in different ratios (human to monkey). The lower limit of detection of human DNA in a mixture was 5% [16].

Ono and colleagues [17] evaluated a nested PCR targeting the cytochrome *b* gene of 7 animal species (human, mouse, rat, rabbit, cat, cow, and pig). In this method, the amplicons generated for the different animal species have differing molecular weights and, therefore, migrate different distances on gels, conferring the ability to identify the species. The assay was used to evaluate mixtures of DNA (mouse [WEHI-3b] plus human [A549], mouse plus rat [Py-3Y1-S2], and rat plus human) to estimate the sensitivity for detection of interspecies cell mixtures. The DNA proportions tested for each species pair varied between 10,000:1 and 1:10,000. The sensitivity of the method for detecting the contaminating cell DNA depended on whether the species-specific primers were used in monoplex or multiplex

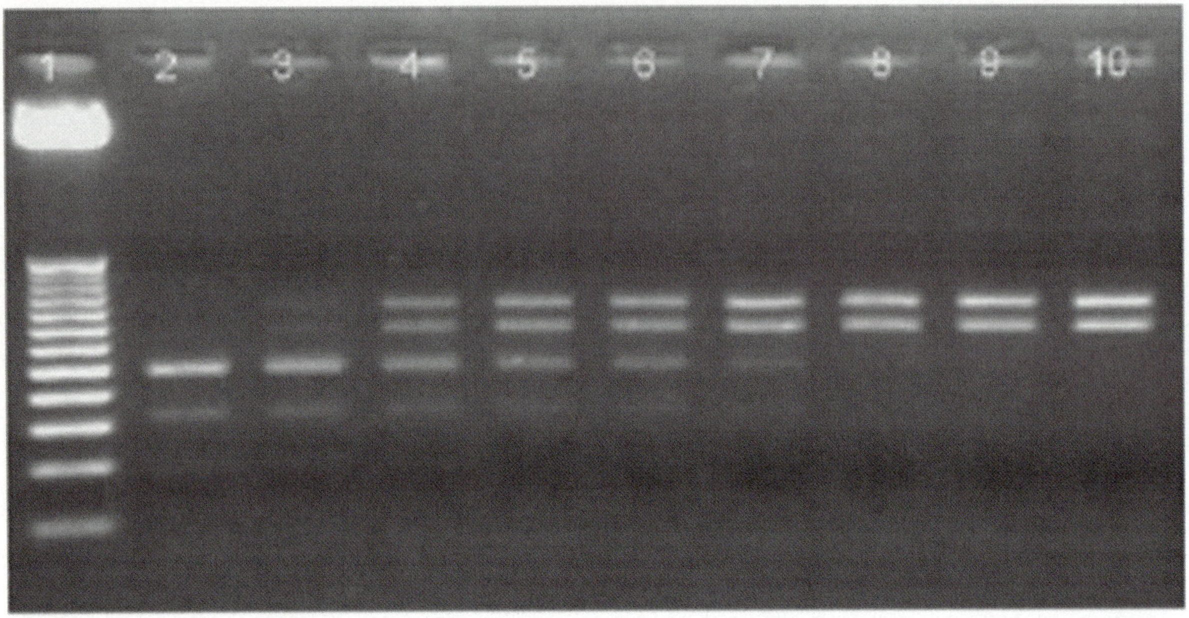

Cat	100	90	50	33	25	10	5	2.5	0
Goat	0	10	50	67	75	90	95	97.5	100

FIG. 4 Cytochrome *b* PCR-RFLP analysis of mixtures of cat and goat DNA representing a hypothetical cell mixture. Lanes were loaded with the ratios of cat and goat DNA indicated below the figure. (Reprinted by permission from Springer Nature: Losi CG, Ferrari S, Sossi E, et al. An alternative method to isoenzyme profile for cell line identification and interspecies cross-contaminations: cytochrome b PCR-RLFP analysis. In Vitro Cell Dev Biol Anim 2008;44(8-9):327.)

mode. In the latter case, which would typically be used in an assay designed to detect interspecies cell mixtures, the sensitivity for detecting human, mouse, and rat DNA differed. The investigators did not report the lowest proportions detected in the different mixtures; however, from examination of the figures, it seems that the human DNA was detected at the 1:10,000 and 1:1000 levels in the presence of mouse and rat DNA, respectively. Mouse DNA was detected at the 1:10 and 1:1000 levels in human and rat DNA, respectively. Rat DNA was detected at the 50:50 and 1:99 levels in human and mouse DNA, respectively. The differences in sensitivity noted were attributed to differing amplification efficiencies for the species-specific primers used [17]. Another explanation could be the mitochondrial genome copy number between the different samples due to extraction efficiencies or biological differences. The investigators acknowledged that further optimization of the method is needed.

Ramya and colleagues [6] also used a nested PCR targeting the mitochondrial cytochrome *b* gene to evaluate different interspecies cell mixtures (canine [MDCK] contaminated with Syrian hamster [BHK-21], African green monkey [Vero] contaminated with bovine [MDBK] or canine [MDCK], primary cattle kidney [PCK] contaminated with Syrian hamster [BHK-21], and Syrian hamster kidney [BHK-21] contaminated with primary cattle kidney [PCK]). In these mixtures, the contaminating cell was present at 1% to 5% proportion. These cell mixtures were not apparent by isoenzyme analysis but the presence of the contaminating cell was detected in each case by the nested PCR [6].

A multiplex PCR method that included primers targeting the genes encoding cytochrome *c* oxidase subunit 1 of human, cat, dog, mouse, rat, horse, rabbit, and African green monkey, and cytochrome *b* of Chinese hamster, was described by Parodi and colleagues [18]. The method was found to be capable of detecting contaminating African green monkey (Vero) cells in a mixed culture containing 99% rat (RBL-1) cells and 1% Vero cells [18].

This level of sensitivity for detecting interspecies cell mixtures was also achieved with a different multiplex

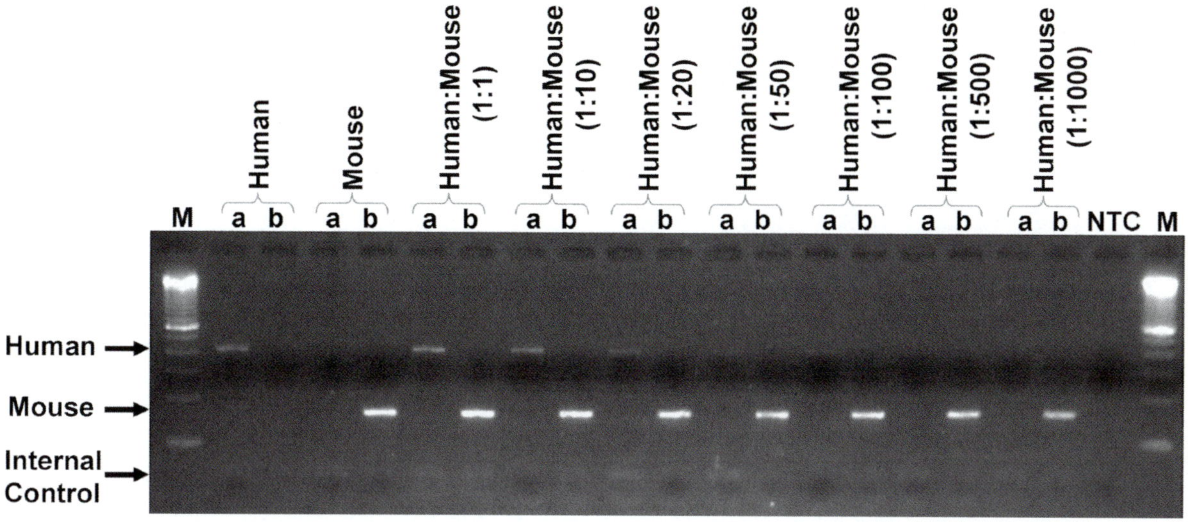

FIG. 5 Human (H522) cells and mouse cells (LL/2 [LLC1]) and various mixtures of the 2 were analyzed by cytochrome *c* oxidase I (COI)-specific PCR amplification. The presence of human cells was detected using a set of primers specific for the human COI target (lanes a), whereas the presence of the mouse cells was detected using a multiplex PCR targeting 11 nonhuman species (cat, Chinese hamster, rhesus monkey, horse, cow, African green monkey, rat, goat, dog, New Zealand rabbit, and mouse) (lanes b). Detection of the contaminating human cells was achievable down to the 1% level. Lanes indicated as M contain molecular weight marker only, lane indicated as NTC was loaded with no template control. (Reprinted by permission from Springer Nature: Nims RW, Sykes G, Cottrill K, et al. Short tandem repeat profiling: part of an overall strategy for reducing the frequency of cell misidentification. In Vitro Cell Dev Biol Anim 2010;46(10):811-9.)

PCR method described by Cooper and colleagues [19] that targeted the gene encoding cytochrome *c* oxidase subunit 1 of human, mouse, rat, horse, Chinese hamster, and cow. It was designed to yield differently sized amplicons to facilitate interpretation of the resulting gels. In this case, mixtures of human (HeLa) and mouse (*M musculus;* [L929]) cells were evaluated. Cell mixtures containing 1% mouse in 99% human cells or 1% human cells in 99% mouse cells were detected [19].

A similar multiplex PCR targeting cytochrome *c* oxidase was used by Nims and colleagues [5] to evaluate human (NCI-H522) and mouse (*M musculus;* LL/2 [LLC1]) cell mixtures in different proportions. The human cells could be detected in this DNA assay if present at as low as 1% (Fig. 5).

Bian and colleagues [2] detected 5 instances of interspecies (human and mouse) cell mixtures among 482 human cell lines evaluated in their study. The mixtures were identified using a multiplex PCR method that included primers targeting the genes encoding cytochrome *c* oxidase subunit 1 of human, mouse, rat, Chinese hamster, Syrian hamster, rabbit, cow, dog, African green monkey, and pig.

Cytochrome *c* oxidase subunit 1 barcoding has been proposed as a method for determining the identity of animal cells to the species level, and an American National Standards Institute (ANSI) standard has been published for this method and purpose [20]. The sensitivity of this approach for detecting an interspecies cell mixture has not been reported in the literature. A study performed for informational purposes indicated that cell mixtures containing ratios of human to mouse cells of 1:9 and 9:1 generated amplicons, in a barcoding assay for species identification, that were detected as mixed sequences, which would trigger an investigation into a potential mixed culture [21].

Nuclear DNA Analysis

Jordan and colleagues [22] designed a PCR assay targeting the highly conserved microtubulin-actin crosslinking factor 1 (MACF1) gene for detecting species of origin of cell lines. The method discriminated between human, African green monkey, hamster (species not provided), Muscovy duck (*Cairina moschata*), and fruit bat (*Rousettus aegyptiacus*) based on amplicon size and resulting differences in migration on gels. The investigators used this assay to demonstrate the kinetics of overgrowth and replacement of a fruit bat cell line (R06E) by African green monkey (Vero.GFP) cells, when the latter were added at a low number to the R06E culture

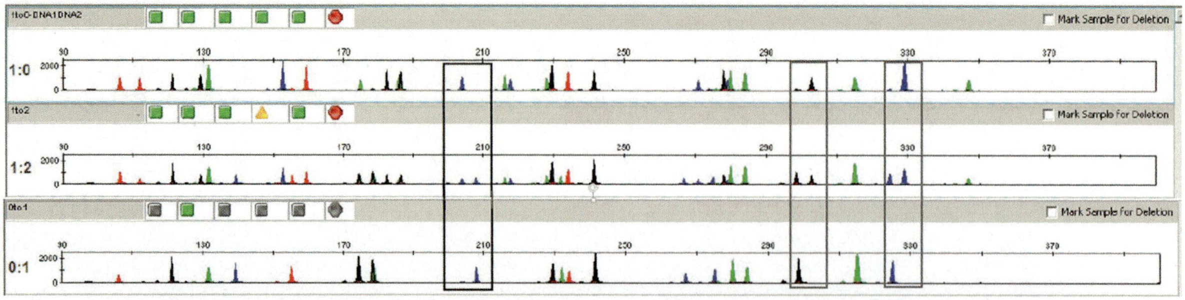

FIG. 6 STR profiling of mixtures of human cell DNA representing a hypothetical intraspecies cell mixture. The rows, from top to bottom, represent analysis of mixtures of the indicated proportions of HCT15 and ACHN cell DNA. Changes at the alleles within the boxed areas are especially useful for detecting the mixture. (*From* Fang R, Shewale JG, Nguyen VT, et al. STR profiling of human cell lines: challenges and possible solutions to the growing problem. J Forensics Res 2011;S2:005. doi: 10.4172/2157-7145.S2-005; with permission.)

and the resulting coculture was passaged at a 1:20 split ratio once weekly. The Vero cell DNA was first detected by passage 4, when the culture was estimated by fluorescence activated cell sorting to be approximately 20% Vero.GFP cells. Only the Vero.GFP cell DNA was detected by passage 7 of this culture [22].

Short Tandem Repeat and Single Nucleotide Polymorphism Profiling

Short tandem repeat (STR) profiling involves the PCR-amplification of variable microsatellite regions from a genomic DNA template, followed by separation of the PCR amplicons on a genetic analyzer [13]. Single nucleotide polymorphisms (SNPs) are single-base sequence variations between individuals occurring at certain points in the genome. Several SNP genotyping methodologies are available [14]. Commercial kits are available for performance of tests and analysis of results, and an ANSI standard for performing STR profiling analysis of human cell lines is available [23]. The detection of multiple (ie, >2) alleles at 1 or more loci is generally interpreted as evidence of a cell mixture because individuals are expected to be either homozygous or heterozygous at any given locus. In addition, mismatched repair defects in cell lines can give rise to microsatellite instability that can manifest through multiple peaks that differ by plus or minus 1 repeat unit.

Although primarily used for identifying human cells to the individual donor level, STR and SNP profiling have also been characterized for their abilities to detect intraspecies cell mixtures. For instance, Fang and colleagues [24] evaluated mixtures of DNA from the human cell lines CHT15 and ACHN, using STR analysis (Fig. 6). They concluded that it was possible to detect mixtures of the 2 different cell lines based on unshared alleles if the contaminating cell DNA made up at least 10% of the total DNA [24].

Liang-Chu and colleagues [25] characterized the sensitivity of SNP analysis using the Illumina (Illumina, Inc., San Diego, CA) and Fluidigm (Fluidigm Corporation, South San Francisco, CA) platforms for detecting intraspecies human tumor cell mixtures (THP-1/SK-MEL-1, AU565/SK-MES-1, and MCF-7/LOX-IMVI) in ratios ranging from 1:99 to 99:1 of the 2 cell lines. The sensitivity of the Fluidigm SNP Trace assay for detection of 1 of the cells in the pair depended on the cell type. In some cases, as low as 2% contamination could be detected, whereas, in the worst case, the contamination could only be detected at 50%. These investigators also conducted DNA mixing studies for human male and female diploid cell samples in different proportions of male or female DNA from 1% to 20% and the reciprocal mixtures. In this case, the contaminating cell type could be detected if the DNA was present at 5% or greater. The investigators concluded that degree of aneuploidy and copy number at a given locus for the contaminating cell influenced the sensitivity of the method for detecting the intraspecies contamination [25].

Bian and colleagues [2] detected, using STR profiling, 3 instances of intraspecies cell mixtures among 482 human tumor cell lines evaluated. Another case of an intraspecies cell mixture was identified recently by Korch (C. Korch, personal communication 2018). In this rather complicated case, the stable cell mixture BHP18-21 was found by STR profiling (Table 3) to comprise the human M14 melanoma cell line and the human papillary thyroid cell line TPC1. The STR profile indicates 9 STR loci in which the mixed cell line BHP18 possesses alleles corresponding to each of the 2 cell lines composing the mixture.

TABLE 3
Detection of an Intraspecies Human Cell Mixture Using Short Tandem Repeat Profiling

Cell Line	Passage	Description	STR Locus									
			Amelogenin	**D3S1358**	**D5S818**	**D7S820**	**D8S1179**	**D13S317**	**D18S51**	**D21S11**	**FGA**	**vWA**
M14 [26]	14	Melanoma cell line with lost Y-chromo some	X	*14*, 16	*11*, *12*	*8*, *10*	*13*	*12*	13, *17*	30	20	*16*, 18
BHP18 (C. Korch, personal communi cation 2018)	21	Mixed M14 + TPC1	X	*14*, 16, **17**	**8, 10,** *11*, *12*	*8*, *10*, **11**	**11,** *13*, **17**	**11,** 12	13**, 16,** *17*	30, **31.2**	20, **21**	**14,** *16*, 18
TPC1 [27]	—	Thyroid cell line	X	16, **17**	**8, 10**	**11**	**11, 17**	**11,** 12	13, **16**	30, **31.2**	20, **21**	**14,** 18

Italicized values are contributed exclusively by M14, while bolded values are contributed exclusively by TPC1.

STR or SNP profiling of human cells is, however, not informative of the presence of an interspecies contaminant [2,5]. To address this issue, Almeida and colleagues [28] designed a mouse STR panel that contains 2 human STR loci in addition to 9 mouse loci. This method is therefore able to detect the specific mouse or human interspecies cell mixture in addition to detecting intraspecies (mouse) cell mixtures.

Didion and colleagues [29] used SNP arrays to distinguish among different mouse cell lines. The investigators also characterized the sensitivity of the method for detecting an intraspecies DNA mixture. Detection of an intraspecies contaminant in this method is facilitated by a computational approach that evaluates markers with allelic ratios falling outside of the expected range for the given cell line. The investigators estimated that the minimum level of contamination that would be detectable using this method ranged from 5% to 10% contaminating DNA, depending on the specific commercial SNP array used [30]. A new version of the array (GigaMUGA, Neogen Genomics, Lincoln, NE) is now available commercially that can distinguish between mouse species, subspecies, and strains [30].

Next-Generation Sequencing

Mitchell [31] has recently developed a species-level cell purity assay that detects 19 mammalian and insect species using next-generation sequencing (NGS) of 3 mitochondrial gene PCR amplicons for each species. With Chinese hamster ovary (CHO) cell DNA spiked with DNA from the 18 other species in different ratios of CHO or non-CHO species from 0.1% to 10%, the method detected and confirmed each of 3 species-specific amplicons down to 0.1%, with no false positives. A cell mixing study was also performed, with test samples including DNA from pure CHO cells or CHO cells spiked with Syrian hamster (BHK) cells and *Spodoptera frugiperda* (Sf9, fall armyworm) cells at the following ratios: 98% CHO spiked with 1% BHK plus 1% Sf9, or 99.8% CHO spiked with 0.1% BHK plus 0.1% Sf9. The 3 BHK-specific and Sf9-specific amplicons were detected and confirmed for each spiked sample, demonstrating that this method can detect multiple contaminating species at levels as low as 0.1% of the total cell population (C. Mitchell, WuXi AppTec, unpublished data, 2018).

DISCUSSION

The term cell line cross-contamination has often been used in the literature interchangeably with cell line misidentification, despite that there are causes of cell line misidentification that do not involve cross-contamination (eg, mislabeling of flasks or cryovials) [5]. Intraspecies cell line misidentification is best addressed through cell line identity testing, which is beyond the scope of this article. (see Christopher Korch and Marileila Varella-Garcia's article, "Tackling the Human Cell Line and Tissue Misidentification Problem Is Needed for Reproducible Biomedical Research," in this issue.) Cross-contamination of cultures may also lead to a misidentified culture but also may lead to transient or stable cell mixtures. Stable cell mixtures are likely to be rare but are occasionally detected [1,2]. Detection of a transient cell mixture depends on the stage of the cross-contamination because this determines the proportions of the various cells in the mixtures and the sensitivity of the detection method. To detect the earliest stages of cell cross-contamination, 1 of the methods designed specifically for this purpose with the greatest sensitivity will therefore be needed to detect cell mixtures containing the lowest proportion of contaminating cells.

As previously described, there are a variety of approaches for detecting interspecies or intraspecies cell mixtures. The sensitivities of these methods for detecting cell mixtures range from less than or equal to 1% to as high as 50%. Not all of the methods are available as commercial kits, although many of the methods are available at contract testing laboratories. Unfortunately, currently, there is not a molecular method that is capable of detecting both interspecies and intraspecies cell mixtures with adequate sensitivity. The most promising approaches for detecting interspecies cell mixtures are the multiplex PCR and NGS assays targeting mitochondrial genes, such as cytochrome *b* or cytochrome *c* oxidase subunit 1. When optimized, these have sensitivities for detecting contaminating cells that make up as low as 0.1% of the cell population. Intraspecies human or mouse cell mixtures are detectable using STR profiling and SNP analysis, though sensitivities for this purpose may vary widely, depending on the specific cell contaminant and the SNP technologies used.

SUMMARY

The species-level and donor-level identity testing methods currently available for cell line authentication are not really designed for, or very sensitive for, detection of interspecies or intraspecies cell mixtures. Therefore, there is always a risk of a small population of an interspecies or intraspecies cross-contaminant escaping detection during routine identity testing of cell lines. This point needs emphasis in the modern era of sequence-based cell line identity testing. This article states the problem and describes the historical and the currently preferred methods for detecting interspecies and intraspecies cell mixtures and the relative sensitivities of these methods for this purpose.

ACKNOWLEDGMENTS

This article is dedicated to the memory of our colleague, Dr Roland Nardone, who passed away in June 2018 at the age of 90. I was one of many who were enlisted by Roland into his army of crusaders against cell line misidentification. His leadership in this regard will be sorely missed.

REFERENCES

[1] Nims RW, Herbstritt CJ. Cell line authentication using isoenzyme analysis. Strategies for accurate speciation and case studies for the detection of cell line cross-contamination using a commercial kit. Int J Biopharm 2005;18(6):76–82. Available at: http://www.biopharminternational.com/cell-line-authentication-using-isoenzyme-analysis?id=&sk=&date=&pageID=2. Accessed September 10, 2018.

[2] Bian X, Yang Z, Feng H, et al. A combination of species identification and STR profiling identifies cross-contaminated cells from 482 human tumor cell lines. Sci Rep 2017;7(1):9774.

[3] Nims RW, Shoemaker AP, Bauernschub MA, et al. Sensitivity of isoenzyme analysis for the detection of interspecies cell line cross-contamination. In Vitro Cell Dev Biol Anim 1998;34(1):35–9.

[4] International Cell Line Authentication Committee (2017) Register of misidentified cell lines. Available at: http://iclac.org/databases/cross-contaminations/. Accessed September 10, 2018.

[5] Nims RW, Sykes G, Cottrill K, et al. Short tandem repeat profiling: part of an overall strategy for reducing the frequency of cell misidentification. In Vitro Cell Dev Biol Anim 2010;46(10):811–9.

[6] Ramya R, Nagarajan T, Sivakumar V, et al. Identification of cross-contaminated animal cells by PCR and isoenzyme analysis. Cytotechnology 2009;61(3):81–92.

[7] Cabrera CM, Cobo F, Nieto A, et al. Identity tests: determination of cell line cross-contamination. Cytotechnology 2006;51(2):45–50.

[8] Drexler HG, Dirks WG, MacLeod RAF. False human hematopoietic cell lines: cross-contaminations and misinterpretations. Leukemia 1999;13(10):1601–7.

[9] White AD, Sweeney MC. Detection of male cells in mixtures containing varying proportions of male and female cells by fluorescence in situ hybridization and G-banding. Cytometry 1993;14(1):9–15.

[10] Defendi V, Billingham RE, Silvers WK, et al. Immunological and karyological criteria for identification of cell lines. J Natl Cancer Inst 1960;25(2):359–85.

[11] Nelson-Rees WA, Flandermeyer RR, Hawthorne PK. Banded marker chromosomes as indicators of intraspecies cellular contamination. Science 1974; 184(4141):1093–6.

[12] Pereira F, Carneiro J, Amorim A. Identification of species with DNA-based technology: current progress and challenges. Recent Pat DNA Gene Seq 2008;2(3): 187–200.

[13] Reid YA, Storts D, Riss T, et al. Authentication of human cell lines by STR DNA profiling analysis. In: Sittampalam GS, Coussens NP, Brimacombe K, et al, editors. Assay guidance manual. Bethesda (MD): Eli Lilly & Company and the National Center for Advancing Translational Sciences; 2004. https://www.ncbi.nlm.nih.gov/books/NBK144066/. Accessed September 10, 2018.

[14] Butler JM. Single nucleotide polymorphisms and applications. In: Advanced topics in forensic DNA typing: methodology. Amsterdam: Academic Press; 2011. p. 347–70.

[15] Losi CG, Ferrari S, Sossi E, et al. An alternative method to isoenzyme profile for cell line identification and interspecies cross-contaminations: cytochrome b PCR-RLFP analysis. In Vitro Cell Dev Biol Anim 2008;44(8–9):321–9.

[16] Mohammadi A, Farzinpoor M, Lotfi M, et al. Comparative sensitivity analysis between two methods for species differentiation and interspecies cross contamination in animal cell culture. Arch Med Lab Sci 2016; 2(3):84–8.

[17] Ono K, Satoh M, Yoshida T, et al. Species identification of animal cells by nested PCR targeted to mitochondrial DNA. In Vitro Cell Dev Biol Anim 2007;43(5–6): 168–75.

[18] Parodi B, Aresu O, Bini D, et al. Species identification and confirmation of human and animal cell lines: a PCR-based method. BioTechniques 2002;32(2): 432–40.

[19] Cooper JK, Sykes G, King S, et al. Species identification in cell culture: a two-pronged molecular approach. In Vitro Cell Dev Biol Anim 2007;43(10):344–51.

[20] Cooper JK, Almeida JL, Bauer BA, et al. ANSI/ASN-0003-2015, Species-level identification of animal cells through mitochondrial cytochrome c oxidase subunit 1 (CO1) DNA barcodes. 2015. Available at: http://webstore.ansi.org/RecordDetail.aspx?sku=ANSI%2fATCC+ASN-0003-2015. Accessed September 10, 2018.

[21] Nims RW. Suitability of the CO1 barcode assay for animal cell identity testing. BioReliance White Paper 2015. Available at: https://www.bioreliance.com/assets/deepweb/assets/bioreliance/content/pdf/rua-o-1030815-co1-white-paper-rn-05aug2015-final/rua-o-1030815-co1-white-paper-rn-05aug2015-final.pdf. Accessed September 10, 2018.

[22] Jordan I, Munster VJ, Sandig V. Authentication of the R06E fruit bat cell line. Viruses 2012;4(5):889–900.

[23] ANSI/ATCC ASN-0002-2011. Authentication of human cell lines: Standardization of STR profiling. Available at: https://webstore.ansi.org/RecordDetail.aspx?sku=ANSI%2FATCC+ASN-0002-2011. Accessed September 10, 2018.

[24] Fang R, Shewale JG, Nguyen VT, et al. STR profiling of human cell lines: challenges and possible solutions to the growing problem. J Forensics Res 2011;S2:005. https://doi.org/10.4172/2157-7145.S2-005. Accessed September 10, 2018.

[25] Liang-Chu MMY, Yu M, Haverty PM, et al. Human biosample authentication using the high-throughput, cost-effective SNPtrace™ system. PLoS One 2015;10: e0116218.

[26] Korch C, Hall EM, Dirks WG, et al. Authentication of M14 melanoma cell line proves misidentification of MDA-MB-435 breast cancer cell line. Int J Cancer 2017; 142(3):561–72.

[27] Schweppe RE, Klopper JP, Korch C, et al. Deoxyribonucleic acid profiling analysis of 40 human thyroid cancer cell lines reveals cross-contamination resulting in cell line redundancy and misidentification. J Clin Endocrinol Metab 2008;93(11):4331–41.

[28] Almeida JL, Hill CR, Cole KD. Mouse cell line authentication. Cytotechnology 2014;66(1):133–47.

[29] Didion JP, Buus RJ, Naghashfar Z, et al. SNP array profiling of mouse cells identifies their strains of origin and reveals cross-contamination and widespread aneuploidy. BMC Genomics 2014;15: 847.

[30] Morgan AP, Fu CP, Welsh CE, et al. The mouse universal genotyping array: from substrains to subspecies. G3 (Bethesda) 2016;6(2):263–79.

[31] Mitchell C. Cell line authentication: species identity and purity analysis using next generation sequencing. ISBioTech 2017 Fall Meeting, Virginia Beach, VA, December 11–13, 2017.